Neural Transplantation

Cellular and Molecular Neuroscience
Charles F. Stevens, editor

Neural Transplantation

An Introduction

William J. Freed

A Bradford Book
The MIT Press
Cambridge, Massachusetts
London, England

The views expressed in this book do not necessarily represent the views of the National Institutes of Health and/or the Department of Health and Human Services.

This book was set in Sabon by Achorn Graphic Services, Inc., and was printed and bound in the United States of America.

Library of Congress Cataloging-in-Publication Data

Freed, William J.
  Neural transplantation : an introduction / William J. Freed.
    p. cm. — (Cellular and molecular neuroscience)
  "A Bradford book."
  Includes bibliographical references and index.
  ISBN 0-262-06208-9 (hardcover : alk. paper)
  1. Nerve tissue—Transplantation—Technique. 2. Central nervous system—Transplantation. I. Title. II. Series: Cellular and molecular neuroscience series.
  [DNLM: 1. Brain Tissue Transplantation.   WL 368 F853n 1999]
  RD124.F74   1999
  617.4'80592—dc21
  DNLM/DLC
  for Library of Congress   99-20115
                                                                      CIP

Contents

Preface

Why should we study the brain at all? One reason for studying the brain is simply to understand how it works. Developing a complete understanding of the processes of brain function is a task of almost infinite complexity. This simple and straightforward motivation has been the principal motivator for much of brain research during the life of the discipline. Other motivations for brain research are more philosophical, such as "to understand the brain is to understand ourselves" or "the brain is the ultimate frontier." Not being a very philosophical person, I do not find these reasons to be sufficient. It seems to me that the most compelling reason to study the brain is to be able to do something to alter it; specifically, to be able to repair the brains of individuals with nervous system injury or disease. Over the years, ideas on how to repair the brain have included removing parts of it, the use of mechanical devices, infusing chemicals and drugs, performing genetic modifications of cells within the brain (chapter 24), and—maybe the most promising—inserting new cells into the brain.

Since about 1970, enormous advances have been made in the understanding of brain function. Increasingly sophisticated methods for unraveling the molecular structure of brain cells have led to an increasingly detailed knowledge of the processes through which brain cells operate, and the molecular defects responsible for nervous system disorders are gradually being deciphered. Tools that can now be applied to studies of brain function include methods for investigating the electrical and biochemical processes through which cells of the nervous system communicate, analysis of the protein molecules that are responsible for neuronal structure and function, techniques to study biochemical and anatomical interactions between brain cells, and application of molecular techniques such as cloning and PCR (the polymerase chain reaction) to finding the genes responsible for neural form and function. It has been recognized that, in many respects, the rate of acquisition of knowledge about brain function has exceeded the rate at which that knowledge can be assimilated into coherent models of overall brain function. Thus, steps are being taken to develop improved means of incorporating this vast amount of information into meaningful models.

This book describes the relatively new technology of brain tissue transplantation, which has formed the basis for—if not quite the practice of—a new discipline within brain research: a technology of repairing parts of the brain that, at one time, would have been considered to be permanently damaged. What is rendered possible by this technology, as well as what may not be possible, will be discussed. A book that describes neural transplantation and the possibilities for brain repair in a manner that is accessible to the general public has not, so far, been available. My goal is to explain the subject in a manner that can be understood by the average person, but without oversimplification. In addition to the interested non-scientist, the intended audience includes students in various fields related to biology and medicine, students in psychology and philosophy, and perhaps patients with neural degenerative disorders or their relatives, who would benefit from some knowledge about this area and the prospects for human clinical use.

A bit of orientation may be useful. For anyone reading this book who has no background knowledge about brain function, I would suggest reading chapters 1–9 in sequence, and using the glossary extensively. After chapter 9, the chapters do not have to be read in any particular order. For any neuroscientists reading this book: I would welcome hearing about errors and omissions. This book was not really intended for other scientists in this field, but perhaps even they might find a few things in here that are interesting, amusing, or at least irritating!

The discipline of neural tissue transplantation has developed along two largely parallel but mainly separate lines. One line of research involves attempts to replace neuronal cell bodies by the transplantation of particular cells to repair or augment specific neuronal systems. This line of research started with, and is exemplified by, studies in Parkinson's disease.

Currently, research is being pursued in many additional areas, including Huntington's disease, chronic pain, and epilepsy. A second line of research is historically related to studies of regeneration and recovery from injury, especially of the spinal cord. This work originated with attempts to promote spinal cord regeneration and, following a long series of incremental developments, is currently focused on attempts to promote neuronal regeneration through transplantation of cells and the use of various materials that encourage the regrowth of central nervous system pathways. The history of neural transplantation in these two areas of study comprises the major part of this book. A third area of neural transplantation research is related to experimental studies of developmental mechanisms rather than nervous system repair, and for the most part is not considered. No attempt has, however, been made to make this book complete. Supplementary sources should be consulted by the reader interested in the entire range of topics encompassed by the field of neural transplantation. A brief discussion of some of the topics that are not included is at the end of chapter 4. However, my goal throughout is to be thought-provoking, not in any sense to provide a comprehensive review of the scientific literature.

The brain was flashburned and the ashes saved for burial; but all the rest of the body, in slabs and small blobs and parchment-thin layers and lengths of tubing, went into storage in the hospital's organ banks. (Larry Niven, "The Jigsaw Man," in *Three Books of Known Space,* pp. 64–65)

Acknowledgments

I am extremely grateful to Joseph Mendelson, my first scientific mentor, without whose help I would have been either a musician or a social worker, I'm not sure which (after having become disillusioned with electrical engineering)—but certainly not a scientist. Thanks are also due to Fiona Stevens, earlier with MIT Press, for helping me to get started with this book, and Michael Rutter of MIT Press for helping me to complete it. I especially appreciate the assistance of Brita Elvevåg, who read the entire first draft and provided me with encouragement and many useful suggestions, and Julie Gorey for reading and commenting on parts of the book. Thanks are due to the anonymous reviewers for their suggestions. The research described that was done in my laboratory would not have been possible without the help of my longtime friends and coworkers, including Eleanor Krauthamer, Lannie Cannon-Spoor, Ora Dillon-Carter, Sharyn Crump, and especially Cynthia Rodgers, who died in 1989 but will not be forgotten, as well as the recent staff in my laboratory and colleagues, including Marquis Vawter, Mary Ellen Truckenmiller, Maciej Poltorak, Magda Giordano, Hidetoshi Takasmima, Concepcion Conejero-Goldberg, Mark Coggiano, and Peisu Zhang.

It is my pleasure to express my appreciation for a few scientific colleagues, especially John R. Sladek, Jr., for his consistent support and his outstanding work as editor of the journal *Experimental Neurology;* Barry J. Hoffer, for being a steadfast friend and ally over the years; Lars Olson and Ake Seiger, for showing me how to dissect fetal rat brains; and Herb Geller, for his consistent support and encouragement.

I am indebted to my wife, Lois, for her help and encouragement, not to mention being my original inspiration for getting serious about a scientific career and for helping in other ways too numerous to mention; my daughter, Melanie, for helping with the illustrations and for listening to explanations of things; my son Ben, for helping with computer workings, and my son Billy, for help with drawings.

Finally, I acknowledge the important role of the American Society for Neural Transplantation and Repair, and the members who attend its meetings every year. Through small contributions from the membership, each of whom does his or her own small part, I think that, as a group, we will be able to sustain the endeavor of learning how to repair the brains of patients with neurodegenerative disease. I strongly believe that the atmosphere of cooperation fostered by our meetings does far more to sustain the field than the contributions of any one individual. As noted before, this book is not comprehensive, and thus I have neglected to mention many important contributions from individual members of our group.

I

Introduction

1

Introduction to Transplantation in the Nervous System

What Is Brain Tissue Transplantation?

The words *brain transplantation* evoke science fiction of an earlier era: diabolical professors keeping brains alive in jars and such things. These words tend to elicit a sense that it is something bizarre, or at least a mysterious and arcane enterprise. In part because of this historical reference, the current usage of "brain tissue transplantation" has tended to provoke a great deal of interest, possibly related to a sense that something from science fiction has come to pass. In a way this is true; a form of brain transplantation has become a reality.

In one sense, the form of brain tissue transplantation that has become a reality is something far less shocking, and far less likely to change our concepts of say, individuality, than the "Frankenstein" type of brain transplantation. In another sense, brain tissue transplantation as it is currently being considered and practiced, is something far more elegant than—and technically goes far beyond—anything that had previously been conceived of by science fiction novelists or filmmakers.

Prior to 1979, a few scientists had studied transplantation of brain tissue, as well as various other types of tissues, into the mammalian brain. There is actually a long history of studies of brain tissue transplantation in submammalian species. Harrison (1929, 1933), for example, using salamanders, employed neural tissue transplantation to study development early in the twentieth century.

One curious paper, published in 1969 by David Bresler and M. E. Bitterman, contained results that came the closest to a "science fiction" usage of neural tissue transplantation of any study before or since. In that experiment, Bresler and Bitterman found that normal fish that had received transplants of additional brain tissue (from other fish) became capable of mastering a type of learning task that fish could not otherwise perform. This task involved learning to press a red or green Plexiglas panel in order to receive food. When the animals had learned to press the correct panel, the panels were reversed, so that it became necessary to press the opposite panel to obtain food. Fish can learn this task, but they do not become progressively better at it when the panels are repeatedly reversed. Normally, this form of learning can be mastered only by birds and other higher animals. Some of the fish with transplants mastered the reversals progressively better with repeated trials, a phenomenon characteristic of higher animals!

This study has not been followed up or otherwise pursued since that time (so far as I know), but it certainly—if the phenomenon can be reliably replicated—would create ground for speculation! Can brain transplants allow creatures to behave at higher orders of functioning? Thus, worms could behave like crabs, crabs could behave like fish, fish could behave like birds, birds could behave like mammals, rats could behave like man, and human beings could become like—what? Is this possible, and is it even something that we ought to worry about? Probably not; it does not even seem likely that this phenomenon represents a generalized enhancement of the learning ability of fish. In humans and higher animals, which have undergone millennia of evolutionary pressure toward increased learning ability, enhancement of learning ability in normal individuals seems highly improbable (figure 1.1). This is a topic that will be considered indirectly in various contexts later in the book (chapters 7 and 24).

Nonetheless, to forestall speculation—if it is not clear already—it should be emphasized that brain tissue transplantation is not a method that can be or is intended to be used to alter personalities, create superhumans or automatons, or alter our concepts of what makes us uniquely individual. It is, and should be, limited to the repair of specific neuronal circuits. The use of neural transplants to produce fundamental alterations in human nature is not being pursued by any serious scientist, and in all probability such procedures will not be possible. Inherent limitations in the plasticity of the brain and the degree to which it can be remodeled

THE FAR SIDE By GARY LARSON

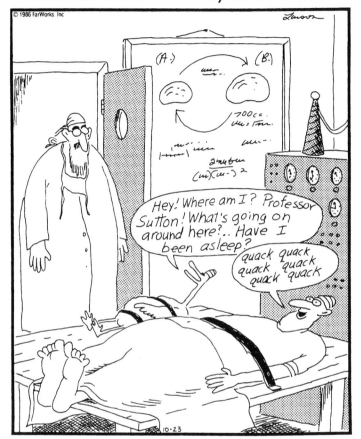

The operation was a success: Later, the duck,
with his new human brain, went on to become
the leader of a great flock. Irwin, however,
was ostracized by his friends and family
and eventually just ambled south.

Figure 1.1
"Brain transplantation" is fundamentally a technique employed for repairing localized defects in neural function. Use of this technique for changing fundamental properties of human cognition is not likely. (Reproduced from THE FAR SIDE, © 1986 FARWORKS, INC. Used by permission. All rights reserved.)

are likely to frustrate any attempt to produce fundamental alterations in the nature of brain function.

The Chronic Nature of Neurological Disease

In the "heyday," so to speak, of infectious disease, it was possible for a substantial portion of the population of a city or village to die during an epidemic. In the black plague epidemic of 1346–1350, the most dramatic example, it has been estimated that approximately one-third of the population of Europe and western Asia died, and there were additional population losses during periodic recurrences until 1665. Entire villages disappeared during these epidemics. Smallpox had a similarly devastating effect on populations of American Indians following European contacts; in some cases entire tribes disappeared. Diseases including measles, diphtheria, and influenza resulted in substantial death rates among children until quite recently (McNeill 1976).

The impact of infectious disease upon the individual was usually a short period of incapacity, followed by either recovery or death. The impact of infectious disease upon society as a whole was, therefore, largely demographic. Shortages of particular types of skilled labor might develop, or frequent loss of children might cause larger families to become customary, as insurance against probable loss.

As infectious diseases have decreased in their impact, diseases of the brain and nervous system have become much more prominent, in part because more people are living long enough to experience them. These diseases produce a very different form of incapacity and a very different type of impact upon society. In many or most instances, individuals with brain injury or central nervous system (CNS) disease do not die in the short term, but experience long periods during which they are able to live, and in some cases even to work, but are partially or almost entirely incapacitated. For example, typical individuals with stroke or traumatic brain injury may suffer from aphasia (loss of ability to use/comprehend speech), agnosia (loss of ability to recognize familiar objects), or ataxia (loss of motor coordination) for many years. Such individuals may be partially or greatly incapacitated, and suffer from a greatly impaired quality of life, but may survive with the sequelae of the illness for many years.

Because of the long periods of incapacity, such illnesses may also be extremely costly.

A few of the most common disorders that involve nervous system function are mentioned below; it is impossible to provide a comprehensive list. If taken together, however, the number of individuals with disorders of nervous system function is very large. Especially if drug and alcohol abuse are included in this list, it can be seen that the cost to society is vast. Not including drug and alcohol abuse, it has been estimated that about 50 million people in the United States are afflicted with some form of neurological or psychiatric disorder. An extensive recent survey on the prevalence of mental disorders, performed by the Institute for Social Research at the University of Michigan, examined affective disorders (e.g., major depression), anxiety and panic disorders, and schizophrenia. It was concluded that 48 percent of Americans at some time during their life experience some form of psychiatric illness (Kessler et al. 1994). Of course, many of these diseases can be treated effectively by drugs, and in many or most cases invasive treatment measures such as brain tissue transplantation would not be justified.

The reader is almost certain to know someone who suffers from a disorder of brain function, and who is thereby impaired or unable to fully experience a normal life. In estimating cost of these disorders, usually two types of costs are considered: direct costs, for medical care and assistance of the patient, and indirect costs, including lost wages, lost wages of caretakers, and costs to society. The cost to the nation, including direct and indirect costs, has been estimated by the Dana Alliance for Brain Initiatives to exceed $300 billion per year, more than $1,000 per individual per year.

Estimates of the costs of brain disorders have varied somewhat, and of course depend upon what diseases are included. The National Foundation for Brain Research (1992) has estimated the cost of diseases of the brain in 1991 in the United States to be about $400 billion, with $160 billion of that attributed to alcohol and other substance abuse. A more recent estimate by the Dana Alliance for Brain Initiatives (1995) put the total cost at $579 billion, with $160 billion of that attributed to addictive disorders. Interestingly, the Dana Alliance estimated that about 200 million people in the United States are affected by a brain disease, although the actual number of individuals is less because patients with more than one disease were counted twice. Even if this estimate is too large, however, it is clear that brain dysfunction is extremely common.

A few examples of diseases relevant to neural transplantation are given below.

Parkinson's disease. This disorder has an onset in late middle age, usually the fifties or sixties, and involves a slow, progressive loss of motor function. Patients with Parkinson's disease may be affected for 20 years or more. The incidence of Parkinson's disease is substantial; approximately 1 percent of the population over 50 years of age is affected. The Dana Alliance estimates that there are 500,000 patients with Parkinson's disease in the United States, costing $6 billion per year.

Spinal cord injury. There are approximately 250,000 individuals in the United States, and many more worldwide, who are incapacitated by spinal cord injury. These individuals may live for many years with severe impairments, and almost always require at least some medical and maintenance care. Analogous impairments occur in individuals with traumatic brain injury (e.g., due to motor vehicle accidents). The Dana Alliance estimates the costs of spinal cord injury to be $10 billion per year, and the National Foundation for Brain Research estimates the direct costs to be $22 billion per year. Both spinal cord injury and head injury turn out to be extremely costly because the victims are often young adults and live for a long time subsequent to the injury. Of course, prevention is the best alternative, but even if prevention is greatly improved, there will be a significant potential benefit from improved treatment methods.

Epilepsy. The incidence of epilepsy, in some form, is estimated to be between 0.25 and 1 percent of the population. In nearly one-third of these patients, seizures are not adequately treated by existing drugs. There are an estimated 2.5 million patients in the United States with epilepsy, costing the nation an estimated $3 billion per year.

Alzheimer's disease. This disorder, which becomes increasingly prevalent with increasing age, causes progressive mental deterioration and affects approximately 15 percent of the population over 65 years of age. Many patients with Alzheimer's disease require continuous inpatient care. There are an estimated 4 million patients with Alzheimer's disease in the United States, costing an estimated $60 billion per year.

Huntington's disease. This is a relatively rare disorder that has nonetheless received considerable attention in relationship to neural transplantation, because the neural circuitry involved in the disease is quite well understood and perhaps is amenable to modification through neural transplants. Patients with Huntington's disease are usually healthy until early adulthood, and then begin to develop motor abnormalities. The Dana Alliance estimates that there are 25,000 patients in the United States with Huntington's disease, costing an estimated $250 million per year.

Schizophrenia.   This is a widely misunderstood, but severe and incapacitating, form of brain dysfunction. Although classified as a psychiatric disorder, it certainly should not be trivialized as a sort of psychosocial maladjustment or personality disorder. In fact, schizophrenia is unquestionably a disease of the brain. There is no specific reason to believe that it can be treated by brain tissue transplantation at the present time; however, such a possibility is not unthinkable.

The Dana Alliance estimates that 2 million patients in the United States have schizophrenia, costing $30 billion per year. The National Foundation for Brain Research estimates that all psychiatric diseases cost $136 billion per year, with direct costs (e.g., treatment, psychiatric hospitals) of $59 billion, indirect costs (e.g., morbidity and mortality, loss of productivity) of $72 billion, and other costs (e.g., legal costs, family caregiving, incarceration) of $5 billion. A more detailed analysis of the costs of schizophrenia (Wyatt et al. 1995) for 1991 estimated the direct costs at $19 billion and the indirect costs at $46 billion. In any case, this is a considerable amount of money.

In addition, there are dozens or hundreds of less common illnesses that adversely affect brain function, including various mental retardation syndromes, inborn errors of metabolism, damage due to maternal drug abuse or disease, brain injury related to heart attack, and many other relatively unusual illnesses, such as striatonigral degeneration, amyotrophic lateral sclerosis ("Lou Gherig's disease"), Tourette's syndrome, Lesch-Nyhan syndrome, and many others. There are also demyelinating disorders such as multiple sclerosis. Psychiatric disorders, including depression, obsessive-compulsive disorder, manic-depression or bipolar mood disorder, and panic and anxiety disorders, are unquestionably disorders of brain function. Even alcohol and drug abuse, which are often thought of mainly as targets for legal or social/reeducational intervention, or problems of individual lack of self-control, are likely to be brain disorders, at least in some sense. Genetic factors contribute strongly to susceptibility to drug addiction, and drug addition is likely to be related to underlying brain dysfunction.

It has long been hoped that science could do something about some of these disorders, and in fact, something has been done for many of them. For the most part, until about 1980, only two means of manipulating brain function were known. The first is the use of drugs, a classical example being the treatment of Parkinson's disease with L-DOPA (discussed further in chapter 8). For some diseases, such as Parkinson's disease, schizophrenia, depression, and obsessive-compulsive disorder, drugs that are partially or even remarkably effective are available. For other disorders, such as Huntington's disease and Alzheimer's disease, little or no effective means of drug treatment has yet been found. The second major means of treatment involves removal of tissue, a classical example being the surgical removal of epileptic foci (discussed further in chapter 4, section "Grafts in Epilepsy"). Neither treatment modality—drugs or surgical ablation—can be considered in any sense to comprise repair of the underlying deficit. The field of brain tissue transplantation allows for the possibility of actually—at least in part—repairing the brain in certain cases of neural dysfunction.

2

Brain Structure and Development

Although this book will not provide a comprehensive description of how the brain is put together, some basic and essential information that is needed for understanding the concepts to be presented will be given. We will describe the general structure of the nervous system and of neurons, how neurons communicate with other cells, and primitive and more complex types of brain circuits.

Components

The brain is not very much like a computer; nevertheless, it is useful to think of the nervous system (for this one paragraph anyway) as a control circuit that receives sensory inputs from various parts of the body (through channels such as hearing, touch, pain, taste, and proprioceptive information); processes, stores, and integrates this information, using the brain, spinal cord, and to some extent smaller collections of nerve cells called ganglia; and forwards instructions to the body through effectors such as skeletal muscle, the heart, and the digestive system. Some of the sensory information is stored and reorganized (using memory and cognition) for later use.

The brain and spinal cord comprise the central nervous system; the major regions of a rodent and human brain are shown in figure 2.1. The complex circuitry of the brain and spinal cord requires connections with the outside world in order to receive sensory information and act upon its decisions, so to speak. Sensory input and motor output occur through the peripheral nervous system, via cranial nerves (these exit directly from the brain) and spinal nerves (which exit from the spinal cord). The cranial

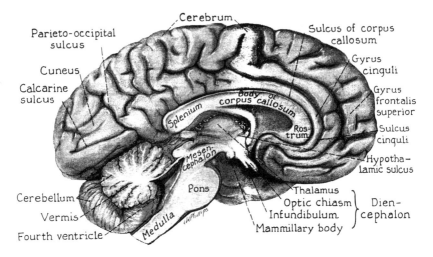

Figure 2.1
Diagram showing some of the major regions of the human brain. The views are saggital sections (i.e., a side view) consisting of slices oriented so that anterior or rostral is to the left, and superior or dorsal is at the top of the page.

nerves perform a variety of functions, including many sensory and regulatory functions (e.g., they convey taste and auditory information, and control heart rate, salivation, digestion, facial muscles, and eye movements). The optic and olfactory nerves are considered to be cranial nerves, although these two structures are contiguous to the brain and can be considered part of the central nervous system (CNS).

Over the short term, the brain initiates many responses of which we are unaware, including postural adjustments, adjustments in internal functions (blood pressure, digestion, etc.), and motivations (e.g., initiating a drive to seek food or, colloquially, determining whether one is hungry or not). Other processes, of which we are more aware, we conceive of as being the major functions of the brain. These include learning, memory, thinking, imagining, decision making, and conceptualizing. These latter functions do in fact occupy a major part of the capacity of the human brain. Such cognitive processes can also be thought of as an aspect of the integrative and processing functions of the brain, providing instructions to body systems based on primary sensory input, over a very long time scale.

Based on these general divisions of brain function, the circuitry of the nervous system can be divided into several categories, at least for this chapter. These include circuits of the following types:

a. Primary sensory systems (the sensory systems themselves and the first relay systems that receive their information)

b. Systems that control homeostatic functions (lowest level)

c. Systems that control emotional functions and motor functions (intermediate level)

d. Integrative functions (higher level)

e. Primary motor systems.

The division of the brain into three parts (b, c, and d above) is a concept that was originated by Paul McLean. He coined the term "triune brain" to describe division of the brain into "reptilian" (homeostatic functions), "mammalian" (controlling emotional functions), and "human" (integrative systems and memory) parts. Although this concept has often been criticized as being an oversimplification, since the various parts of the brain interact in a very complex manner that cannot really be reduced to three separate functions (which is certainly true!), it remains a useful way of thinking about the general organization of the brain and the types of functional systems that exist.

This division, although not absolute, will become of importance later in this chapter as we discuss possibilities for repairing the nervous system: in a sense, these various types of circuits are differentially amenable to being repaired. Before discussing this issue, however, it will be necessary to discuss some elementary concepts of nervous system organization.

Sensory Input

Primary sensory input is acquired through a large number of specialized cell types located in areas including the eye, skin, skeletal joints, the retina, the inner ear, and the tongue. Cells in these areas contain specialized components that allow them to translate outside events into cell signals. The means through which outside events are detected varies with the type of cell, but in general, sensory cells contain protein molecules that are specialized to detect environmental or internal events. In the retina, the rod cells are light-sensing cells. They contain the protein rhodopsin, which is sensitive to light and translates illumination to a change in cell metabolism.

Sensory information is relayed to the brain through bundles of nerve fibers called by the general term "nerve." These include the optic nerve (part of the central nervous system) and two types of peripheral nerves: cranial nerves, which relay information directly to the brain, and spinal nerves, which relay information to the spinal cord.

Information Processing
Once information is received by the central nervous system, it is processed in a progressively more complex manner. For example, visual information is initially received by the retina, which itself contains a fairly complex network of neuronal connections. The ganglion cells of the retina send processed visual information from the retina to the brain. The ganglion cells' axons proceed to the lateral geniculate nucleus (a part of the thalamus) and to a nucleus called the superior colliculus. In primates particularly, the cerebral cortex plays a crucial role in the processing of visual information; there, information relayed through the lateral geniculate nucleus is integrated with other information. The superior colliculus is relatively more important in lower animals (e.g., rats), and processing through the lateral geniculate nucleus and cerebral cortex is considered to be more important in primates and especially human beings.

There is apparently a considerable amount of overlap and plasticity in the mapping of (for example) visual information from optic nerve through thalamus to cortex. It has been shown that removal of certain forms of sensory input results in expansion of nearby areas of the cortex that are devoted to other forms of sensory input. In a landmark experiment, Timothy Pons and coworkers found a remarkable alteration of cortical representation areas when sensory inputs from the periphery were removed; thus removal of some sensory inputs to the cortex resulted in expansion of adjacent areas responding to intact sensory inputs (Pons et al. 1991). Therefore, even in the cerebral cortex, which is probably the most complex and highly organized part of the brain in higher mammals, circuits are not fixed and immutable even in adults.

One category of information processing, the regulation of homeostatic information and functions, is highly dependent on a small subcortical region located at the base of the brain, the *hypothalamus*. Nuclei in the hypothalamus are important in the control of blood pressure, thermoregulation, metabolism, thirst, and endocrine functions. Such processes are mainly controlled automatically, without conscious thought, but at times are influenced by higher centers, that is, the cerebral cortex.

Other functions can be thought of as intermediate between the higher (thought, conscious) functions (which are mainly the province of the cerebral cortex) and the more basic homeostatic functions, for which the hypothalamus and other more primitive regions are mainly important. An example of such an intermediate function is the control of automatic aspects of motor functions, a process that involves, among other regions, the caudate putamen and the cerebellum. Thus, the initiation of the process of moving one's hand to pick up a coffee cup originates in the cerebral cortex, but the mechanics of the movement itself are organized by subcortical regions including the caudate putamen. Damage to these subcortical motor regions therefore usually results in specific patterns of abnormal movement, such as tremor, choreiform (spasmodic, uncoordinated "dancing") movements of the limbs, inability to start or stop movements accurately, or ballistic movements (large amplitude flinging or flailing).

Effectors

Execution of the commands of the nervous system involves mainly the control of skeletal muscles, smooth muscle, and hormonal secretions. Effectors are activated via cranial and spinal nerves, through which sensory inputs also travel. The circuits that are directly in control of effectors are relatively fixed, so that they are not much modified by experience and use. This makes a certain kind of sense: it would not be useful for fibers that normally activate contraction of the thumb to be modified by practice so that they activate contraction of the index finger. In the same manner, primary sensory circuits also are relatively fixed.

Cellular Components

The solid matter of the brain is composed of cells, as well as of deposits of protein and carbohydrate that lie outside the cells (extracellular matrix). Spaces outside of cells, within the extracellular matrix (extracellular space), are filled by water containing soluble molecules, which provides a medium through which soluble molecules, some of which serve as messengers, can diffuse from cell to cell.

The cells of the brain are thought of as two types: neurons, or "nerve cells," and glia, or "support cells" (figure 2.2). Neurons provide the complex interconnections between cells, and perform the primary functions of communicating and processing information. The term *glia* is derived from the Greek word for "glue"; glia perform many important functions involved in communication between cells, although the function of rapid, complex, and long-range communication between cells is reserved for neurons.

In some cells, the cytoplasm is extended to form branches that are called "processes" or sometimes "cytoplasmic extensions." In neurons, these processes may be very long and thin, and often are branched; they are called "neurites." Neurites are of two types: "dendrites," which receive inputs, and "axons," which send information to other cells (figure 2.3). The major part of the neuron, excluding the processes, is called the "cell body," "soma," or "perikaryon." Glia also may have processes, but these are not as extensive as those of neurons.

Axons may be very long, to communicate with widely separated parts of the brain and with peripheral effectors. At their terminals, axons form specialized structures called *synapses,* sites of connection between neurons (figure 2.4). At synapses, axons usually send messages by means of chemical signals, although in a few cases direct electrical communication occurs. The chemicals that convey information across synapses, called neurotransmitters, are stored in small packages called "synaptic vesicles." When a neuron sends an electrical signal along the axon, it results in the release of neurotransmitter from synaptic vesicles into the synapse. The "decision" when to send such signals (i.e., the formation of an "action potential") is made in response to the summation of various inputs that the neuron receives.

Dendrites, by contrast, are mainly specialized for the purpose of receiving signals. These structures are highly branched, and branch relatively close to the cell body. The branches often terminate in structures called "dendritic spines," small protrusions that are the sites for formation of one or two synapses. In addition, synapses may be found on any part of the dendrite.

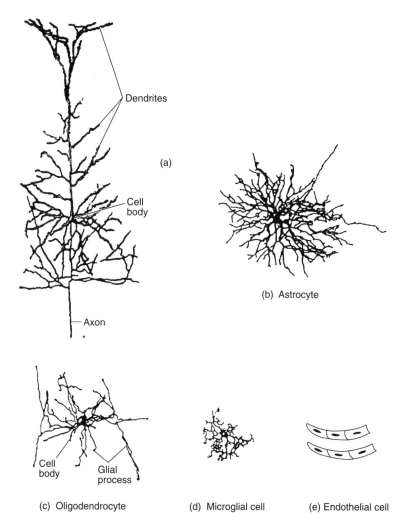

(a)

(b) Astrocyte

(c) Oligodendrocyte   (d) Microglial cell   (e) Endothelial cell

Figure 2.2
Major cell types of the central nervous system (CNS). (a) A neuron, which performs the major functions of rapid and especially long-range communication of information. (b) Astrocytes, which are responsible for numerous support, trophic, and communication-related functions. Astrocytes sometimes have processes that look like those of neurons. (c) Oligodendrocytes, which produce myelin in the CNS, as they appear when grown in culture. (d) Microglia, which perform support and immunological functions. Microglia have a variety of forms depending on maturity and environment, the more complex branched shapes being predominant in mature, resting microglia. (e) Endothelial cells, which line blood vessels.

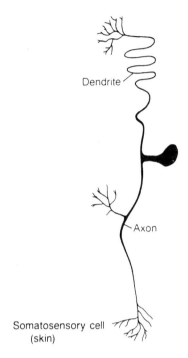

Dendrite

Axon

Somatosensory cell
(skin)

Figure 2.3
A typical neuron and its major features. Dendrites often have small extensions, called "dendritic spines," which receive synaptic inputs. Each neuron has only one axon, but axons may extend for considerable distances, and may branch extensively before terminating at synapses.

Each neuron employs a characteristic neurotransmitter. In many cases, there are cotransmitters, substances released in combination with the primary neurotransmitter. A considerable number of substances appear to act as neurotransmitters. Of the many substances that are currently thought to act as neurotransmitters, there are 12 "classical" neurotransmitters, most of them amino acids and other small molecules (amines). They are the primary neurotransmitters for most neurons. Most of the remaining neurotransmitters are peptides, chains of several (usually five or more) amino acids. Often one or more peptide neurotransmitters are released in combination with a classical transmitter. Finally, there are certain gases (e.g., nitrous oxide) that appear to serve as agents of com-

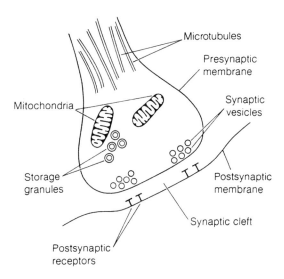

Figure 2.4
Major features of a synapse.

munication between neurons. And there probably are as yet undiscovered neurotransmitters.

Our current, probably inadequate, knowledge seems to suggest that some of the classical neurotransmitters are especially important in the control of behavior and disease-related abnormalities. These important classical neurotransmitters include dopamine, norepinephrine, acetylcholine, γ-aminobutyric acid (GABA), glycine, serotonin, and glutamate (table 2.1). Some of these neurotransmitters are organized into pathways in such a manner that they can be considered "systems" with cell bodies clumped into discrete regions of the brain and organized pathways that terminate in defined locations. The distribution of systems in the brain that use acetylcholine as a neurotransmitter are shown in figure 2.5.

Neurons can be classified in various ways. Earlier, they were classified according to the shape of the cells (such as "stellate," "pyramidal," or "fusiform") and their location in the brain. Currently, in neuronal classification, the emphasis is more on chemical *phenotypes*. Most neurons are thought to produce a single classical neurotransmitter, as well as an array of other chemical substances. Therefore, today neuronal phenotypes are

Table 2.1
Examples of neurotransmitters and neuromodulators; associated behaviors, neural functions, and disease states in which these may be abnormal; and drugs that may mimic or influence these neurotransmitters

Neurotransmitter/ Neuromodulator	Associated Behaviors and Disease States	Associated Drugs
Acetylcholine	Learning, memory, and motor dysfunction, Alzheimer's disease	Early anti-Parkinson's disease drugs, proposed anti-dementia drug Tacrine
Adenosine	Activation, arousal	Caffeine
Dopamine	Parkinson's disease, schizophrenia, drug abuse	Amphetamine, cocaine, L-DOPA for Parkinson's disease, neuroleptics for treating psychosis
γ-aminobutyric acid (GABA)	Epilepsy (GABA is inhibitory, dysfunction may cause overexcitation)	Antianxiety drugs, some anticonvulsants (Gabapentin and Depakene)
Endorphins	Pain	Opiates
Glutamate/ aspartate	Neurotoxicity, seizures, possibly Huntington's disease	No commonly used drugs: proposed anticonvulsants (maybe Depakene), phencyclidine
Norepinephrine	Possibly posttraumatic stress disorder	Several drugs that have mainly peripheral effects
Serotonin	Obsessive-compulsive disorder, depression	Antidepressants (Prozac), appetite suppressants

defined predominantly by these biochemical properties, as well as by characteristics such as shape.

Glia are of several types and serve functions such as insulating parts of neurons, responding to injury, performing immunological functions, and guiding the positioning of neurons and the formation of connections. Glia may also communicate with neurons. In most cases, communication between neurons and glia probably occurs only over a relatively long time scale, that is, on the order of a second or so, and mostly only over short distances, with adjoining cells. The four major types of glia cells are (1) microglia, which are believed mainly to perform functions related to limiting the extent of, and responding to, CNS injury; (2) astrocytes,

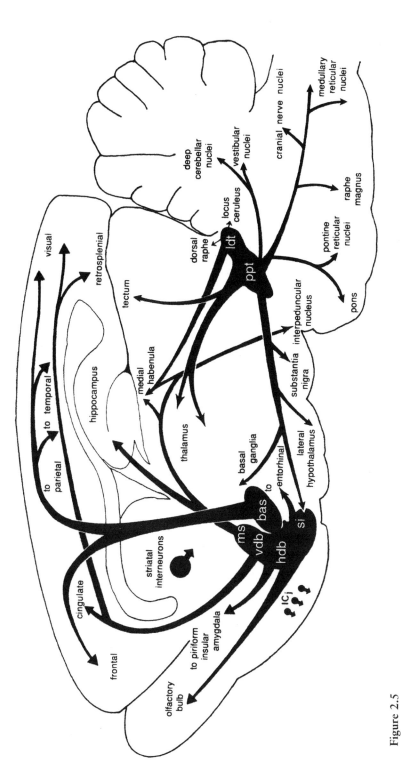

Figure 2.5
Distribution of acetylcholine-containing systems in the brain. The diagram illustrates the distribution of one particular neurotransmitter in the rat brain; a similar diagram is shown for dopamine systems in figure 8.1. (From Woolf 1991; reproduced with permission.)

which perform a number of cellular support-related functions; (3) oligo-dendrocytes, which produce myelin in the CNS; and (4) Schwann cells, which produce myelin in the peripheral nervous system. Although myelin serves a similar purpose in both the central and the peripheral nervous systems, aiding in the propagation of action potentials along axons, there are important differences between the organization of central and peripheral nervous system myelin, which are discussed below.

Although long-range and rapid information processing is probably almost entirely the province of neurons, it is important to note that communication between neurons and glia may be quite extensive and complex. The role of glia in information processing by the brain is currently not well understood, and its importance is often greatly underestimated. Glia, especially astrocytes but other types as well, communicate with neurons by using strategies that include the release of chemical substances as well as cell-to-cell contacts. Glia can release neurotransmitters, small peptides, larger peptide mediators known as cytokines and neurotrophic molecules, and other mediators such as nitric oxide. They also communicate with neurons through cell-to-cell contacts. Molecules on the surface of glia known as cell recognition molecules can interact with other proteins on the surface of neurons to produce changes in neuronal function. Finally, glial cells produce neurotransmitter receptors and can respond to several neurotransmitters, in addition to releasing neurotransmitters through a process that does not involve synaptic vesicles (Attwell et al. 1993).

An example of the kinds of interactions that may occur between neurons and glia is provided by the studies of Patricia Whitaker-Azmitia, Colin Clarke, and Efrain Azmitia (Whitaker-Azmitia et al. 1993). These investigators found that certain types of glia, from certain regions of the brain, secrete a protein molecule called S100β when stimulated by serotonin (these glia contain a certain type of serotonin receptor, the 5-HT$_{1A}$ receptor). This protein, in turn, stimulates serotonin-containing neurons to extend neurites. Thus, glia can serve as intermediaries that are required for neuronal development.

Another interesting form of communication between neurons and glia has been described by Tweedle and coworkers (1993). In a part of the brain called the hypothalamus, one of the functions of which is to regulate homeostatic functions related to thirst and fluid balance, changes were seen in astrocytes and nearby neurons when the animals were infused with saline at concentrations slightly above the normal physiological concentration (this triggers a chain of physiological events, the end result being that the animal becomes thirsty). The saline infusion caused the processes of astrocytes to withdraw from between adjacent neurons, allowing synapses and direct contacts to form between these neurons. This process took place quite rapidly, within 30 minutes. In this circumstance, therefore, the astrocytes apparently were regulating the ability of adjacent neurons to communicate. These studies are mentioned here simply to point out that there probably is still much that we do not understand about how the brain processes information.

Although Schwann cells and oligodendrocytes both produce myelin, and in both cases the myelin serves a similar function (aiding in the propagation of action potentials along axons), there are very important differences between these cell types. It is important to understand these differences for later discussions. Schwann cells, which again are located in the peripheral nervous system, are dedicated to individual axons, so that each Schwann cell myelinates only a single axon. In fact, each axon encounters a series of Schwann cells, all of which are dedicated to that single axon. In contrast, a single oligodendrocyte extends processes that contact several axons (figure 2.6). Schwann cells in peripheral nerves are aligned within a tubular structure called the basal lamina. Thus in a peripheral nerve, when the axon is severed from the cell body and therefore degenerates, the myelin disappears, but the Schwann cells and the tube of basal lamina remain in place to re-form new myelin and guide a regenerating axon. In contrast, there is no corresponding supportive scaffolding in the CNS for oligodendrocytes (figure 2.6). Thus, when axons in the CNS are destroyed, the myelin disappears and no trace of the former structure remains. This greatly complicates efforts to repair long-distance connections in the brain and spinal cord.

Second, Schwann cells have the general property of promoting axonal growth, whereas oligodendrocytes have the general property of inhibiting axonal growth (for further information, see chapter 18). In fact, substances produced by oligodendrocytes that inhibit axonal growth have been identified, and this information has been employed to develop

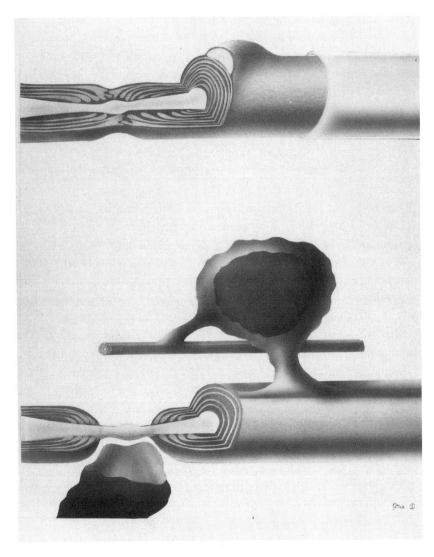

Figure 2.6
An illustration of myelin production in the central and peripheral nervous systems. In the peripheral nervous system (top) each single peripheral nerve fiber is myelinated by a collection of Schwann cells, which are contained in an outer membrane called the basal lamina. When the axon itself degenerates, if the remainder of the structure is not severed, the Schwann cells and basal lamina remain, and can guide regrowing axons. In the central nervous system (bottom), in contrast, a single oligodendrocyte may extend processes that myelinate several axons. When the structure degenerates, no trace remains. (Adapted from Bunge, 1968, and reproduced from Freed, de Medinaceli, and Wyatt, 1985.)

strategies for using neural transplantation for promoting regeneration in the spinal cord (see chapter 18). Schwann cells produce several substances, each of which promotes axonal growth in isolation, such as the cell surface protein L1, nerve growth factor, and laminin. When they are produced in combination by Schwann cells, these materials provide a strong stimulus for axonal regrowth. Given the structure of central and peripheral myelin, it makes sense that CNS myelin would not be conducive to axonal growth. Since the structure to guide newly growing axons is not present, this new growth would be chaotic, compared with that in peripheral nerves, where structure remains in place to guide new growth.

Types of Circuits

The entire brain and nervous system develop together, as a single unit. Thus, the final form of each circuit of the brain is not "cemented" together until all of the components are in place. Certainly, interconnections between neurons are highly complex, so that each network in the brain involves thousands of neurons and various networks are connected to each other. In fact, it is probably the case that each neuron in the brain is connected, through a chain of synapses, to each and every other neuron. In the adult mammal, the mechanisms for development of the brain no longer exist, and they do not reappear when the brain is injured. Moreover, even if it were possible to reactivate these mechanisms for brain development for certain damaged circuits, the remainder of the brain would not be reactivated; thus the reactivated parts would not become integrated with the remainder. In all probability, no single component of the brain can be replaced in isolation, with a complete restitution of all its connections with other components. In other words, a complete repair of any individual circuit or circuit component of the brain would require replacement of the entire brain. This issue will be discussed further in the concluding chapter (chapter 25).

This problem notwithstanding, it appears likely that repairs of the CNS can be made in certain circumstances. How is this conclusion consistent with the conclusion that the entire CNS is more or less interconnected, so that damage to one component interrupts a massive network of interconnected links? First, there appears to be a great deal of redundancy and overlap between circuits. There also appears to be considerable excess capacity. These factors allow relatively minor corrections to be made without noticeable deficit. One might say that the interconnectivity is so vast that damage of a single link is usually not catastrophic.

Second, although mechanisms for major circuit alterations and "rewiring" do not persist to adulthood, mechanisms for more minor adjustments in brain circuitry continue to function. Throughout the life of the adult, changes in brain circuitry are constantly taking place. Synapses between adjacent or nearby neurons are continually changing, involving the growth of axonal sprouts and formation of extensions of dendrites, especially dendritic spines. In addition to structural adjustments, biochemical adjustments of synaptic function occur constantly. These changes occur mostly over relatively small distances, on the order of tenths of a millimeter up to a millimeter or two. The changes in circuitry that do not occur in the adult are especially those involving large distances, several millimeters or more, including regrowth or alterations in major fiber tracts and especially in myelinated tracts. As a general rule, existing pathways can make adjustments in detail, but the pathways themselves do not change in form. The capacity of the brain to make these minor adjustments can potentially be exploited and built upon in order to make more significant repairs. In my opinion, however, the brain will impose upon us limitations that prevent the type of major rewiring that would grossly alter major brain functions.

To give some specific examples of how we might take advantage of the normal plasticity of the brain, we might consider either (1) augmenting this local circuit adjustment capacity to enable short-range restructuring, or (2) artificially building replacement long-range circuits while depending on endogenous mechanisms to adjust the details of the connections.

In the "Components" section of this chapter, it was mentioned that the brain includes circuits that perform a variety of functions related to controlling homeostatic mechanisms, emotion, and integrative processes, as well as primary sensory and motor circuits. Although these various systems are not completely separate, the capacity for plasticity in these circuits varies widely. At the input and output ends of the nervous system are primary motor and sensory circuits terminating in peripheral nerves that connect the nervous system with the remainder of the body. These pathways traverse, for example, the optic nerve and spinal cord. More centrally located are the brain regions and circuits that control emotional and integrative functions. The capacity of the brain for self-repair and the obstacles to induced repair vary greatly among these different kinds of circuits. As a generalization, it appears that primary sensory and motor circuits, those connected directly to inputs and outputs, are subject to limitations related to accuracy: new connections must be exact. More centrally located systems are more plastic, perhaps not requiring exact point-to-point connections. On the other hand, these more centrally located circuits may have a greater complexity of integration with other circuits.

Let us consider a peripheral nerve that controls the muscles of the hand (in reality, the situation is more complex; peripheral nerves also include sensory and autonomic functions). Minor adjustments in this circuitry, in contrast with more central integrative circuitry, are not continually taking place. This can be viewed as essential; in other words, it would not do for the synapses between adjacent fingers to continually be changing. In that case, one morning you might wake up and find that when you tried to move your thumb, your index finger moved instead. Thus, primary sensory and motor circuits are essentially fixed: the same neurons always make exactly the same connections with the same targets. Such circuits are sometimes referred to as "point-to-point" circuits. Thus, strategies used for repair of integrative circuits in the brain may not be applicable to peripheral nerves, and perhaps also not for primary sensory and motor circuits closely connected to the periphery.

On the other hand, there are other strategies that can perhaps be used to repair such circuits. In contrast with centrally located circuits, peripheral nerves terminate. Thus, the synapses at the end of peripheral nerves do not connect to other synapses. Perhaps that is the reason peripheral nerves can spontaneously regenerate, even over long distances and without our help, such as surgical intervention. The subject of peripheral nerve regeneration is beyond the scope of this book. Nonetheless, it should be made clear that in the case of peripheral nerves, the problem is not to induce regeneration; rather, the problem is to promote regeneration to the correct targets, so that the original "point-to-point" mapping is retained (cf. W. J. Freed, de Medinaceli, and Wyatt 1985 for further details). Maintaining specific details of circuit organization may also be an issue for circuit repair in the CNS, especially when primary sensory or motor systems are involved.

Conclusion

What degree of repair is possible? We believe that certain kinds of minor adjustments and corrections might be made. Could it then be possible to add repairs and adjustments bit by bit, along with developmental substrates and scaffolding, until a large part of the brain has been replaced? Something like this might be possible, although a normal brain might not be the result. This topic will be considered in detail in the concluding chapter (chapter 25).

The individual—character, personality, and so on—is a composite of genetic information and life experience. Suppose any degree of brain repair were possible. Say an individual lost 75 percent of his or her brain tissue as a result of a motor vehicle accident. Suppose it were possible to replace all of this tissue. In this case, one would have to assume that the repaired individual would differ in personality from the original. If we were to continue making more and more intrusive kinds of brain repairs, replacing more and more of the brain, at some point we presumably would start to see major personality alterations. Would more minor, and more feasible, repairs also alter personality? Could such alterations present problems for society, or could the technology for making such alterations be subverted for diabolical purposes? This book will consider both the reality and the fantasy of brain repair, and from explanations of brain repair in the context of the normal organization of the brain, I hope to make it clear what might and might not be possible.

Further Reading

Brodal, P. (1992). *The Central Nervous System*. Oxford University Press, New York.

Churchland, P. S., and Sejnowski, T. J. (1992). *The Computational Brain*. MIT Press, Cambridge, Mass.

Cooper, J. R., Bloom, F. E., and Roth, R. H. (1996). *The Biochemical Basis of Neuropharmacology*. Seventh edition. Oxford University Press, New York.

Freed, W. J., de Medinaceli, L., and Wyatt, R. J. (1985). Promoting functional plasticity in the damaged nervous system. *Science* 227: 1544–1552.

Haines, P. S. (editor). (1997). *Fundamental Neuroscience*. Churchill-Livingstone, New York.

Levitan, I. B., and Kaczmarek, L. K. (1997). *The Neuron: Cell and Molecular Biology*. Second edition. Oxford University Press, New York.

Nicholl, J. G., Martin, A. R., and Wallace, B. G. (1992). *From Neuron to Brain*. Third edition. Sinauer Associates, Sunderland, Mass.

Shepard, G. (1994). *Neurobiology*. Third edition. Oxford University Press, New York.

II

General and Background Information

3

History of Neural Transplantation

The "modern era" of brain tissue transplantation began in 1979, with the reports that brain tissue transplants could, in part, reverse functional deficits seen in animals following brain injury. These experiments involved the nigrostriatal dopamine system, which will be described in chapter 10 in detail. Since this particular brain system was already known to be important in the control of behavior, and the circuits involved were quite well mapped, the idea of transplanting tissue to repair it was hardly far-fetched. The "reasonableness" of this idea which has led to the development, and even the excitement, that has been attached to this field. More outlandish ideas—such as diffuse transplantation of brain tissue into the brains of mentally retarded individuals (which is rumored to have been performed in China), or the idea of keeping the heads of monkeys alive in jars—are not only less useful but also ultimately far less interesting.

Prior to 1970, several researchers had reported on more or less successful attempts to transplant brain tissue. Even though the general idea of these experiments was often to repair the brain, the experiments were unavoidably very nonspecific by today's standards. That is, pieces of brain tissue were transplanted, but markers to identify particular types of cells, the connections that they made, or the functional importance of these connections were lacking. Therefore, these early experiments could do little more than investigate whether or not the transplanted tissue survived. Details of early experiments on brain tissue transplantation have been reviewed by both Gash (1984) and Bjorklund and Stenevi (1985), and these sources can be consulted if the reader is interested in greater detail on the early literature than appears below.

The Earliest Experiment

The very earliest published report on brain tissue transplantation appeared in 1890, when W. Gilman Thompson described attempts to transplant pieces of cortex several cubic centimeters (cc) in size (quite large pieces!) from adult dogs or cats into cavities in the cortex of adult dogs. The very brief report of the results stated that the graft site healed nicely, and it appears that some type of tissue was present at the implantation site after six weeks. Although a photomicrograph was shown, no surviving neurons can be positively identified. We now know that under the conditions used (transplantation of large tissue fragments from one adult animal to another—of a different species, in some cases), it is probable that most of the original transplanted tissue was resorbed, and that little more than scar tissue remained by six weeks. Thompson nevertheless considered his experiment to have been a success; in fact, the paper was titled "Successful Brain Grafting." This paper was published only seven years after the germ theory of disease had become firmly established, as a result of the work of Robert Koch in the Egyptian cholera epidemic. Although this was not much of an experiment by today's standards, it is interesting how early it appeared. The paper by Thompson also predated, by almost 50 years, the studies of Medawar, who established that graft rejection is an immunological phenomenon!

Even more astonishing is the fact that the "neuron doctrine"—the principle that the nervous system is organized as a network of separate cells that communicate at synapses—was first proposed only shortly before, in 1889, and elaborated in 1891. The Golgi technique, which allowed neurons to be distinguished histologically, was developed in 1883. Thus, curiously, the study of brain tissue transplantation has been in existence almost since the neuron doctrine, the beginnings of modern neuroscience (table 3.1).

Insofar as it is important what was "first," it seems that Thompson's report was indeed the first study of transplanting brain tissue. Nevertheless, his study seems to have had little impact upon subsequent investigators in this field. Apparently, it was unknown to later experimenters until somehow unearthed by Don Gash (1984) for his review. Saltykow, for

Table 3.1
Early history of neural transplants in the context of early neuroscience

---

1883 Camillo Golgi develops stain for neurons, using silver nitrate.

1886 William His and Alfred Florel propose "neuron doctrine," suggesting that the nervous system is made up of individual cells (neurons) that communicate with each other.

1888 Santiago Ramón y Cajal's anatomical studies of the structure of the brain are first published.

1890 W. Gilman Thompson reports on attempt to transplant brain tissue.

1891 Neuron doctrine is elaborated by Wilhelm Waldeyer.

1900 John Forssman implants brain tissue to peripheral nerve.

1905 Sergije Saltykow reports studies of removal and reimplantation of cortical tissue in young rabbits.

1906 Publication of Ramón y Cajal's classic studies on nervous system regeneration.

1906 Ramón y Cajal and Golgi share Nobel Prize for the discovery that the neuron is the basic communicating unit of the nervous system.

1907 G. Del Conte reports on (mostly unsuccessful) implantation of various embryonic tissues into the brain.

1917 First scientific report on successful transplantation of immature brain tissue by Elizabeth Dunn.

---

example, who published his work in 1905, believed his own study to have been the first.

For the most part, modern neuroscientists consider the work by Elizabeth Dunn, published in 1917, to have been the first meaningful experiments on transplantation of brain tissue. When I began working on neural transplantation, I knew of neither Thompson's, nor Saltykow's, nor even Dunn's work. From searching the literature, I found papers published by Greene and Arnold (1945), Le Gros Clark (1940), and R. M. May (1955). I was surprised to find these, and assumed that nothing on neural transplantation could possibly have been done any farther in the past. Thus, I didn't even look.

Since Thompson's work has been considered to be little more than a historical curiosity, and did not stimulate additional experiments at the time, it might be interesting to see if we can learn anything from it now, perhaps by comparing it with more recent work. First of all, we could enumerate the ways in which the techniques of neural transplantation have changed, by comparing Thompson's experiment with present techniques. There certainly have been technical improvements. Neurons can be identified and classified into specific types, both on the basis of shape (e.g., pyramidal or stellate) and more recently on the basis of chemical properties. In fact, in Thompson's time, it was not entirely established what neurons were! The "neuron doctrine,"—that neurons are responsible for most of the information processing by the nervous system—became firmly established only subsequent to 1888, when Ramón y Cajal began to publish the results of his anatomical studies of the brain.

There are now many methods through which interconnections between neurons can be identified. More important, these and a host of other techniques, as previously discussed, have been used to study interconnections, biochemical properties, and the functional importance of many discrete neuronal systems, so that transplantation is not used only as a way of diffusely "patching up" holes in the brain following injury, but can instead be applied with very specific goals of reconstituting the function of discrete neuronal systems. This is the first and most important difference between Thompson's study and most current experiments on neuronal tissue transplantation. The goals of his experiment were not well defined, because the tools required to establish them were not available at the time. As will be seen in the following pages, specific functional goals of neural transplantation were not developed until the late 1970s.

A second difference between then and now relates to the outcome of the experiment. Thompson described his experiment as "successful"; yet he was content to have observed a tissue mass at the site where it was placed, considering this to be a success. What current investigators may consider to be success may vary somewhat—possibly the formation of new connections, correction of some behavioral/functional deficit, or at least survival of neurons. In Thompson's time, however, it was sufficient to have observed that the tissue as able to survive for seven weeks without having "wholly lost its identity as brain substance" (1890, 702).

Another interesting difference is the style in which the results were presented. Thompson's paper was published in the *New York Medical Journal*, a general-purpose publication. It did not publish the results of experiments on brain anatomy or physiological function. Since Thompson's time, there has been a great deal of expansion and specialization in this field of research. There are now entire journals that are devoted to experimental studies of brain function, and even to scientific studies of neural transplantation and related topics.

As might be expected, there were many differences in technique. Thompson transplanted rather large pieces of tissue (from 1.5 to 8 cc). Currently, solid tissue fragments larger than about 2 or 3 mm in size (in any dimension) would rarely be used; that is, the size of current neural transplants is between 100 and 4,000 times smaller. Thompson transplanted tissue from adult donors, and we now know that neurons from adult donors usually will not survive transplantation. Also, Thompson transplanted tissue from one species to another (from cats to dogs) in some cases. This involves two different species that are quite widely separated. Such grafts, called xenografts, would not usually survive without potent immunosuppressive treatment, using drugs such as cyclosporin. Only recently have effective immunosuppression methods been developed.

Another minor detail is that the surgical technique was suboptimal. Thompson implanted the tissue at the same time the cortical lesion was made. Currently, when grafts are implanted using roughly similar techniques, a "bed" for receipt of the graft is generally prepared some time before (at least seven days). This procedure serves to promote vascularization (i.e., entry of blood vessels into the graft) and, as discovered by Nieto-Sampedro and coworkers in 1982, it also may promote the formation of trophic substances (substances produced by the surrounding brain that promote graft survival). Note, however, that this latter piece of information was not reported until 92 years after Thompson's experiment! There have, of course, been additional developments, including such major advances as the development of specialized strains of animals that can be used for laboratory experiments (e.g., the laboratory rat), and developments in general surgical technique and improvements in methods that might be used for studying such grafts.

Despite all of these differences, there is one very noteworthy similarity that can be viewed as fundamental and in some sense as overriding all of the differences. Thompson apparently understood—or at least the form of his experiment suggests that he had some understanding of—the basic premise upon which the entire field of neural transplantation is currently based. That is, the goal of brain tissue transplantation must be to make relatively small corrections in brain circuits, to repair existing damage. Thompson did not, for example, attempt to transplant an entire brain, an entire hemisphere, or even an entire brain nucleus. Rather, he produced a discrete brain lesion and implanted tissue similar to what had been removed into the site of the lesion. This is, in concept, surprisingly similar to what is being done now. He also appreciated the limitations of his methodology, as evidenced by the following statement: "Of course, I had no expectation of being able to restore abolished function by the operation, but the question of vitality of the brain tissue and the course of its degeneration is a subject of very wide interest" (1890, 701). This is a remarkable statement for 1890!

Furthermore, the general notion of transplanting small fragments of brain tissue into essentially intact structures is not self-evident, and is not the only possible path that "brain transplantation" might follow. For example, there was a famous experiment by a student of Pavlov (the Russian brain scientist who developed the principles of classical conditioning—remember the salivating dog experiments?) around 1917, in which a supernumerary head (an extra head) was transplanted to a dog. This might have been a predecessor to an entirely different kind of "brain transplantation." More recently, Robert J. White (1968) investigated the possibility of transplanting entire brains. He was able to obtain electrical activity from intact brains of dogs and monkeys, either transplanted to the neck vasculature or kept alive in jars. (For what possible purpose, I cannot imagine!) Even though this concept now seems to be useless, a paper on this concept formed the concluding chapter for a major text on transplantation (covering all organ systems) published in 1968. This sort of brain-in-jars thing has periodically been mentioned in the popular press, the notion being to keep brilliant minds alive after death. White and his associates were able to remove the head from one monkey, transplant it to the neck of a second monkey, and keep it alive in this manner for about a week. In a more recent speculative article in the popular press (Jacobsen 1997), a specific potential use for this technique was to preserve the brain of the famous physicist Steven Hawking, who suffers from a neurodegenerative disorder, by "severing Hawking's head and re-attaching it to a headless donor body" (Jacobsen 1977, 6). White, the neurosurgeon who developed the procedure, was quoted as saying (in reference to monkey experiments), "For the first time in the history of medicine . . . we proved that the body was nothing more than a power pack" (Jacobsen 1997, 6). This peculiar idea also appeared, in a more fanciful manner, in *Time* magazine ("Frankensteins 'Я' Us," May 11, 1998, pg. 19).

There also have been several experiments in which extra tissue has been implanted to the cortex or forebrain, the idea being to supplement intelligence. Experiments of this type have been performed in fish (see introduction), and perhaps even in mentally retarded human patients in China. Thus, the use of transplantation to repair discrete circuits or areas of damage is not the only path that neural transplantation might have followed. It is interesting that the present course was foreshadowed as early as 1890.

Thompson in 1890 had touched upon the concept of brain tissue transplantation almost precisely as we know it now; that is, as a way of repairing malfunctions in small, discrete parts of the brain. Admittedly, a great deal remained to be developed and refined, both technically and conceptually. The idea of specific widely distributed systems, such as the dopaminergic system, which has been the focus of much of the research on brain tissue transplantation, remained to be uncovered. Nonetheless, all of the subsequent work can be thought of as progressive developments and refinements of this basic technique. Thompson concluded his study with a statement that is often quoted: that his finding ". . . suggests an interesting field for further research, and I have no doubt that other experimenters will be rewarded by investigating it" (1890, 702).

Subsequent Early Studies

It is also important to mention that another line of research involving neural transplantation involves its use for the study of brain development. This work began with experiments on salamanders and other nonmammalian species. Often this research has involved juxtaposition of neural ganglia, brain regions, or other body parts to study the specificity and mechanisms of brain and nervous system growth and development. This form of brain tissue transplantation has made major contributions to the study of nervous system development, and has proceeded somewhat independently of brain tissue transplantation as a "repair" technique, although the two lines of research often have been connected and are quite interdependent. The more general topic of neural transplantation in embryology and developmental biology will not be covered in this book. It should be noted that very sophisticated studies of vertebrate development which employed transplantation of both neural and nonneural tissues were conducted long before neural transplantation was anything more than a mere curiosity. Of particular note are the studies by Ross Granville Harrison in the late 1920s and 1930s (Harrison 1929, 1933; see also Twitty 1966).

There were several interesting studies on neural transplantation of one sort or another published in the early 1900s. Saltykow (1905), for example, implanted small pieces of tissue into the brain to examine effects on scar formation. His technique involved removal of fragments of cerebral cortex and immediate replacement into the same site. As described in Bjorklund and Stenevi's review (1985), Saltykow concluded that brain tissue implants of this type reduced the formation of scar tissue. However, this experiment does not fit a strict definition of "transplantation"— transplantation connotes removal of tissue from one location or individual and implantation into a different individual or location. Nonetheless, it is clearly related to the topic. Another interesting work was that of Forssman (1900), who was studying implants of brain tissue to peripheral nerves. He also performed control experiments in which brain tissue implants were compared with implants of other tissues (spleen and liver), examining the histological features of the various implants.

Following the studies by Saltykow and Forssman in 1900–1905, there were a number of studies of transplantation of autonomic ganglia to brains, peripheral nerve transplants, and peripheral tissue transplants to brain. These experiments are primarily of historical interest, and the interested reader may consult the excellent reviews by Gash (1984) and Bjorklund and Stenevi (1985) for further information. The next important step in the field was the work of Elizabeth Dunn, published in 1917 but apparently initiated in 1903 (see Gash 1984). In these experiments, Dunn transplanted immature (neonatal) rat cerebral cortex into other neonatal animals, and in a few cases a small number of surviving neurons were found. This is considered by most to have been the first bona fide study of brain tissue transplantation, for several reasons: (a) brain tissue was, in fact, transplanted; (b) some (albeit, not many) of the transplanted cells actually survived; (c) details of the experiment were described in a scientific journal.

The study by Dunn (1917) was actually quite significant, because the important idea of using *immature* brain tissue for transplantation was first developed. Although there are some exceptions, immature brain tissue, usually fetal tissue, is essential to allow neurons to survive transplantation. Moreover, this report by Dunn was connected in the literature to subsequent work in the field. The later study by LeGros Clark (1940), for example, which bridges the "ancient" world of neural tissue transplantation to the modern era, drew upon the work of Dunn. Thus, the important idea of using fetal material as a source of tissue can be traced to the study by Dunn.

Experiments on Specific Systems

In 1970, a study was published by Lars Olson and Torbjörn Malmfors that represented a very significant change in the field. Olson was interested in the interrelationship between the autonomic fibers of the periphery and the central neuronal systems that contain similar catecholamine neurotransmitters. In order to examine these interrelationships, he adopted an old technique, transplantation to the anterior chamber of the eye. At first, Olson and his coworkers apparently conceived of this technique as a means of studying peripheral nervous system development (figure 3.1). In later experiments, Olson and his coworkers, including Ake Seiger of the Karolinska Institute and Barry J. Hoffer at the National Institute of Mental Health at St. Elizabeths Hospital in Washington, D.C., used the same method to examine development of neurons from the CNS and their properties in relationship to transplantation. This eventually provided the technical basis for most later studies of neural transplantation as a means of repairing the brain.

Another important step came in 1971, when Gopal Das and Joseph Altman exploited the method of labeling cells with radioactive thymidine

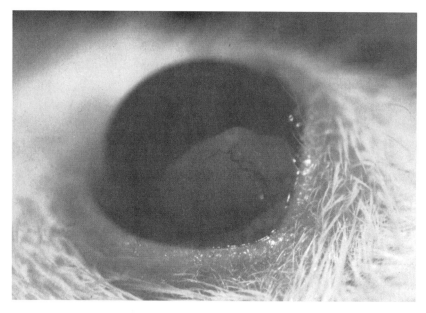

Figure 3.1
A graft of fetal hippocampus in the anterior chamber of the rat eye. The transplant is highly vascularized with numerous blood vessels, and the pupil (above the transplant) is unobstructed, allowing normal vision. Hippocampal transplants of this type become organized so that the basic features of hippocampal cell structure are retained. (Photograph courtesy of Lars Olson, Department of Neuroscience, Karolinska University, Stockholm.)

to differentiate transplanted neurons from host neurons. Thymidine is one of the building blocks of DNA, the genetic material of the cell. If a cell is provided with external thymidine while it is dividing, that thymidine will be incorporated into the cell's genetic material. If that thymidine is radioactive (this is done using a relatively harmless form of radioactivity), the cell that has been exposed to the radioactive thymidine can thereafter be detected through the presence of radioactivity. This technique was used to study cerebellar grafts in young animals, and it was shown that the transplanted cells became integrated with cells of the host cerebellum.

The studies of Das and Altman (1971) and of Olson and Malmfors (1970) formed the technological basis, in a sense, for the subsequent development of neural transplantation. They were the first to identify specific cells and clearly describe interactions between the transplanted and host cells. Technically and surgically, these experiments showed a degree of refinement sufficient to allow interactions and integration to occur, and technically were similar to even quite recent experiments. Subsequently, Lund and Hauschka (1976) found that transplanted neurons could develop connections with the host brain, and Rosenstein and Brightman (1978) described the favorable properties of the ventricles as a site for transplantation. Their studies and some in the early 1970s formed the basis for the development of neural transplantation as a technique capable of being used to repair circuits in the brain.

Further Reading

Bjorklund, A., and Stenevi, U. (1985). Intracerebral neural grafting: A historical perspective. In *Neural Grafting in the Mammalian CNS*, A. Bjorklund and U. Stenevi (eds.), pp. 3–14. Elsevier Science Publishers, Amsterdam.

Corsi, R. (1991). *The Enchanted Loom: Chapters in the History of Neuroscience*. Oxford University Press, New York.

Gash, D. M. (1984). Neural transplants in mammals: A historical overview. In *Neural Transplants: Development and Function*, J. R. Sladek and D. M. Gash (eds.). pp. 1–12. Plenum Press, New York.

4

Transplants and How They Are Used

The idea of using transplants to repair the brain is one facet of the more general goal of promoting brain repair and recovery of function. Repairing almost anything—for example, bridges, air conditioners, automobiles, lawns, human skin, bone, eye, or brain—almost always involves a combination of preserving or enhancing the function of what is already there and replacing certain parts. Rarely does repair involve a precise reproduction of the original. Brain transplants are the "replacement parts" of CNS repair.

To give an example, an automobile engine that is not running well can sometimes be repaired by adjusting the carburetor to control the mixture of air and gasoline, or by adjusting the timing of the ignition to synchronize the explosions in the cylinders with the rotation of the engine, or it might run better with a better lubricant or when a gum-dissolving chemical is added to the fuel; sometimes it needs new spark plugs—or maybe a new carburetor. But since replacing the entire engine (the whole brain) is not an option (let's just say that we don't have the money for that!), replacing various components is the only possibility.

Parts may be used in the conventional manner, as direct replacements for parts that have deteriorated, or they may be used in novel ways. Relatively simple parts may sometimes be used to enhance the performance of other parts or systems that have deteriorated but are not so easily replaced. For example, at one time spark plug extenders were used to recess spark plugs, and thereby keep them from being fouled by oil, in engines that were worn in such a way that oil leaked past the piston rings into the chambers. A much better repair could be accomplished by replacing the piston rings, but this was a complex and expensive job.

Moreover, spark plug extenders caused poorer performance in engines that were in good condition. Or consider a bridge, where steel supports might be used to reinforce a concrete structure that has deteriorated. The concrete itself cannot be replaced, or the bridge would fall down. So it is with the brain: transplants cannot be used to restructure the brain entirely, but may be used to enhance the function of remaining intact elements or to replace certain missing functions of circuit links.

This analogy has limits; it probably has already been stretched about as far as it can go, but there is a point: once we have a means of installing "spare parts" in the brain, it may be possible to employ these spare parts in more than one way. At first, brain tissue transplantation was conceived of as a way of installing new inputs to restricted brain sites. That is, as a means of replacing single circuit components consisting of *inputs* to restricted regions of the brain (W. J. Freed 1985). Neural tissue transplantation is still most often used in this way—for example, to replace dopaminergic inputs to the striatum or noradrenergic inputs to the hippocampus. This is accomplished either through the formation of new synapses—with the presynaptic sites being parts of the graft and the postsynaptic sites belonging to the host—or through the release of neurotransmitter into the *extracellular space,* followed by diffusion to host neurotransmitter receptors. Although this type of application still predominates, there are a number of ways in which brain grafts can potentially be used for repairing the brain and spinal cord (figure 4.1).

How Is Tissue Transplanted into the Brain?

In transplantation of organs, or intact parts of organs such as the kidney, heart, liver, skin, or cornea, a complex surgical procedure is involved. In most cases, the tissue must be carefully matched for histocompatibility; transported carefully and very delicately, using special precautions; used rapidly; and transplanted by means of a complex surgical procedure involving reconnection of blood vessels. One can imagine a similar scenario for brain tissue transplantation: teams of world-renowned surgeons conferring on the best approach to the particular patient's case, considering the complexities involved in the surgery, and so on. Although, of course, no surgery is routine, the reality of brain tissue transplantation is

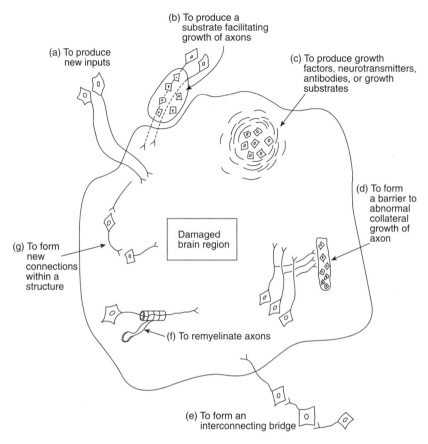

Figure 4.1
Some of the ways that transplants might be used in repairing the brain: (a) to produce new inputs to a deafferented region, either forming new synaptic connections or releasing neurotransmitter into the extracellular space; (b) to deposit a substrate, thereby facilitating new axonal growth; (c) to produce neurochemically active substances, such as neurotransmitters, growth factors, growth substrates, and antibodies; (d) to produce a barrier preventing abnormal collateral growth of axons; (e) to form an interconnecting bridge, receiving inputs from one brain region and providing modulated inputs into a damaged part of the brain; (f) to remyelinate axons; (g) to form new interconnections, replacing damaged interneurons within a structure.

relatively mundane: usually—more or less—the tissue is simply injected into the appropriate site through a metal needle.

Many factors must be considered in the procedural realm of transplanting tissue into the brain, and some of the approaches that have been used are relatively complex. Unlike transplantation of entire organs (e.g., the kidney), however, brain tissue transplantation involves fragments of tissue that are relatively quite small. Often such fragments will survive without reconnection of blood vessels, and therefore they can sometimes be transplanted simply by injection or insertion into the appropriate place in the brain.

It is important to note that brain tissue transplantation has not yet been envisioned, for the most part, as a procedure that would be customized for individual patients, on a case-by-case basis. The notion of learned doctors examining the details of a particular case and conferring about the type of transplant that might be useful for this particular patient—for example, "Dr. Smith, this patient seems to have some difficulty walking, with slight impairment of vestibular function and weakness on the left side." "Yes, Dr. Jones, but he is clearly an asocial individual, and quite obese. I would recommend a substantia nigra transplant, with a touch of ventromedial hypothalamus on the right side, and a small graft of glia from the lateral geniculate nucleus into the prefrontal cortex to assist in dealing with his obnoxious personality"—is far-fetched (to say the least). Nonetheless, this kind of possibility has been discussed somewhat indirectly in the scientific literature (Stein 1991; W. J. Freed 1991) and will be considered to some extent in chapters 16 and 25. Brain tissue transplantation is, instead, a procedure designed and developed to treat a particular disease or diseases with a specific cause and a relatively uniform localization. Currently, brain tissue transplantation is being performed using research protocols that specify particular and fairly uniform types of cases for inclusion.

In general, procedures are usually based on studies in animal models, from which a specific procedure is developed in detail. Usually, or ideally, the first experiments are performed in rodents, refined in subhuman primates (such as rhesus monkeys), and then applied to human subjects. This is somewhat of a generalization, however, and there are exceptions. In many cases, methods have been developed in rodents and applied directly to human patients. In other cases, there have been a few intervening experiments in monkeys. Other procedures have been tried in humans without any directly relevant preceding trials in animals. For some human trials, very extensive experiments in subhuman primates have been performed prior to employing procedures in human patients. Factors that have influenced the course of development of these procedures include the availability of applicable animal models, the availability and effectiveness of alternative treatments, the norms of the country in which the experiments are being performed, and the degree of caution of the investigators.

Since this entire book deals with the subject of transplantation of tissues into the brain, it might be useful to paint a detailed picture of exactly how this is done. I will describe below some of the methods that have been used for transplantation of fetal tissue in rats, in a model of Parkinson's disease, with some references to the methods used in human patients with the actual disease. Several variations of the procedures will be described.

The first step in transplantation of fetal tissue into the brain involves obtaining the tissue. In rats, this is generally done by anesthetizing and subsequently euthanizing the pregnant animal, then removing the entire uterus, which typically contains between 8 and 16 fetuses. The uterus is stored on ice or at room temperature while the remainder of the procedure is performed (figure 4.2). Individual fetuses are then removed and placed in petri dishes containing a physiologic saline solution. These solutions contain salts that mimic those of body fluids: mostly sodium chloride and potassium chloride, with small amounts of other substances, such as calcium. Culture media containing nutrients are often used as well. In humans, fetal tissue is obtained from abortions. Current rules in the United States do not permit the abortion procedure to be modified in any way to accommodate tissue transplantation, which places limits on handling the tissue specifically for transplantation (see chapter 6).

In the rat (which has been used for most experimental transplantation studies), the period of gestation is 21 days, but the fetuses are born very immature—pink, hairless, and a little more than an inch long. Tissue for transplantation is usually obtained from fetuses at between 12 and 17

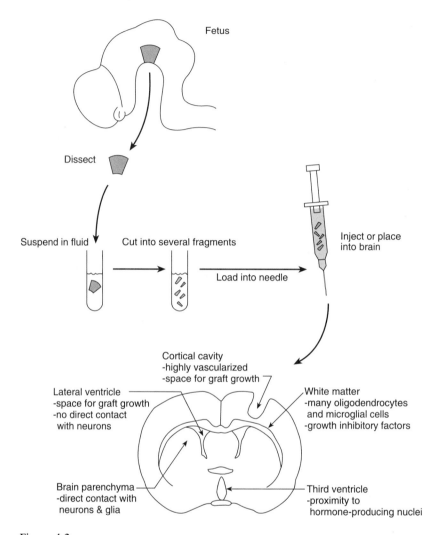

Figure 4.2
The general procedure used in transplanting fetal brain tissue into the brain. A
small region of the fetal brain is dissected, placed in a small container, and either
cut into small pieces or dissociated into individual cells (figure 4.3). The tissue
fragments are then injected or placed into one of a number of possible locations
in the brain. Each location has advantages and disadvantages as a transplantation
site.

days of gestation; let's say we are using tissue from a 14-day gestational fetus, which is typical. These fetuses are less than half an inch in length. For human transplantation, tissue is obtained from fetuses at a similarly early stage of development, about 7–8 weeks' gestational age. The fetuses are dissected, first removing the brain and then dissecting the desired region of the brain. In virtually all cases, the part of the brain that is transplanted comprises a minute portion of brain tissue. The fragment of tissue that is used, in the current example, is the one that will develop to contain the neurons of the same type as those which degenerate in Parkinson's disease. These neurons are located near a fold on the lower surface of the brain called the *mesencephalic flexure.* The dissection must be performed under a microscope, and the final piece of tissue which is used is approximately 1 mm by 1 mm by 0.5 mm for rats. The size of the corresponding tissue fragment for humans is about 2 mm by 2 mm by 1 mm. This tissue fragment is stored for varying periods in a saline solution or tissue culture medium.

In all cases, transplantation of tissue into the brain employs pieces of tissue that are small enough to be nourished by diffusion of nutrients into the graft from the surrounding host brain, until new vessels can grow in from the surrounding host brain. Because of this nourishment limitation, the fragments of tissue that are transplanted can be no more than about 1 mm in thickness. Tissue fragments are often broken up into smaller pieces, or even "dissociated" into individual cells because of this nourishment limitation (see below). This is an additional reason that fetal tissue is generally used, since adult neurons usually cannot survive dissociation. No known examples of brain tissue transplantation employ anastomosis (reconnection) of blood vessels, as is done for organ (e.g., heart or kidney) transplantation.

In the meantime, the rat that is to receive the graft is anesthetized and placed in a device called a *stereotaxic instrument.* Human subjects are immobilized in a similar instrument, generally using magnetic resonance imaging to determine the precise location in the brain where the transplant is to be made. In general, these stereotaxic instruments consist of a solid frame and attachments that immobilize the head in a fixed position in relation to the frame, so that locations in the brain can be found using coordinates measured in reference to the frame. In animals, the head is usually fixed in position by insertion of bars into the ears and under the front teeth, while in humans the skull is usually immobilized by screws that press against the skull. Other attachments hold metal needles that can be lowered into the brain.

The fragment of tissue can be treated in either of two ways. In some cases, it is simply aspirated (sucked up) into the end of a small metal (or glass) tube or needle, along with a small amount of fluid. The needle is then lowered into the brain, and the tissue is ejected from the needle in the appropriate location. Several kinds of devices have been developed to minimize the trauma of ejecting the tissue into the brain. Grafts made in this manner are sometimes called "solid grafts"; these have been used in human patients as well as in many animal studies. There are variations in this procedure that involve the location into which the tissue in grafted. The tissue may be placed into the ventricles, into various locations within the brain, or into sites from which some tissue has previously been removed.

In other cases, the tissue can be "dissociated" (figure 4.3). When first removed from the brain, the piece of tissue does not consist of individual, loose cells, but is a clump of cells interconnected through a protein matrix, forming a semisolid mass. When the tissue is gently agitated, usually by aspirating and ejecting it from a glass pipette repeatedly, it can be broken up into individual cells. This process is called "trituration." This can facilitate injecting the tissue into the brain into discrete sites through small metal needles or smaller glass tubes. If the tissue is taken from fetuses at an early enough stage of development (in the rat, about embryonic day 13–14 or earlier, or in humans about 8 weeks' gestation), it can be dissociated by trituration only. If more mature tissue is used, enzymes that break the protein matrix interconnecting the cells must be added; otherwise, the degree of agitation needed to break apart the cells causes damage. Most of the time, it works better to use the youngest tissue and avoid the enzymes.

In general, most studies use either solid fragments or dissociated cells. A further variation, however, involves the cutting or extrusion of tissue into the brain in narrow strands or ribbons, placing these ribbons so that they contact the host brain along an extended surface. Sometimes the interior of a large graft may not survive because of problems with blood

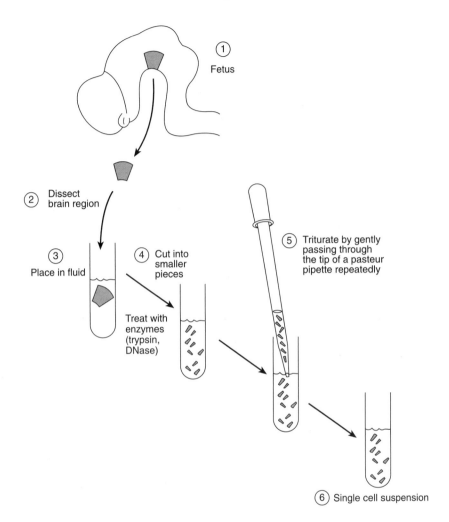

Figure 4.3
Illustration of the process by which cells are dissociated for use in transplantation. Tissue is dissected and cut into small pieces, as in figure 4.2. In many cases it is necessary to use tissue from slightly less mature fetuses for the preparation of dissociated cells. The tissue is often treated with enzymes, usually trypsin and DNAse, which makes the tissue easier to dissociate, and thus less easily damaged. The dissociation to form a suspension of individual cells is accomplished by trituration, repeatedly passing the fragments through the tip of a glass pipette.

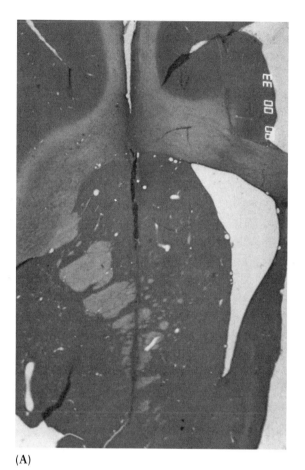

(A)

Figure 4.4

An example of a graft implanted into the brain of a monkey as a continuous ribbon. It appears that the improved contact between graft and host brain resulted in a substantial increase in the survival of the grafted adrenal chromaffin cells. The graft is a long, continuous band of darkly stained tissue extending vertically through the brain in (A), and shown at higher magnification in (B). Immunohisto-chemical staining for tyrosine hydroxylase was used. (Photograph courtesy of Mark Dubach, University of Washington, Seattle. From Dubach and German 1990, 10.)

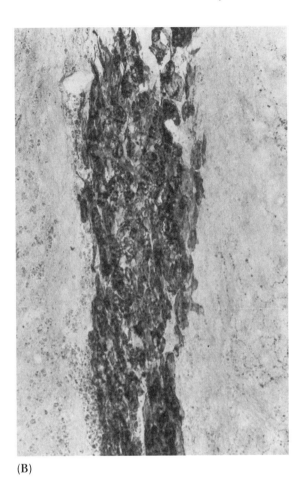

(B)

supply; extension of the tissue in a ribbon form may prevent this problem by maintaining better contact between the graft and host. Several variations of this idea have been described, most extensively by M. Dubach and D. C. German (1990) for adrenal medulla grafts in monkeys (figure 4.4), and a similar procedure has been used for fetal substantia nigra grafts in humans by C. R. Freed and coworkers (1991) (see chapter 13). The use of adrenal medulla for human clinical transplantation, which will be discussed in chapter 11, in many cases involved implantation of tissue under direct visual guidance rather than stereotaxically. In these studies, an opening was made through a cortical fissure, to allow the lateral ventricle to be accessed directly. A fragment of the patient's brain was removed, and the tissue was placed into the cavity thus created and secured with metal clips.

In human patients, in most cases, fetal tissue has been transplanted into the brain using procedures that closely resemble those used in animals. There are, of course, many adjustments that must be made to meet the requirements of human surgery. Some of these modifications are related to preventing disease transmission through the graft tissue, greater sophistication of the anesthesiology and general surgery, measures to deal with the relative difficulty of obtaining and sometimes storing human tissue, and the complications resulting from the ethical concerns of isolating donor from host.

Maturational State of the Donor Cells and the Host

One general principle of neural transplantation is that in most circumstances, the best donors of tissue are the most immature. Similarly, the best results are obtained with relatively immature hosts. The transplanted neurons usually develop more completely when transplanted into the brains of immature animals, for example, into newborn rats.

Immature neurons often survive transplantation and show a greater ability to form connections with the host brain. There are limits to this rule, however; if the donor tissue is too immature, it may be impossible to isolate the exact population of neurons that one wishes to transplant. Another drawback is that very immature neurons may develop very slowly after transplantation, so that improvement or therapeutic effects are seen only after a very long time has elapsed. A more subtle problem is that the appropriate neuronal population may not yet have developed. In extremely immature tissue, cells may not have yet become committed to particular phenotypes. That is, cells present in the very immature tissue may not yet have "decided" whether to become (for example) oligodendrocytes, astrocytes, dopamine-producing neurons, or GABA-producing neurons. After transplantation, when the cells are in a damaged or diseased brain, or are located through transplantation in places other than their normal environment, signals from the surrounding tissue that would normally guide cellular development are altered, so that the cells may become something other than what is desired. Conceivably, transplanted cells might develop properties that could be detrimental to alleviating the disease being targeted for treatment. Although this has not been a problem, it is certainly within the realm of biological possibility.

The best integration of graft with host occurs when the host is immature. In an immature host brain, mechanisms that guide development of the brain structure (e.g., molecules on the surfaces of glial cells that guide neurite growth) are still present, even if not to their maximal extent. Thus, a small remnant of a glial cell population that permits neurite growth may make a large difference in the degree to which a graft becomes integrated into the structure of the host brain. In many rat experiments, relatively large degrees of graft-host interconnection are often seen when grafts are implanted into newborns. There are some examples of graft-induced behavioral restoration that can, apparently, occur only when both donors and hosts are quite immature—that is, when fetal neurons are transplanted to newborn rats.

How Can Cells Be Used to Repair the Brain?

There are several quite different strategies or modes in which we might imagine that grafts could be used to repair the brain; some of these are illustrated in figure 4.1. Most have been used, while others are more hypothetical. The examples that will be described are the following:

1. Release of neurotransmitter at synapses
2. Release of neurotransmitter into the extracellular space
3. Release of a growth factor, such as nerve growth factor
4. Release of an antibody, toxin, enzyme, or cell surface/extracellular matrix protein
5. Deposition of substrate
6. As a substrate for growth or as a bridge to allow the growth of processes
7. As a bridge to receive inputs and make outputs, or to restore parts of a damaged circuit (Huntington's disease models)
8. To provide physical or metabolic support for surrounding cells
9. As a growth barrier, to prevent abnormal growth
10. To degrade a toxin
11. Remyelination

Below are examples of how grafts have been or might be used in each of the above modes.

1. Release of neurotransmitter at synapses. Substantia nigra grafts, taken from fetal tissue donors and implanted into or adjacent to the striatum, have been shown to produce new connections with the host brain. Fibers not only grow into the host brain but also form synapses with host neurons. These grafts reduce some of the consequences of substantia nigra lesions, including relieving abnormalities of motor function, apparently due to release of neurotransmitter at these newly formed synapses.

2. Release of neurotransmitter into the extracellular space. Grafts of several cell types that do not form new synapses with the host, including adrenal medulla (see chapter 11) and encapsulated tumor cells (chapter 22), also can attenuate some of the consequences of substantia nigra injury, at least in small animal models. Cell grafts capable of producing this effect share the property of releasing large amounts of catecholamines. It appears that these grafts produce their effects by release and diffusion of dopamine to synapses that are some distance from the cells, without the assistance of axons and synapses. Another effect of transplants that appears to be entirely mediated by release of chemical mediators, and is actually a better example, is the alleviation of pain by adrenal medulla grafts, discussed in chapter 14. This latter effect, produced by the release of opioid peptides and catecholamines from chromaffin cells of the adrenal medulla, appears to involve diffusion of biochemicals from the grafts into the host brain. There is evidence that these grafts are effective in human patients.

3. Release of a growth factor, such as nerve growth factor (NGF). A number of ways of employing tissue grafts to release a growth factor, thereby producing a beneficial effect, have been described. In a classic example, M. B. Rosenberg and coworkers (1988) showed that cells genetically modified to produce NGF were capable of preventing the death of certain types of neurons that would have otherwise been killed by severing their axons.

4. Release of an antibody, toxin, enzyme, or cell surface/extracellular matrix protein. Schnell and Schwab (1990) employed a monoclonal antibody, IN-1, directed to a protein produced by oligodendrocytes that inhibits neurite growth. Cells that produce this antibody were transplanted

into the spinal cord in a nitrocellulose filter matrix, as a means of continuously delivering the antibody into the spinal cord over a long period of time. Through this method, regrowth of damaged spinal cord axons was greatly increased.

5. Deposition of substrate. Many cells secrete proteins into the extracellular space, and some of these proteins, such as laminin and fibronectin, can promote neurite extension. Transplanted cells might be used to deposit a material, such as laminin, that promotes the growth of processes from other cells.

6. As a substrate for growth, or as a bridge to allow the growth of processes. A series of experiments by Albert Aguayo and coworkers at McGill University in Montreal showed that the axons of many CNS neurons, which do not normally regenerate, would grow over considerable distances if they encountered peripheral nerve (Aguayo et al. 1983; Bray et al. 1981, 1987; Richardson et al. 1980). In their work, pieces of peripheral nerve were transplanted into the brain or spinal cord. Axons of CNS neurons grew into these peripheral nerve grafts, extending for considerable distances.

7. As an interconnecting bridge, to receive inputs and make outputs. This is a more complex version of example number 1. In addition to providing outputs to connect to the host brain, an ideal graft might receive inputs as well. There is evidence that certain types of grafts do receive inputs from host brain neurons. This is particularly true of grafts that are implanted into immature animals, but also may occur to some extent in grafts implanted into fully mature hosts. An example is grafts of fetal striatum into the mature striatum, which have been shown by K. Wictorin and coworkers (1989), and others to develop inputs from the host brain as well as outputs to several host brain structures. A graft may exert its effects by releasing neurotransmitter at host brain synapses, but in order to be optimally effective, it might be expected that inputs from the host brain would also be necessary.

This kind of scenario has received considerable attention as a possibility for repairing spinal cord injury. In this case, the idea is that a graft located in an area of spinal cord injury might make connections both above and below the injury site, thereby restoring some communication between spinal cord and brain.

8. To provide physical or metabolic support for surrounding cells. It has been reported that effects of striatal lesions can be attenuated somewhat by grafts of fetal striatal tissue, and that smaller protective effects can be produced by implantation of nonneuronal tissues, and even Gelfoam and adipose tissue. These grafts do not form connections with the host brain, and are implanted prior to the induction of injury, so that they are not serving the function of restructuring brain circuits (Levivier et al. 1995; Pearlman et al. 1993a, 1993b). Although the mode of functioning of these grafts is unknown, it may be that they provide some sort of metabolic support for surrounding cells.

9. As a growth barrier, to prevent abnormal growth. I cannot think of a concrete example of this possibility. Nevertheless, a realistic possibility might be proposed. Several studies have reported that patients with long-term epilepsy develop psychological abnormalities. In addition, it has been noted that some patients with epilepsy who are treated by removal of the temporal lobe develop behavioral abnormalities, including psychosis, over the long-term (a year or more) (Stevens 1990). Because of the nature and time course of these changes, the possibility that the abnormalities were due to sprouting of new abnormal connections is suggested by Stevens. It might be possible to attenuate such sprouting by transplantation of cells with growth-inhibitory properties (such as oligodendrocytes) into the site of the lesion. Thus, rather than simply removing the temporal lobe in epileptic patients, it might be better to remove the temporal lobe tissue and fill the lesioned area with cultured oligodendrocytes. These transplanted cells might be able to prevent adjustments in synaptic connectivity in the area of tissue removal that would otherwise cause long-term psychiatric problems. This suggestion, although hypothetical, is consistent with the available data, and would probably be quite a reasonable approach if further studies confirm a high frequency of psychiatric problems in epileptic patients following temporal lobe surgery.

Another conjectural example of this possible mode of graft functioning would be phantom limb pain. Amputation of a limb often results, after a period of time has elapsed, in pain that is perceived as originating in the limb which is no longer there. One theory is that this phenomenon is related to inappropriate adjustments in synapses in brain regions that had previously received inputs from the amputated limb. Neurons in these areas may be hyperactive, or inappropriate connections may develop (see Harwood et al. 1992; Postone 1987; Sherman 1989). Perhaps oligodendrocytes or other cells that inhibit the growth of neural circuits could be transplanted into sensory areas which would have received inputs from the damaged limb, to inhibit aberrant synaptic adjustments.

It is conceivable that abnormal axonal growth and the formation of abnormal neuronal connections following injury will turn out to be a more general source of dysfunction following brain injury. There are indications that injury-induced sprouting or synaptic restructuring plays a role in the initiation or progression of some forms of seizures (see, e.g., Van der Zee et al. 1995). Injury-induced sprouting has also been suggested as a hypothetical cause of schizophrenia (Stevens 1992). Thus transplantation as a means of preventing synaptic growth and restructuring might conceivably be widely used. Such use is, however, highly speculative, and there have been no experiments on this topic in animal models.

10. To degrade or attenuate effects of a toxin. The experiments mentioned under topic 8 reported that tissue grafts into the striatum attenuate damage induced by an excitatory neurotoxin (quinolinic acid). The way these grafts worked was not clear, but another possibility is that the tissue grafts may have assisted in the absorption or degradation of the toxin. A sham transplantation procedure (performing the surgical procedure without implantation of tissue), implantation of liver, and implantation of fetal striatal tissue were all found to be effective in preventing impairments due to administration of the neurotoxic substance 6-hydroxydopamine into the striatum (Przedborski et al. 1991). This protection is likely to be due in part to effects of glial cells (see Mattson and Ryuchlik 1990).

11. Remyelination. An interesting possibility is that oligodendrocytes, the CNS-myelin-producing cells, might be implanted into the brain to replace myelin. There are certain disorders, notably multiple sclerosis, in which CNS myelin is lost through degeneration in localized regions, causing motor dysfunction. It is possible that transplantation of oligodendrocytes into local regions of demyelination could produce improvements.

Thus, in addition to the most obvious possibility—using grafts to restucture the brain by directly replacing lost cells, there are other ways in which cells or tissue might be implanted into the brain to improve the outcome of injury or disease. Of these alternative mechanisms, the use of grafts to produce and secrete biochemical substances—especially peptides, which are active in small amounts, such as nerve growth factor (chapter 23) or endogenous opiates for treatment of pain (chapter 14)—seems especially appealing and might eventually be widely used. Chapters that follow will discuss several examples of the use of grafts for various forms of brain injury or disease. There are, however, additional possibilities for the use of neural transplantation to influence the outcome of brain injury that as yet have been only minimally explored.

Diseases and Possibilities Not Covered in This Book

Since it is not possible to comprehensively discuss all, or even most, of the diseases and conditions for which neural transplantation has been used experimentally, I have limited myself to a few topics. The greatest amount of attention (several chapters) is devoted to Parkinson's disease, since that is by far the most studied disorder in relationship to neural transplantation. Far more human subjects have received transplants for Parkinson's disease than for any other disorder. Three other conditions for which the effects of transplants appear to be primarily (although not exclusively) secretory were selected for inclusion. These are (1) cortical injury, for which effects of grafts on behavior that have been found so far are probably mostly secretory, although more complex effects also may occur; (2) of pain, for which effects of grafts are exclusively secretory; and (3) hypothalamic function, for which effects of grafts are also mainly secretory, although in a more complex fashion than is the case for pain.

Three sites at which brain grafts are used mainly to reconstruct circuits in various ways also were chosen for inclusion. These are (1) the visual system, (2) the spinal cord, and (3) the neostriatum in Huntington's disease models. Other possibilities include (1) transplantation of cerebellar cortical cells to deep cortical nuclei, to repair cerebellar degeneration, as described by Triarhou and coworkers (Triarhou 1996; Triarhou et al. 1995), (2) transplantation of *cholinergic* neurons in Alzheimer's disease or other cognitive disorders; (3) transplantation of hippocampal neurons to repair the hippocampus; (4) transplantation of inhibitory neurons to suppress seizures in epilepsy; and (5) transplantation of oligodendrocytes into the CNS to repair demyelinating conditions. Additional details on the above possibilities can be found in the list of resources for further reading.

Transplantation also has been employed for a surprisingly large number of human disorders, in many cases with little or no experimental justification. These disorders include cerebellar atrophy (Cheng-Yuan et al. 1992), schizophrenia (Kolarik et al. 1988), spinal cord injury (see chapter 18), and progressive supranuclear palsy (chapter 11). I wish to make it clear that, at the present time, I believe clinical use of neural transplantation is justified in only a few specific circumstances such as chronic pain, Parkinson's disease, and possibly Huntington's disease, that are described later in this book.

Grafts in Epilepsy

Among the relatively less explored possibilities for neural transplantation in disease states, I find the potential for use in epilepsy especially appealing (even though epilepsy does not have a chapter to itself). Epilepsy can be serious and debilitating, and frequently drug treatment is not effective. In fact, despite the availability of numerous anticonvulsant drugs, it is often necessary to resort to neurosurgery for the treatment of epilepsy. This often involves the quite crude procedure of removing a large part of one temporal lobe. It seems to me that if one is going to remove a large piece of tissue anyway, why not try to transplant something there first? We could hardly do worse than just suck it out; and if the transplant did make things worse, then go ahead and remove the tissue, as was going to be done anyway.

Although there has been some work on transplantation in animal models of epilepsy, this topic has received considerably less emphasis than other areas. One problem is that unlike Parkinson's disease, epilepsy is not known to be caused by a defect in a specific neural circuit. Thus, most studies of neural transplantation in epilepsy have involved induction of seizures accompanied by transplantation of inhibitory neurons in a related pathway.

Several transplantation studies have employed a model of epilepsy known as kindling. In the classical kindling epilepsy, first discovered by G. Goddard and coworkers in 1969, animals repeatedly receive electrical stimulation of the amygdala or hippocampus. There is initially a small response to this stimulation, without overt seizures. The response gradually increases, and after several days of stimulation the animals experience major generalized seizures, eventually culminating in spontaneous seizures without electrical stimulation. Of the various epilepsy models that might be used for neural transplantation experiments, this model is the most appealing in some ways, since the location in the brain from which the seizures are elicited is known. In contrast, for some other types of seizures, the part of the brain that is responsible for generating the seizures is not as clear. Kindling seizures also have several properties in common with epilepsy in humans (McNamara 1984).

In the kindling seizure model, the rate at which animals develop seizures is greatly accelerated by lesions that deplete brain noradrenaline (McIntyre et al. 1979). The most successful experiments on transplantation and seizures have used this model: animals were depleted of noradrenaline by locus ceruleus lesions, then received grafts of locus ceruleus into the hippocampus (Barry et al. 1987, 1989; Bengzon et al. 1990, 1991). Kindling seizures were then produced by stimulation of the hippocampus. It was found that the rate of development of seizures was slowed by these grafts; thus, the kindling-enhancing effect of noradrenaline depletion could be reversed by grafts that produce noradrenaline. These studies did not show a suppression of seizures that had already been established, and effects were seen only in animals with noradrenaline depletion.

Several other avenues have been explored, at least partially, in developing techniques for the use of neural transplantation in epilepsy. One useful piece of information is that seizures of several types can be suppressed by microinjections of GABA-like compounds into the substantia nigra (Iadarola and Gale 1982). Kokaia and coworkers (1994) found that seizures induced by kindling could be suppressed by implanting a polymer matrix that released GABA into the substantia nigra. Loscher and coworkers (1998) reported that transplantation of fetal striatum, which contains GABAergic neurons, produced a temporary (a few weeks) and partial suppression of kindled seizures. Therefore, in the future it might be possible to effectively suppress seizures by transplanting cells into the substantia nigra, especially if cells that make very large amounts of GABA can either be found or made in the laboratory.

Another study found lasting reductions of seizure severity in genetically epilepsy-prone rats, which had depletions of serotonin, by transplants of serotonin-containing neurons (Clough et al. 1996). Thus, there may be a number of transplantation techniques that can be used to reduce seizures, depending of the type of seizures or their cause. In general, I would think that methods which involve transplanting cells producing inhibitory modulators or neurotransmitters will eventually become effective in decreasing seizure activity. Perhaps all that is needed is a cell line (see chapters 22 and 23) that produces large amounts of GABA.

In some cases of epilepsy, neurosurgery that involves tissue removal is performed. In cases where tissue removal is going to occur anyway, transplantation can be tried first, once an effective method is developed (assuming that we can find a procedure which involves cell transplantation into the temporal lobe). This circumstance (impending neurosurgery) provides an ideal opportunity for initial clinical studies with a very minimal potential for transplantation to produce adverse consequences. Transplanting cells into the substantia nigra is more problematic—there are major risks involved, since damaging the substantia nigra would have serious consequences—but eventually this may become a possibility as well.

Disorders of Central Nervous System Demyelination

A second very interesting possibility that does not have its own chapter, but should be described somewhat, is the possibility of transplanting oligodendrocytes into the brain to repair areas of demyelination, as in multiple sclerosis. In the CNS, when oligodendrocytes are lost, there may be considerable functional deficits even though the neuronal pathways remain intact. In multiple sclerosis, oligodendrocytes are lost in fairly well circumscribed regions. It is then conceivable that transplanted immature oligodendrocytes might be able to remyelinate CNS axons, and partially restore conduction patterns. A number of animal studies have demonstrated that transplanted oligodendrocytes have the capacity to myelinate CNS axons in myelin-deficient animals (Archer et al. 1994; Tontsch et al. 1994; Utzschneider et al. 1994). Moreover, oligodendrite precursor cells have been shown to remyelinate axons in the spinal cord in experimentally induced areas of demyelination (Groves et al. 1993). This is something that could, conceivably, become practical. Presumably, areas of demyelination in multiple sclerosis could be identified by MRI scanning, and oligodendrocytes or oligodendrite precursors could be transplanted into the lesions. A major problem would be that there are many areas of demyelination in multiple sclerosis, and the large number of needle penetrations required might pose an unacceptable risk.

Immunology

The immunology of brain grafts is a controversial and technical topic. Although the issues of whether or not grafts will be rejected, and how rejection can be avoided, do not tell us much about the potential for brain restructuring with grafts, it is important for understanding the discussion in some parts of this book.

There is a long-standing idea that the brain is an "immunologically privileged site." This term originally meant that grafts placed in the brain would not be rejected at all, but has come to mean that grafts in the brain are *relatively* less likely to be rejected than when placed elsewhere, such as under the skin.

Generally, this remains true to some extent, but there are so many caveats and conditions that the "immunological privilege" of the brain has not turned out to be very useful in clinical procedures. The probability of graft rejection turns out to depend on the type of donor tissue, specific immunological properties of the donor tissue and the host, the specific location to which the tissue is transplanted, whether other transplantation procedures using the same tissue have been performed previously, and so on. There also seem to be conditions that involve immunological reactions which may damage, but not completely destroy, the graft. Thus, it is not really possible to state unequivocally that grafts of brain tissue from one human subject to another will not be rejected. Probably rejection won't occur, but rejection could have serious adverse consequences in a human patient. Thus, hardly anyone is entirely confident that brain graft rejection will never occur. Therefore, in human patients, immunosuppression to prevent any possible immune reaction is almost always used at least for a few months after transplantation.

Grafts can be categorized as *autografts,* which are grafts within a single individual. For example, when adrenal chromaffin cells are removed from the adrenal gland and transplanted into the brain, or fibroblasts are removed from the skin and transplanted into the brain of the same person, these would be considered autografts. Autografts do not provoke immune reactions per se. Nevertheless, the brain can react to the presence of foreign tissue by producing a glial scar around the graft even without a specific destructive immune reaction to the graft. In experimental situations, *syngrafts* or *isografts* are grafts between two genetically identical animals. Genetically identical animals are produced by repeated inbreeding; in humans, the analogous situation would involve monozygotic (identical) twins. Syngrafts behave like autografts, and do not produce specific immune reactions.

Allografts are the most common type of graft; they are between two individuals of the same species that are not genetically identical. Allografts of peripheral organs (e.g., kidney or heart) produce strong immunological reactions that destroy the graft unless potent immunosuppressive measures are used. Allografts of fetal brain tissue into the brain usually do not lead to destructive immune reactions. Some immune reactions to brain tissue allografts have, however, been seen. In some cases, these immune reactions do not entirely destroy the graft but may impair tissue survival.

At the opposite extreme are *xenografts,* which are from one species of animal to another (e.g., from pig to human; see chapter 13). Xenografts of peripheral tissue—such as heart or kidney—are virtually always rejected, and sometimes very rapidly. In brain tissue xenografts, some survival of tissue occurs occasionally in grafts from closely related species, for example, from mouse to rat, although there is usually a considerable immune reaction. For xenografts of brain tissue from widely disparate species, such as from human to rat, there is a strong immune reaction and the graft is invariably destroyed unless immunosuppressive measures are used.

The reasons for the immunological privilege of the brain are complex, and probably involve a combination of factors. For one thing, the absence of rejection of brain tissue grafts is probably due in part not to the immune privilege of the brain per se, but to the fact that the fetal brain is not a potent immunological stimulus wherever it is transplanted. Other factors that contribute to the immune privilege are mainly related to the fact that immunological stimuli in the brain are not generally recognized by the immune system, for a variety of reasons that will not be discussed here. Often it is said that potential immunological stimuli are *sequestered* in the brain, so that, for whatever reason, the immune system often does not "notice" a graft in the brain. When the brain is injured, as occurs during the surgery used to transplant cells into the brain, there is an interruption in this sequestration, so that immune stimuli can then be recognized. This has two implications. First, immunosuppression is most important during the first few weeks or months after transplantation surgery. Second, repeated transplantations of cells into the brain may sensitize the immune system, and any procedure that requires multiple transplantation surgeries may therefore be dangerous and requires special consideration of this problem. The degree to which immunosuppression is required for brain tissue grafts, the optimal amount and duration of immunosuppression to be used, and the variations in type and degree of immune reactions that occur for fetal brain tissue grafts in various places in the brain are issues which are presently not well understood. Ultimately, it will be important to learn more about the kinds of immune reactions that occur in the brain, and sequences of cellular reactions to brain grafts that can occur in various circumstances.

Further Reading

Bjorklund, A., and Stenevi, U. (eds.). (1985). *Neural Grafting in the Mammalian CNS.* Elsevier Science Publishers, Amsterdam.

Dunnett, S. B., and Bjorklund, A. (eds.). (1994). *Functional Neural Transplantation.* Raven Press, New York. Adv. Neurosci. 2.

Dunnett, S. B., and Richards, S.-J. (eds.). (1990). *Neural Transplants: From Molecular Basis to Clinical Applications.* Elsevier Science Publishers, Amsterdam. Prog. Brain Res. 82.

Freed, W. J. (1993). Neural transplantation: Prospects for clinical use. *Cell Transplant.* 2: 13–31.

Freed, W. J. (1996). Cell transplantation: Brain. In *Yearbook of Cell and Tissue Transplantation 1996/1997,* R. P. Lanza and W. L. Chick (eds.), pp. 163–173. Kluwer Academic Publishers, Dordrecht.

Gash, D. M., and Sladek, J. R., Jr. (eds.). (1988). *Transplantation into the Mammalian CNS.* Elsevier Science Publishers, Amsterdam. Prog. Brain Res. 78.

Lindvall, O. (1991). Prospects of transplantation in human neurodegenerative diseases. *Trends Neurosci.* 14: 376–384.

Lindvall, O., Bengzon, J., Elmer, E., Kokaia, M., and Kokaia, Z. (1994). Grafts in models of epilepsy. In *Functional Neural Transplantation,* S. B. Dunnett and A. Bjorklund (eds.), pp. 387–413. Raven Press, New York.

Poltorak, M., and Freed, W. J. (1997). Transplantation into the CNS. In *Immunology of the Nervous System,* R. W. Keane and William F. Hickey (eds.), pp. 611–641. Oxford University Press, New York.

Sladek, J. R., Jr., and Gash, D. M. (eds.). (1984). *Neural Transplants: Development and Function.* Plenum Press, New York.

Stein, D. G., Brailowski, S., and Will, B. (1995). *Brain Repair.* Oxford University Press, New York.

5

Control Groups and Experiments

The effect of an experimental treatment on any behavior, disease, or phenomenon is defined by a comparison: that is, to determine that a treatment is effective, it is compared with something. In science, this comparison involves experiments, or intentional, systematic comparisons. The manner in which these comparisons are made is termed *experimental design.*

The most primitive kind of comparison involves an observation before and after treatment. For example, a caveman (Og) has a fever. He tries drinking birch bark tea—or praying to Ishmon, the god of fever—and recovers. This leads to the idea that birch bark tea, or the goodwill of Ishmon, cures the fever. Such methodologies can obviously be misleading at times: he might have recovered anyway. In some cases, the conclusion will be correct, but in other cases, Og's conclusion will be erroneous.

What is the most fundamental way that so-called folk medicine differs from modern medicine? Is it that roots and herbs are used in folk medicine, while chemical compounds are used in modern medicine? No, that is not it. Is it that nowadays medical discoveries are reported in learned journals, while the results of folk medicine are recorded in oral tradition? Also no—but we are getting a little closer. The real difference is experimental design. Quite a few drugs and other therapies employed in modern medicine are actually derived from folk medicine, but we have had the benefit of better experimental design. That is, treatments employed in modern medicine have (or at least under optimal circumstances have) been tested in systematic, controlled experimental trials, using precautions against experimental bias, as described in the following paragraphs. At the very least, treatments have been tested in some systematic fashion.

Thus, we (at least in theory) can be confident in the efficacy of our drugs and treatments.

Why does this matter? It matters because we can be more confident of the efficacy of the treatments that we use, or at least we can be if things are done correctly! Therefore, although the manipulations of modern medicine are certainly on the whole more effective than those of folk medicine, there are ineffective components to modern medicine as well. Ineffectual treatments have crept into modern medicine for at least three reasons. First, treatments have sometimes been adopted without the benefit of careful experimental testing. This occurs for a variety of reasons. For example, in the United States there is no universal standard for medical treatment efficacy for procedures that do not fall under the jurisdiction of the Food and Drug Administration. Second, very frequently there are imperfections in experimental designs, so that unintended factors sometimes influence the results. Third, even under the best of circumstances, a good experiment can be thwarted by error or coincidence. Moreover, although a treatment may be "proven" to be effective in general, for any individual patient, who may differ from the tested cases in some manner, the treatment may not be effective. Thus, the lexicon of modern medicine is on the whole very effective, but we cannot have absolute confidence in the efficacy of every treatment technique for every individual.

The ideal experimental design is the double-blind experiment. What is a double-blind experiment? Perceptions are influenced by our expectations. Scientists (or anyone else, for that matter) thus have an overwhelming tendency to see what they expect, or hope, to see. Thus, if one expects a treatment to work, it often will at least seem to be effective. Clinical evaluation of patients is very subjective, and particularly vulnerable to interpretation. Even measurements that appear to be more objective, or involve mechanical measurement devices, can be subtly influenced by observer expectations in a variety of ways. This is compounded when the enthusiasm of a clinician for a new therapy rubs off on the patient, causing an actual improvement in clinical condition. To overcome this problem, arrangements are made to keep (1) the patient and (2) the person(s) evaluating the patient unaware or "blind" as to whether the patient is receiving active treatment or a control procedure: thus, "double-blind." Sometimes arrangements to maintain the "blindness" of the experiment, by avoiding cues (such as, for example, differences in taste of the experimental and placebo medicines) that would reveal whether the patient is on active treatment, can be quite complex. Such precautions can prevent the expectations of the patient from influencing the outcome, and avoid interpretational bias by those making the measurements.

An effective double-blind experiment requires a control procedure that is, as nearly as possible, indistinguishable from the active treatment. For human patients, this creates obvious problems regarding surgical procedures. We could not, for example, transplant dead tissue into the brain of control subjects. In human patients, the best (i.e., that which would lead to the most conclusive results) experimental design involves administration of control surgery (such as transplantation of some inactive tissue) to a separate group of patients. The patients and the doctors who administer the treatment have to be unaware of whether any individual patient received active or placebo surgery. However, such an experiment is generally considered unethical in human patients. Some compromises are always made, ranging from the use of less stringent controls (e.g., anesthesia only, without surgery, or drilling of the skull without tissue implantation) to not using controls at all (the most common practice). For these reasons, the results from any single human trial of a transplantation procedure will never be entirely conclusive. The manner in which this problem may be overcome, and the interactions with animal experimentation, will be considered further in this chapter.

Experimental Design

The way that treatments and testing conditions are incorporated into a testing scheme, or "experimental design," varies. There are essentially two forms of experimental design: comparisons between, and comparisons within, subjects. *Between-group* designs involve comparison of a group that receives an experimental treatment with a control group, as discussed in the preceding section. *Within-subjects* designs involve comparisons of the same subject or subjects under different experimental conditions. Certain experimental designs, such as the double-blind cross-over experiment discussed in the next paragraph, may incorporate features of both forms.

One of the most effective experimental designs used in human subjects is the double-blind crossover, frequently employed in drug studies. This method randomly assigns patients to either of two treatment groups. One group receives a placebo for a set period (say, four weeks), followed by four weeks of treatment with the active drug. The second group receives the same treatments in reverse order. At the midpoint of the trial, the patients "cross over" from active treatment to placebo or vice versa. Neither the patients nor those administering the drug and evaluating the patients are aware of which group is receiving active or placebo drug: the drug treatments are coded (labeled by number or letter codes), so that the study is double-blind. This type of experimental design effectively eliminates various forms of placebo effect and influence of the observers' expectations, and readily lends itself to statistical analysis.

As is illustrated by the contingencies of the crossover design, there are several reasons why the business of designing methods to test effects of brain transplants poses a difficult experimental design issue. For one thing, between-groups designs require control groups, and the choice of a control group (what kind of transplant, or what procedure, should the control group receive?) is complex in relation to brain tissue transplant studies. Moreover, in human trials, control surgery is not usually possible. There are also problems in using within-subjects designs; such procedures generally require reversal, that is, for a drug trial, a within-subjects design would usually require that some or all of the subjects be tested before drug treatment was initiated, during drug treatment, and after drug treatment was discontinued. Sometimes more than one cycle of drug treatment and discontinuance would be used in each subject, particularly if only a small number of experimental subjects could be obtained. Such would be the case for a rare disease or for intensive studies of individual cases. For any transplantation study, removal of transplants presents difficulties, and for human subjects, transplant removal is not generally feasible. Repeated reversal is more or less impossible. Thus, within-subject experimental designs present special problems for studies of neural tissue transplantation.

Between-Groups Designs and Control Groups

To make a broad generalization, most experiments are of the between-groups type. The essence of a between-groups experimental design is a comparison of the group receiving the active treatment—neural transplantation—and a control group. Several very important principles will be discussed here only briefly: the subjects should be randomly assigned to groups, and both groups should be tested at the same time and under identical conditions. These are fundamental requirements for any statistical analysis of the resulting data. In addition, the issues of blind testing discussed above, although not absolutely essential, greatly improve the confidence that one can have in the conclusions of any experimental study.

Nonetheless, the nature of the control group is the most controversial issue regarding neural transplantation. To repeat, the general principle for a control group in any kind of experiment is that its treatment should resemble that of the active treatment group as closely as possible.

Most experiments on neural transplantation have employed transplantation of fetal brain tissue of one kind or another. In the case of Parkinson's disease, fetal substantia nigra is used for transplantation in the hope that, after being transplanted, it can perform at least some of the functions of the normal substantia nigra. These functions include manufacture of dopamine, formation of synapses with appropriate target neurons in the striatum, release of dopamine, and probably a number of other functions that the dopaminergic neurons of the substantia nigra are specialized to perform. It is presumed that the transplanted neurons are not producing functional effects by doing things that any part of the brain could do, such as releasing fragments of a cell surface protein that is produced by all neurons. The ideal control tissue, for an experiment involving transplants of neurons from the substantia nigra, for example, would not perform specialized neuronal functions (releasing dopamine, etc.) but would do all of the nonspecific things that substantia nigra neurons do (liberating fragments of proteins from damaged cells). Thus, the best control tissue for studies of fetal brain grafts is probably another part of the fetal brain. The use of other parts of the brain as a control tissue allows for ruling out various kinds of nonspecific effects, including relatively mundane problems such as effects related to damage of the brain resulting from surgical manipulations.

One might therefore imagine that all studies of fetal brain grafts would simply employ other parts of the same fetal brain for the controls. As we will see in later chapters, there have been numerous studies of transplantation of a region of the brain called the substantia nigra. Thus, a study of fetal substantia nigra transplants might employ other parts of the fetal brain such as the superior colliculus, raphe nucleus, or cortex for transplantation in the control group. There are, however, some potential problems with using another region of the fetal brain as a control tissue in all cases. There is a degree of plasticity in fetal neurons, so that under certain conditions the attributes of neurons may be altered. For example, neurons in the cerebral cortex, cerebellum, or striatum may have some of the properties of substantia nigra neurons under abnormal developmental conditions. For this reason, it is possible that a control tissue which would not be expected to be effective would become so after transplantation. Second, it may simply be the case (for whatever reason) that any part of the fetal brain would be effective. For instance, transplants might work by doing something that all neurons can do. If so, we would want to know this. For these reasons, it can be risky to use another part of the fetal brain as the only control, at least for an initial exploratory experiment in animals, because it could lead to interesting effects being overlooked. Also, in a human clinical trial, even if it were possible, one would not necessarily want to use a very stringent control, such as another part of the fetal brain, because the issues of specificity should presumably have been worked out in prior animal experiments.

With these above considerations in mind, one might develop a sort of hierarchy of control groups that could be used for animal transplantation experiments. After fetal brain, the next best choice might be another living tissue from an adult donor. In animal experiments, we have often employed peripheral nerve (sciatic nerve) obtained from the same pregnant animals that provided the fetal tissue. Peripheral nerve has the virtue of being neuronal tissue, since it contains axons as well as cellular elements (especially the myelin-producing Schwann cells). However, it contains no neuronal cell bodies, so there is no possibility that it could metamorphose into a collection of dopaminergic neurons, or any semblance thereof. There are other possibilities for control procedures, which are listed in table 5.1. Most of these are generally, at least under most conditions, less desirable. One might consider, however, using injections of fluid alone or of killed cells as a control procedure for some kinds of experiments. For example, such controls may be useful for preliminary exploratory experiments in animals.

For transplantation of tissues and cells other than fetal brain, the possibilities for control tissues are different. In some cases, the choices are relatively simple. Genetically altered cells are especially interesting (for details, see chapters 20 and 23). Typically, a cultured cell of some type is genetically altered by insertion of DNA from some other source. This foreign DNA generally directs the host cell to make a foreign protein. For genetically altered cells, excellent controls are readily available: the original cells without genetic alterations, the original cells with an irrelevant genetic alteration, or altered cells in which the inserted DNA has been scrambled so that there is either no product or a nonfunctional product can be used.

For adrenal medulla transplantation, one tissue that has often been employed as a control is sciatic nerve. Sciatic nerve has the virtue of containing some of the cell types that are present in adrenal medulla (fibroblasts and Schwann cells), but does not contain the catecholamine-producing chromaffin cells of the adrenal medulla. Moreover, sciatic nerve fragments grow to about the same size as adrenal medulla grafts, or slightly larger, when transplanted to the lateral ventricle (Takashima et al. 1993).

One would imagine that the issue of control groups for studies of neural tissue transplantation would not even be in question, in this day and age. We now have advanced technologies, molecular biology, and so on. Basic concepts such as the use of control groups by now must have been thoroughly mastered, one would think. Emphatically, this is not so. Problems related to the use of control groups, or the lack thereof, have plagued studies of the functional effects of neural tissue transplantation since their beginning, and continue to be a problem.

Table 5.1
Types of control procedures used to identify effects of neural transplants in animals

Procedure used for control group	How good? (ability to discriminate "real" effects of transplants when used for the control group)	Is the expected reaction of the brain to tissue implantation similar?	Is the general surgical trauma to the brain similar?	Is the general surgical trauma to the body (anesthesia, incision, etc.) similar?
Another region from the same brain	Best	Yes	Yes	Yes
Comparison of donor tissue of different ages	Almost as good	Usually	Yes	Yes
Another living tissue	Almost as good	Sometimes, depends on tissue used	Yes	Yes
Killed tissue	Less satisfactory	No	Yes	Yes
Injection of fluid medium	Unsatisfactory	No	Yes	Yes
Sham procedure	Very unsatisfactory	No	No	Yes
No procedure	Very unsatisfactory	No	No	No

The procedures are ranked, roughly, from best to worst in terms of their ability to discriminate specific from nonspecific effects. Specific effects are defined as effects related to the expected physiological functions of the transplanted tissue. Nonspecific effects are changes related to brain injury or reactions of the brain to injury or the presence of foreign tissue. The third, fourth, and fifth columns concern whether or not each control procedure is similar to the actual transplantation of tissue, in terms of the three listed experimental complications.

The choice of a control group can have a profound influence on the outcome of an experiment, particularly in studies of neural tissue transplantation. Any direct manipulation of the brain can produce effects by itself; insertion of tissue transplants into the brain inevitably produces damage. The damage itself or cellular reactions to damage may produce changes erroneously interpreted as improvement, or even are improvement per se. There are quite conclusive data showing that several human diseases can be improved, at least in some respects, by removal or injury of brain tissue. These diseases include epilepsy, Parkinson's disease, schizophrenia, and obsessive-compulsive disorder. In addition to effects of the surgery, improvements that take place over time may be interpreted as being changes produced by the experimental surgical manipulation, unless the results in the surgical patients are compared with an appropriate control group.

Therefore, a transplantation may appear to produce improvement in a patient group without repairing the brain at all. Improvement in clinical condition may be caused simply by expectations of the patient or of the doctors, or may be related to more complex changes, such as reactions of the brain to minor injury of the affected region. Separating real, physiologically meaningful effects of brain transplants from these other effects is one of the major challenges in this field.

6
Regulations and Guidelines for Fetal Tissue Transplantation

There is a considerable literature devoted to the ethical, religious, and legal issues regarding fetal tissue transplantation. Opinions of interested individuals vary widely, and I do not feel that I have any special qualification to decide what is ethical and what is not. Some references are included at the end of this chapter for further reading, and I will outline some of the issues here.

Regulations for neural transplantation exist, in one sense, to protect the occurrence of practices that society would find objectionable. One might imagine unscrupulous doctors performing all sorts of gruesome procedures. The most useful way of thinking about such regulations, however, is that they exist mainly to protect the various participants. That is, regulations regarding the use of fetal tissue exist for the benefit of the donor (the pregnant woman) and the fetus itself. The recipient of the tissue also needs to be protected from being used as an experimental guinea pig. Patients should not be used in place of animals to develop methods and should not be subjected to surgical procedures that have little chance of success. There are regulations regarding the use of fetal tissue, which will be discussed first, and issues about surgical research on human subjects, which will be discussed later in the chapter.

Fetal Tissue Research and Use

The use of fetal tissue for research purposes, especially research for therapeutic procedures in human subjects, raises a number of unique issues. Some facets of regulations in this area touch on issues that are controversial and cannot be neatly resolved by any sort of argument or experiment.

A good example is the following: Should a fetus be considered a *cadaver*, implying that it is an independent human, or should it be thought of as a *tissue specimen* that is donated by the mother, and thus deserving no special consideration of its own?

Neither view is entirely satisfactory. Dealing with the fetus as a cadaver is unsatisfactory for the simple reason that the fetus cannot itself either give or withhold consent for its use. Yet dealing with the fetus as a tissue specimen also is not entirely satisfactory, for at least two related reasons. First, a fair percentage of the population is opposed to abortion in any form, on the grounds that the fetus is a human being and deserving of consideration on those grounds. Second, dealing with a fetus as a tissue specimen, as though it deserved no more consideration than, perhaps, a skin biopsy, leads to possible scenarios that most people would find objectionable, as will be described later in this chapter. Since this problem cannot be resolved to everyone's satisfaction, the general approach to regulation has been a conservative one: that regulations should be more, rather than less, protective of both the pregnant woman and the fetus.

For example, the issue has been raised as to whether a woman may become pregnant for the purpose of donating the fetus to a specific individual, perhaps her husband or father. Or might a wealthy individual with Parkinson's disease pay one, or even several, women to become pregnant for the purpose of donating the tissue to himself? (Most current procedures for fetal tissue transplantation in Parkinson's disease employ several fetuses.) And we can carry this still further: Might this wealthy individual pay several women to become pregnant for the purpose of donating tissue and, to increase the genetic similarity between the donor fetuses and himself (the host), impregnate the women himself? Most people would find this repugnant, I believe. If you, the reader, don't find this objectionable, I will carry the scenario still farther just to make sure. Perhaps the donor could have him/herself cloned, and pay women to become pregnant and carry the cloned embryos in place of, or in addition to, their own embryo until the embryo has developed sufficiently for transplantation. Such a cloned fetus would be an ideal source of tissue, since it would be genetically identical to the recipient.

Would this be repugnant? I would think so!! Again, the most productive way to think about this systematically is to consider who is being taken advantage of, or victimized, in these scenarios, although for these extreme situations the whole business would be repugnant and unnatural.

Mainly, in these scenarios, it is the fetus, or at any rate the concept of a fetus, that would be treated without sufficient respect. If one presumes that the pregnant woman is not coerced, why should she not be allowed to use her body in any way she wishes, including becoming pregnant in order to donate, or to sell, the fetus, or even to incubate an artificially generated (cloned) fetus? If the fetus is no more deserving of consideration than, say, hair, selling it should be acceptable. Granted, selling a fetus does seem to be an unnatural, peculiar, and disturbing perversion of the way things ought to be. But it is hard to say why, exactly, unless one simply acknowledges that a fetus deserves some consideration independent of that given to the pregnant woman. Even donating a kidney under similar circumstances (that is, growing a kidney for the purpose of later transplantation) might seem acceptable, and it would almost certainly seem acceptable if the donor was able to regenerate a new kidney. Thus, the way that this issue has generally been addressed is by presuming that a fetus requires some consideration—perhaps respect is a better word—greater than that given to a kidney.

Even so, there are problematic aspects to this issue. For example, there are those who believe that a woman *should* be allowed to become pregnant in order to donate the fetus to her father, or to sell it. Interference with that potential right might seem, to some, to be an excessive use of governmental powers and interference with individual liberty. Conversely, there are others who believe that the use of fetal tissue for therapeutic research ultimately encourages abortion, and that all fetal tissue research, especially clinical therapeutic research, should therefore be banned. In fact, governmental support of fetal tissue research (therapeutic transplantation research) was banned in the United States until 1992. In contrast, current policy in many countries permits fetal tissue transplantation with provisions to protect both the pregnant woman and the fetus (Gervais et al. 1992).

Fetal Tissue Use Regulations

Despite the potential for controversy, it has been possible to adopt regulations that are generally satisfactory to most of the concerned parties. The regulations in each country differ slightly, but there are similarities. These regulations have been summarized succinctly by Gervais and coworkers (1992). First, there is the cadaver donor framework (category [a] below), which is used as a basis. Added to that are provisions (b) to protect the aborted fetus; (c) to protect the living fetus; (d) to protect the pregnant woman.

Various countries have employed various combinations of the provisions listed below:

a. Cadaver donation provisions include the following:
   (1) Next of kin must give explicit written consent for tissue use.
   (2) Next of kin may designate recipients.
   (3) One next of kin may veto another's consent decision.
   (4) Users may not be involved in care of the deceased or in the determination of death.
   (5) Tissue may not be bought or sold.
b. Additional provisions are based on the belief that the aborted fetus deserves special consideration different from other cadavers. These include:
   (1) Tissue may be used only for biomedical purposes.
   (2) Information must be unobtainable by other means.
   (3) An institutional ethics committee must oversee the research.
c. A second type of provision relates to the belief that the living fetus deserves special protection; these provisions are designed to prevent the use of fetal tissue from encouraging abortion.
   (1) The woman must consent to abortion prior to discussing donation of the fetus, in order to prevent tissue donation from being a motivation for the abortion.
   (2) The woman may not undergo an abortion for the purpose of donating the fetus.
   (3) The woman may not specify how the tissue is to be used, nor designate the recipient.
   (4) There should be an intermediary to transfer tissue and information between the abortion provider and tissue user.

(5) There should be no financial or other inducements for either the pregnant woman or the abortion provider.

d. Finally, provisions have been added to protect the pregnant woman:

(1) The woman's consent is required.

(2) The father cannot veto the woman's decision.

(3) The woman must be given all information requested.

(4) The abortion procedure may not be modified to accommodate tissue donation.

(5) Any known medical or privacy risks must be disclosed.

(6) The pregnant woman's identity must be protected.

(7) The pregnant woman must consent to testing for HIV and other tests used to determine whether the fetus is free of viral and microbial contamination.

(8) Those attending the pregnant woman must not also be conducting research on use of the fetus.

(9) There must be an intermediary between the abortion provider and the tissue users.

(10) The physician's interest in use of the tissue must be disclosed.

(11) There must be no communication between the pregnant woman and the tissue recipient.

The above provisions are used in various combinations and forms by those countries which have adopted provisions for regulation of research that employs fetal tissue.

Possible Problems

Nonetheless, one should not imagine that the existence of regulations has solved every problem regarding the use of fetal tissue. Some people are eloquently opposed to the use of fetal tissue for transplantation studies, in any form. For example: "American Life League urges the distinguished members of this panel to consider very carefully the consequences which the entire human race will face if this experimentation continues. The harvesting of the bodies of these children, executed by design, is so ghoulish that it defies rational thinking" (Brown 1988, D48). This is, obviously, a rationally expressed view that deserves consideration, not a raving tirade that can simply be dismissed.

One can lend further credence to the above opinion by constructing some scenarios that are actually not too far-fetched. Further exploring the possible abuses and difficulties that might arise does not require too much imagination. Let's start by making four or five quite reasonable assumptions. (1) As a result of further research, the procedure of neural transplantation becomes quite routine, so that it can be performed by any reasonably competent surgeon. (2) Neural transplantation becomes applicable (and effective) for several major disorders that occur fairly frequently in individuals with significant financial resources. Let's include Parkinson's disease, Alzheimer's disease, and stroke (or two of those three). (3) Methods for producing cells in culture that can substitute for fetal tissue do not materialize and, further, several fetuses (let's say four) are required to treat each affected patient. (4) Abortion becomes infrequent or illegal, so that supplies of fetal tissue are very limited. Perhaps drugs that terminate pregnancy are used instead. None of these assumptions are all that improbable.

Obviously, the fact that regulations exist does not mean that they will always be followed. A black market in fetal tissue and transplants might conceivably develop. Pregnancies could be initiated and terminated, and transplants provided in one location, for one modest fee! I don't think that this is especially likely, and it would certainly create an uproar. Or some objection from various quarters, at least. But it is indeed a possibility!

My favorite science fiction writer, Larry Niven, imagines a world in which organ transplantation has become quite common, and most parts of the body are used routinely for transplantation. In his book *Flatlander* (1995), demand outpaces supply. To alleviate the problem, capital punishment is adopted even for minor crimes (e.g., false advertising). But these measures are insufficient, prompting the emergence of a new class of criminals called "organleggers" (after "bootleggers"), who traffic in tissues and organs obtained illegally—they sacrifice living persons to harvest their tissues.

In his scenario, Niven imagines that the brain would not be used (see Preface). By changing the conditions slightly, however, the fetal brain becomes the most valuable part, and the illegal trafficking is not in body parts from unsuspecting victims, but rather in fetuses obtained by paying women to provide them. It is not difficult to develop a realistic scenario along these lines! So we indeed need regulations, but we also might need to think in advance about whether there will be major incentives for thwarting such regulations and how to prevent illegal activities. In fact, basic research conducted in the United States and other developed countries could have the effect of promoting illegal or substandard transplantation procedures both in the United States and elsewhere.

Regulation of Transplantation Surgery Research

In regulation of transplantation surgery research, there is really a problem, depending on how hard and where you want to look. The most egregious example that I know of is the fetal tissue transplantation rumored to have been done in mentally retarded individuals in China, in which large amounts of fetal tissue were diffusely injected into the brain. Actually, the entire enterprise of adrenal medulla transplantation (discussed in chapter 11) might well be considered objectionable, on the basis of there having been almost no prior experiments in subhuman primates, and the fact that adrenal medulla transplants performed under similar conditions in lower animals (e.g., when the grafts are obtained from fully mature donors) don't work very well, if at all. In the human subjects, adrenal medulla transplants did help a little bit, so the results weren't entirely catastrophic and we shouldn't be too upset; however, there was an objectionably high incidence of side effects and deaths. In fact, a reasonable individual might question whether the entire area of fetal tissue transplantation in human patients with Parkinson's disease was begun too soon (see chapters 9 and 13). Human clinical trials were not preceded by blind controlled studies of fetal tissue transplants in subhuman primates. Only recently have the first real controlled studies of subhuman primates been published (see chapter 12), after hundreds of transplants have already been performed in humans.

So how are these things regulated? Well, for the most part, not much. In the United States, research studies in humans are reviewed by institutional review boards. Each institution that conducts research sets up a board to review each study in humans before it is started. Although there are requirements for the composition and procedures of these boards, whether a surgical trial will be performed is more or less left up to the individual institution. Whether there has been (for example) sufficient animal research to justify a human trial is not subject to any universal standards of review. Most countries outside of the United States also do not have centralized national procedures for reviewing clinical trials.

It is often asked whether these procedures are reviewed in the United States by the Food and Drug Administration (FDA). The FDA does not review surgical procedures per se. If a fetal tissue transplantation procedure begins to require processing of the tissue, so that it becomes a biological product rather than unprocessed tissue, FDA regulation would be mandated. Similarly, if transplantation required special devices, cell lines, or treatment with growth factors (for example), FDA regulation would probably be required. A major role of the FDA in regulating fetal tissue transplantation is not imminent. Outside the United States, central review of transplantation procedures is done in only a few places (e.g., Sweden).

What is the conclusion? Well, in my opinion, there have been a few misguided trials, and outside of the United States, a few very misguided trials. In the United States, at least, there have not been very many outrageous abuses. In my opinion, the creation of a bureaucracy specifically to regulate surgery is unnecessary. Current institutional review procedures seem to be mostly adequate. Feedback from colleagues, which includes censure for poor judgment, seems to work reasonably well. Professional societies also may institute internal review procedures, which have the potential to improve matters somewhat with a minimum of regulatory complexity. Eventually, neural transplantation procedures will incorporate materials that require FDA review, and that state of affairs is probably satisfactory at least in the United States, for the time being. Nonetheless, there have been some transplantation procedures performed in human patients that were substandard and definitely undesirable, and continued vigilance on the part of both a well-informed general public and the scientific community can help to prevent further abuses. Hopefully, sources of information such as this book and responsible press coverage will keep the public well informed.

Further Reading

Carnahan, W. A. (1984). Legal implications of the use of embryonic cells for transplants. Proceedings of the Colloquium on the Use of Embryonic Cell Transplantation for Correction of CNS Disorders, Chestnut Hill, MA 1983. *Appl. Neurophysiol.* 47: 69–72.

Council on Scientific Affairs and Council on Ethical and Judicial Affairs, American Medical Association. (1990). Medical applications of fetal tissue transplantation. *J. Am. Med. Assn.* 263: 565–570.

Hoffer, B. J., and Olson, L. (1991). Ethical issues in brain-cell transplantation. *Trends Neurosci.* 14: 384–388.

Mahowald, M. B. (1989). Neural fetal tissue transplantation: Should we do what we can do? *Neurolog. Clinics* 7: 745–857.

Murphy, P. J. (1984). Moral perspectives in the use of embryonic cell transplantation for correction of nervous system disorders. Proceedings of the Colloquium on the Use of Embryonic Cell Transplantation for Correction of CNS Disorders, Chestnut Hill, MA 1983. *Appl. Neurophysiol.* 47: 65–68.

Neville, R. C. (1984). Ethics in medical donations. Proceedings of the Colloquium on the Use of Embryonic Cell Transplantation for Correction of CNS Disorders, Chestnut Hill, MA 1983. *Appl. Neurophysiol.* 47: 73–86.

Squires, S. (1993). Congress looks at tissue transplants. *Washington Post Health News,* October 19, p. 7.

U.S. Congress, Office of Technology Assessment. (1990). *Neural Grafting: Repairing the Brain and Spinal Cord.* OTA-BA–462. Washington, DC: U.S. Government Printing Office.

U.S. Department of Health and Human Services, Public Health Service, National Institutes of Health. (1988). *Report of the Human Fetal Tissue Transplantation Research Panel.* Bethesda, MD.: National Institutes of Health.

Vawter, D. E., and Gervais, K. G. (1995). Ethical and policy issues in human fetal tissue transplants. *Cell Transplant.* 4: 479–482.

Vawter, D. E., Kearney, W., Gervais, K. G., Caplan, A. L., Garry, D., and Tauer, C. (1990). *The Use of Human Fetal Tissue: Scientific, Ethical, and Policy Concerns. A Report of Phase I of an Interdisciplinary Research Project Conducted by the Center for Biomedical Ethics.* Minneapolis: University of Minnesota.

7

Mind Control and Other Things to Worry About

A book about brain transplants would seem incomplete without a consideration of whether transplants could be used for "mind control" or some other diabolical purpose. It is difficult to write about this topic realistically. First, I have to point out that, in writing this chapter, I am not going to try to provide definitive answers, but merely to raise questions and point out some probable limitations on what transplants can and cannot do. After discussing details of how transplants are actually used, I will return to this general topic in the concluding chapter (chapter 25).

Can Brain Transplants Be Used to Alter Personality?

Is it possible that by developing techniques for manipulating the brain, we might make it possible for some future dictator to control the population, transforming dissidents into zombies, robots, assassins, or "terminators"? (After all, when I started this book, my youngest son wanted to be a terminator when he grew up!) More realistically, could brain grafts produce changes in personality? Might brain grafts that are used to correct a disease of motor function unintentionally result in personality changes? Or, at the other extreme, might brain grafts be used intentionally to improve the personality of an obnoxious individual, and should something like this be allowed?

At the extremes, the answers are relatively straightforward. No, brain grafts would probably not be useful to a dictator for creating assassins or terminators. For one thing (notwithstanding the dire paranoid visions of the *X-Files* television program), it seems that it is rather easy to obtain such individuals without resort to such drastic means. But more about that later. At the the other extreme, brain grafts probably *can* produce alterations in personality. Examples of this have already occurred. Changes in personality, in fact, accompany many brain disorders, including psychiatric disorders, Parkinson's disease, Huntington's disease, and others. At the very least, if brain grafts are used in these cases, they can be expected to influence these changes in some way.

It would certainly not be surprising if brain tissue grafts could alter certain aspects of personality. Even in diseases that are thought of mainly as disorders of motor function, psychological changes also occur. For example, patients with Parkinson's disease tend to suffer from dementia, and patients with Huntington's disease are frequently depressed, apparently independent of, and often preceding, the motor dysfunction itself (Folstein 1989). Deficits associated with stroke may affect personality. In general, personality is a constellation of numerous characteristics that define the individual. Thus, the possibility that brain tissue transplantation performed to correct brain disease might alter some aspects of personality cannot simply be dismissed.

Have Neural Transplants Already Produced Personality Changes?

In fact, there already are cases in which brain tissue transplantation has produced unintended psychological changes. In the earliest experimental treatments of Parkinson's disease by adrenal medulla transplantation into the brain, by Backlund and coworkers (1985) (this topic is discussed in more detail in chapter 11), only transient changes were seen, presumably because the grafts died within a few days. Even during this short period, one of the patients experienced psychological manifestations (psychosis), presumably due to a combination of the release of dopamine and/or other biologically active substances from dying transplanted cells and effects of therapeutic drug treatments. In the subsequent experiments on adrenal medulla transplantation done in Mexico City by Madrazo and associates, prolonged psychological abnormalities were seen quite frequently. Subsequent experiments using the same technique confirmed the presence of similar psychological abnormalities and described additional psychological changes.

One particularly disturbing problem, seen most often in older patients, was a dissociative reaction; they appeared unresponsive to their environment, did not initiate activity, and remained passive unless directly aroused. In older patients, this dissociative state sometimes persisted for considerable periods. Goetz and coworkers (1991), summarizing a series of studies of adrenal medulla grafting, reported a high frequency of psychiatric complications. Thus, it appears that psychological changes following adrenal medulla transplantation by the Madrazo technique were quite common.

If one also takes into account the fact that the groups performing those procedures were not primarily interested in detecting subtle psychological changes, it seems likely that some very problematic psychological changes may take place when adrenal medulla grafts are used for Parkinson's disease. The general problem of unintended personality changes following brain grafts is particularly serious, since subtle changes in personality cannot necessarily be predicted from studies in rat models, and probably would be difficult to detect even in monkeys. If serious problems were seen in monkey models, they would preclude the use of similar procedures in human patients, but there are many types of personality changes that might not be detectable even in monkeys.

What Might Be Responsible for Unexpected Personality Changes After Brain Grafts?

Is there a more general conclusion that we can draw from the apparent prevalence of psychological side effects after adrenal medulla transplantation? There is at least ground for interesting speculation. Cells produce and release a bewildering variety of chemical mediators; as has been mentioned, these include not only neurotransmitters but also peptides and proteins that induce long-term changes in other cells. Each cell type may be thought of as having a "signature" pattern of chemicals that are released. Thus, dopaminergic neurons release not only dopamine but sometimes also peptides (such as the neuroactive peptide cholecystokinin) and other proteins and growth factors. Adrenal chromaffin cells are superficially similar to dopamine neurons—they contain dopamine and the enzymes required for dopamine manufacture. They also, however, release norepinephrine, epinephrine, and a bewildering array of peptides and proteins, including growth factors, met-enkephalin, L1, tenascin, and many other substances. Brain function might be altered by any of these substances, and changes in psychological function would not be surprising if viewed in this light. When such cells are transplanted to a new location in the brain, where they do not "belong," these chemical mediators are bound to produce some kind of effect. It should be pointed out, however, that some psychological changes have been observed even following transplantation of fetal substantia nigra in Parkinson's disease patients (Price et al. 1995; see chapter 13 of this volume).

Thus, in transplanting adrenal medulla to the striatum, we are introducing a cell type that produces not only dopamine (this is the biochemical we believe we wish to replace) but also many other chemical mediators, some of which perhaps do not belong in the striatum. In contrast, when fetal substantia nigra is transplanted into the striatum, these unwanted changes are likely to be minimized. Although cells from the substantia nigra probably produce many substances other than dopamine, these substances are likely to correspond reasonably well to what "belongs" in the striatum. Nonetheless, even when fetal neurons are used for transplantation, unintended changes are still possible; for example, glia from the substantia nigra may produce unusual effects when relocated to an ectopic region—in this case, the striatum. In the future, we are likely to encounter a number of circumstances that involve transplanting brain cells to locations other than where they originated, as well as circumstances that involve the use of alternative cell types—perhaps cells that do not even originate in the brain. When a great degree of disparity exists between the normal cell population of the target area of the brain and the cells that are to be used for transplantation, increased vigilance concerning potential psychological side effects in humans is certainly prudent. It may even turn out to be the case that the use of nonneuronal cells in human CNS transplantation is more or less impractical—or perhaps should be done only in dire circumstances or instances of extreme debilitation—for this reason.

Can Brain Grafts Be Used Intentionally to Produce Personality Changes?

So, having dealt with the problem of unwanted psychological side effects, is there a problem concerning *intentional* use of brain grafts to produce psychological changes? A short answer is yes—of course there is a potential problem in this area, but it is not much different from problems presented by the availability of drugs that influence mental processes, and bizarre uses of neural transplantation in this realm are unlikely. To consider this issue, we will deal with a range of possibilities.

First, consider a severe form of mental illness. Schizophrenia is a very misunderstood disease. It is emphatically not "split personality"; rather, it is a severe and debilitating disorder. Schizophrenia is unquestionably a disease of the brain, yet it cannot always be treated effectively by drugs. If treatment by brain tissue transplantation became a realistic possibility, schizophrenia would be a reasonable candidate for application of this technique. Especially if it became known that schizophrenia was caused by a specific deficit in a particular neurochemically defined pathway. There have been attempts to treat schizophrenia by neural transplantation (e.g., Kolarik et al. 1988), but the approach used was not, in my opinion, based on any sort of sensible rationale or experimental data. Let us say, for example, that schizophrenia is found to be caused by damage to a pathway from the hippocampus to the nucleus accumbens. Then there would be little objection to repairing this pathway using neural transplantation.

At another level, perhaps, is depression. Depression can exhibit a wide range of severity, and is sometimes debilitating. In contrast to schizophrenia, however, depression can almost always be treated effectively with drugs. Depression is thus a less likely candidate for treatment by brain tissue transplantation, compared with schizophrenia. In contrast to drug treatment, transplantation is a much more invasive, and irreversible, procedure. Thus, the use of neural transplantation in depression would require unusual circumstances. Perhaps depression of life-threatening severity that could not be alleviated by drug treatment would warrant surgical treatment.

What about minor personality problems, or what if transplantation could be used simply to improve mood? In other words, what if a way were found to employ transplantation the way the drug Prozac is sometimes used (Kramer 1993)? In that case, there would be a problem, and in fact the problem would probably require regulations and guidelines limiting the circumstances under which transplantation could be used, much as there are already guidelines for drug use. Current practices regarding the use of Prozac could, in fact, lead to scrutiny of quite similar issues. Certainly a procedure as invasive as transplantation should not be used for a disorder like depression without prior consideration of guidelines and the potential for abuse.

Let us carry this further. If we could change depression with transplants, could we make people generally more (or less) cheerful? Or could we change other personality characteristics? Is it possible that transplantation could be used to completely alter personalities, so that our concept of individuality becomes blurred? Could transplantation be employed for some diabolical purpose? Will a person receiving a brain transplant become a hybrid—part himself, and part donor? Could we induce intrusive memories of past lives or some other weird changes? The short answer to this is no—I don't think this could occur. I think there are limits to the degree of change that can be produced in an individual. The so-called personality is a composite of the entire constellation of brain structure and life experience of that individual. The brain, in the sense of being a personality-producing machine, is a single integrated structure, and cannot be modified to the degree that its overall integrity is changed. It is not likely that intact, complete memories or personality tendencies reside in small fragments of tissue of a size that could be transplanted. Moreover, intact memories reside only in the brains of fairly mature individuals, and for the most part, only fetal brain tissue can be transplanted without destroying the integrity of the transplanted tissue . . . probably. It is, most likely, possible to correct minor problems or to alter certain aspects of personality, but a general restructuring of personality is not likely.

Upon further thought, however, some very peculiar things *might* be possible. We do not know exactly how memories are stored in the brain. We do know a great deal, however. Certain brain areas are important for certain aspects of memory, for example. Exactly how the brain stores information—a recollection of your eighth birthday party for instance—is unknown. What neurons (and glial cells) are involved, and what biochemical changes are responsible for the memory storage events? On a molecular level, where is the information stored? The information we have on this topic is quite incomplete. Suppose, however, that a fragment of cortical tissue is transplanted adjacent to several neurons that play an important role in that particular recollection. These new neurons form connections with some of the birthday memory neurons. One might easily imagine that the memory could be altered—perhaps subtly, perhaps drastically, or perhaps even in minor specific details. Maybe the cake was chocolate in the "real" memory, but became a yellow cake in the "new" memory. Or maybe the "new" memory would simply be blurred. Would the memory then seem to be foreign? Would it seem to be a hallucination? Suppose the cake became yellow with squirming purple and green shapes all over it in the new memory. It is even conceivable that cells could be transplanted into an area that is important for many or all memories, so that many or all memories began to be perceived as hallucinatory. I cannot think of any reason to completely discount this possibility.

Since we do not know exactly how memories are stored in the brain, we cannot discount the possibility that entirely new memories might be formed by brain tissue transplants. To think about this possibility, first perform an introspective self-experiment. Think of your memory of an important event—even a very important event—that took place at least 10 years ago. Perhaps your wedding, the birth of your first child, or a death. One's memory does not consist of a running "video" of the event that one can search for details. Rather, it consists of a series of static and fragmentary images. Very salient memories may contain many closely spaced images, but less salient memories may contain only a few, or even just one. Note that these images lack detail. The amount of information in any one of these images is not very great (perhaps if a similar image were stored in a computer, it would occupy a few thousand bits or so). Thus, could a number of relatively random synaptic connections that are formed between a transplant and the host brain be organized in such a way that a new memory is formed? Would such a memory be perceived as an actual event or, lacking context, would it seem to be a hallucination? Or, to those inclined to such ideas, an intrusion from a past life?

Limits

The brain is often thought of as being fundamentally different from other organs—for example, the liver, in that the liver is a single unit whereas the brain is a grouping of several separate components (e.g., the hypothalamus, cerebellum, cerebral cortex, etc.). It sometimes seems that these components can be dealt with separately, that is, that they can be analyzed or studied as separate individual units. In a very real sense, however, the opposite is true. A part of the liver can be removed without compromising the function of the remainder. No single cell depends on any other cell for its function. In contrast, however, the entire brain is interconnected, and in many ways functions as a single unit. Many parts of the brain serve specific purposes. Thus, the cerebellum is largely involved in motor control, but only in concert with other parts of the brain; it in fact cannot perform any function whatsoever in isolation. In fact, the entire brain is probably interconnected, so that by a circuitous route one could reach any part of the brain from any other part by following interconnections between cells. Although particular functions are concentrated in particular regions, these regions depend on other regions for execution of these functions. Each neuron, wherever it is located, has many connections, and the entire pattern forms during development, as a single unit. Most of the scaffolding for development of interneuronal connections disappears once the connections are formed, and is replaced by other materials (e.g., myelin). Thus, it is probably impossible to entirely reconstitute the complete interconnections of even a single cell, much less a major part of the brain.

How does this pertain to our discussion of personality? It means that the degree of reconstruction that is possible is extremely limited. It will therefore be possible to rewire only a very minor part of the brain in the adult, and the connections of even this part will be incomplete. Thus, limitations of the system will ensure that the host will always remain the same individual, and thus the blurring of individuality will not become a problem.

Finally, there remains the issue of whether brain tissue transplantation can be employed for some diabolical purpose. Can it be employed to produce assassins, or Democrats, or Republicans? Although this is a fanciful suggestion, it is not entirely impossible that brain grafts might be used to produce some particular form of personality alteration, say, increased aggressiveness.

There are many possible forms of mind control that might be conceived. Several have been popularized in movies. For example, one might imagine that highly potent methods of reward or punishment might be devised, so that individuals could be made highly aggressive, placid and compliant, or robotlike zombies. In fact, some of these aims can already be achieved, using relatively primitive and crude technologies. A form of brain surgery, the prefrontal lobotomy was widely used in the 1940s and 1950s, and in more extensive forms could be used to produce individuals with little ability for emotional expression (Valenstein 1973). Several drugs that are readily available produce extremely effective rewarding effects. The crack form of cocaine is thought to produce, in at least some individuals, a state of pure pleasure exceeding that which can be obtained through natural sources (or through brain surgery). In the late 1950s and 1960s, when electrical stimulation of the brain was first being studied, similar fears were aroused. It developed, however, that the pleasure produced by direct electrical stimulation of the brain is relatively mild (Delgado 1969; Heath 1964; Ervin and Mark 1969). The response to hypothalamic stimulation (in one of the regions regarded as being a "pleasure center" in the rat) were described as being "mild euphoria (like two martinis)" (Ervin and Mark 1969, 161). It is not, apparently, sufficient to weaken one's will or to control one's behavior. Drugs such as amphetamine and phencyclidine (or PCP or angel dust) often promote aggressive behavior. Increased aggressiveness also may accompany certain forms of brain injury, for example, injury of the temporal lobe.

The term "physical control of the mind" was coined by José Delgado (1969) to describe the control of behavior through electrical stimulation of the brain. In a famous example, Delgado implanted electrodes into the brain of a bull. He then entered a bullring complete with cape and radio transmitter. The charging bull was stopped in its tracks by electrical stimulation of the brain; however, it has since been questioned whether the bull actually adopted a "pacifist" viewpoint or, rather, the stimulation simply interfered with the motor aspects of the charge. A number of other applications of brain stimulation were considered, including treatment of human patients with psychiatric disorders (Heath 1963; Monroe and Heath 1954). Despite the fact that the electrodes were thought to be capable of stimulating "pleasure centers" and thereby exerting a strong influence on behavior, the effectiveness of these manipulations in controlling human behavior were eventually determined to be minimal. As mentioned above, crack cocaine apparently produces a much more intense feeling of reward than brain stimulation, and there has not been much consideration of useful applications of this substance.

There are certainly earlier examples of the use of neurosurgery for functional brain control. An example that was quite controversial 25–30 years ago is its use in the treatment of violence. Aggressive epileptic patients were treated with neurosurgery. It is interesting to point out that in some cases, neurosurgery was used as a treatment for the violence associated with epilepsy, not for the epilepsy per se (Mark and Ervin 1970; Mark and Neville 1973). Those involved in this controversy rejected the idea that neurosurgery should be used as a treatment for abnormal behavior in the absence of brain pathology, or at least such was their written opinion. Their stated position was that "Medical procedures as drastic as neurosurgery should be used only when behavior is abnormal, and bad, primarily because of an abnormality in the brain. Abnormal violent behavior not associated with brain disease should be dealt with politically and socially, not medically" (Mark and Neville 1973, 768). In their studies, it was claimed that in many cases the tendency to violence could be reduced by ablative surgery while producing little functional impairment. Although the circumstances are slightly different, the principle applies here. Brain tissue transplantation should be used as a treatment for disease, not as a means of altering behavior per se. We need not concern ourselves too much with what might be possible, provided we adhere to this principle. Nonetheless, not everyone would necessarily agree with this principle. And, as Mark and his coworkers experienced, it is not always straightforward to discriminate between "disease" or "abnormal behavior associated with brain pathology," and abnormal behavior that would be convenient to control.

The more general concern is that brain tissue transplantation might ultimately be developed to the point that it could be used as a means of mind control. This possibility also was raised more than 20 years ago. To quote again from Mark and Neville: "It is appropriate to return to the specter of a tyrannical government controlling a submissive population through psychosurgery and electrical brain stimulation. Even though this is technically unlikely now, it is a possibility to be conjured with" (Mark and Neville 1973, 772). More than 25 years later, this scenario is no more imminent than it was then. Then, as now, there are easier ways, such as through the use of drugs, to influence people biologically.

The public, and often scientists as well, have often overestimated the degree of control of the "mind" that can be achieved through biological intervention. Fortunately for those of us who attempt to interfere with brain function through the use of drugs, lesioning, stimulation, transplantation, or other methods, the factors that make up an individual consist of an integrated network so complex and interconnected that it cannot be easily altered in a fundamental sense by any simple medical or physical manipulation. Although the "mind" can be damaged, stimulated, or altered in a variety of ways, an intact brain will be impaired to some degree by such manipulation. Probably only in the case of disease or disorder will it be possible to improve functioning by medical intervention.

As for governmental mind control, the dangers in the misuse of social and psychological manipulation are probably much greater than those inherent in the misuse of medical manipulation. In the Nazi regime prior to World War II, psychological manipulation, with the appropriate contextual and political climate, allowed political manipulators to subvert large segments of the population to execute the most diabolical and necrophilic social program that could be imagined, in a far more effective fashion than is likely to have been possible than if a medical form of manipulation were used. In that case, medical misexperimentation was not used for political control. Rather, the political regime was allowed to divert medicine for diabolical purposes. It is unlikely that hideous and ghoulish behavior, with the degree of pervasiveness and organization comparable with that practiced by the Nazis, could be achieved by "physical control of the mind."

Society and Regulation

Still, after all of this has been considered, it is not out of the realm of possibility that brain tissue transplantation could somehow be used in this manner, to control behavior for nonmedical ends. It is true that technological advances may permit more sophisticated forms of manipulation; perhaps sociopathic behavior could be enhanced by neural transplants. Nevertheless, most forms of manipulation can be accomplished already. If a future dictatorial regime wishes to control your mind, it can be done using current technology: simply remove part of your brain or give you drugs. Doing so might not accomplish much that was useful, even to the dictator, but it could be done. Brain tissue transplantation might result in some more sophisticated types of manipulation, but probably not manipulations that are new in principle.

It is possible, thus, that brain tissue transplantation could achieve similar ends with less compromise of other functions. For example, psychosurgery might, in principle, be used to create a compliant individual who would carry out immoral commands—say, to slaughter innocent civilians. The psychosurgery might also result in impaired decision making, so that this altered individual would execute the commands only literally, with no capacity to make decisions required by arising contingencies. Perhaps brain tissue transplantation could be used more efficiently than other methods (e.g., drugs) in this manner. In the end, however, we are dependent upon the controls imposed by society to prevent abuse.

Many technologies exist that are objectionable in the wrong hands: drugs, guns, kitchen knives, gas chambers, and so on. In some respects, the more sophisticated and efficient the technology, the more damage it can do if abused. Some technologies can be abused in more than one way. Consider drugs: illegal recreational abuse of drugs; improper prescription by doctors; use of Prozac to alter personality; legal but debilitating abuse of alcohol; and the use of drugs to extract information from prisoners of war. Neural transplantation also may be abused in more than one way. Political use is a remote concern, and does not seem very probable at present. Abuse in the form of unjustified medical use, involving experimentation on poorly informed humans or clinical research that does not have a sufficient basis in animal studies, is a much more realistic concern. This is occurring now, and has been occurring sporadically for many years.

Societal controls for all of these technologies can exist at several levels: professional societies, institutional controls, religious proscriptions, conventions of society, and legal restrictions. In the case of guns, for example, when societal conventions fail to control use, as is being observed lately, an outcry for legal control arises. A system for the control of use of neural transplantation is already in place, in the form of institutional review. For some aspects of neural transplantation, especially procurement and use of fetal tissue, there are national standards in the United States and several other countries. The possibility of expansion of these controls, in the form of national or even international standards and review for surgical procedures, has been considered by both professional societies and government agencies. National standards imposed by professional societies, for example, in the form of recommendations that are not legally binding would be a relatively mild form of control. Most of the really egregious abuses seen so far have, however, occurred in countries that are not in close communication with current medical research on neural tissue transplantation. It is not likely that international controls or standards for neural transplantation procedures could be imposed; they would be difficult to monitor and enforce. One realistic possibility would be that an international scientific society could establish standards and a procedure for reviewing clinical protocols. Clinical research that did not meet these standards would not be endorsed by the international scientific community. Something like this would, perhaps, at least discourage egregiously useless procedures.

Two Interesting Things to Think About

To conclude this chapter, we will discuss two scenarios that present different kinds of dilemmas for the use of neural transplantation in human patients. With these examples, I hope to illustrate that there are bound to be future situations that pose quandaries for which there are no clear-cut "right" or "wrong" answers.

A Prisoner Dilemma

Some possible technical issues related to this notion are discussed later, in chapter 15. Reminiscent of the issues surrounding brain surgery for treating violent epileptic patients, discussed earlier in this chapter, imagine the following: First, we will restrict our discussion to criminals who are sentenced either to death or to life in prison without the possibility of parole. These criminals are incarcerated for violent crimes, so their release would place others at risk. Suppose we were able to alter their violent tendencies through some sort of transplantation of cells into the brain; even suppose this occurred at the cost of some modest decrement in intelligence quotient (IQ)—perhaps 10 points. This is reminiscent of the idea of removing brain tissue for treating violence, except that we can now suppose that it would also be possible to remove the transplanted cells, so that the procedure would be permanent but not irreversible. The prisoner could then have an alternative: Would he choose life in prison or release with a cell implant? There is the potential for coercion—and there is the possibility that there would be side effects. But, nevertheless, which is more humane? In the extreme case, if the cell implants had no detectable side effects, and if the prisoner was sentenced to death, and if the cells could be removed, wouldn't implanting cells into the subject's brain be a reasonable alternative to execution or to life in prison?

The Anencephalic Birth

Anencephaly is a congenital malformation in which children are born essentially without a brain, sometimes lacking brain, skull, and scalp. Usually the spinal cord, cerebellum, and brain stem are present, and may exhibit various degrees of reflex activity. Almost all such children die within the first postnatal week. Various other severe forms of abnormal brain development are known; for example, the brain may be very small (microcephaly), or the cortical convolutions may be absent with defects in neuronal migration (lissencephaly) (Adams and Victor 1993). In some of these conditions, the infants may survive indefinitely but in a severely impaired or a nearly vegetative state.

Suppose that we were to try making transplants in such severely malformed infants. We can, perhaps, imagine injecting large numbers of immature CNS cells into the brain, allowing them to develop and organize in whatever way they can. The results would almost certainly be disastrous in one way or another. It is not likely that any semblance of a normal brain could be produced by transplanting cells in this way. Yet, under such circumstances, cogent arguments might be made for performing transplants, and there might well be people who would be desperate for such things to be done. Take the most extreme example, the anencephalic child who would normally survive for only a few days. Quite possibly, a transplantation procedure could improve brain function somewhat and prolong the life of such a child, perhaps indefinitely. But would a procedure like this have the potential to transform a child like this into a normal child, or a child with anything like a normal life? Almost certainly not, because by the time of birth, the brain has matured to such a degree that complete integration of the transplanted cells with the rudimentary brain that is present, or with other parts of the body, would not occur. Thus, what would be produced by such a procedure would most likely be unpredictable, and would be some sort of severely dysfunctional and malformed infant. Such a procedure is not likely to be used, therefore, to any significant extent.

There is, however, another possibility that is somewhat more feasible and thus much more problematic. Suppose that anencephaly (or other severe developmental arrest) could be detected considerably *prior* to birth, at perhaps seven to nine weeks of gestational age. To complicate things, we could suppose even further that the ongoing political climate (or, perhaps, the religious beliefs of the parents) was strongly opposed to abortion, to the degree that termination of the pregnancy was not an option (fetal tissue would still be available, at least from spontaneous abortions, or maybe we could use genetically engineered cells). Neither supposition seems entirely improbable. Then, one might be faced with the prospect of an impending and inevitable birth of a child that would be severely disabled but might survive with the disability for a long time.

I'm sure that the reader can see where this is heading. At seven to nine weeks' gestation, transplantation of a mixture of fetal brain cells into the brain of a severely microcephalic or anencephalic infant might very well improve brain function somewhat. For this kind of procedure, the earlier it was performed, the better the probable outcome. Nonetheless, it is not likely that an entirely normal infant could be produced in this manner. (At least not in the foreseeable future; prevention is more likely.) In the process of developing such a technique, it is also likely that some severely malformed and perhaps monstrously malformed children would be produced, perhaps to survive for many years. I will leave it to the reader to consider the possibilities, ethics, and repercussions of such a procedure. Certainly, I think that this is something that should not be tried. It is possible that it will be, nevertheless, and perhaps things like this need to be considered before they become realistic possibilities. I certainly would not have expected cloning of humans to be proposed as a realistic possibility, but all of a sudden, seemingly, it has been!

III

Parkinson's Disease

8

Neural Systems and Parkinson's Disease

Notwithstanding the quite substantial earlier work on neural transplantation, the technique remained of interest to only a handful of specialists until 1979, when the first studies showing that brain grafts could be used to reverse a functional deficit induced by brain injury similar to Parkinson's disease in animals were published. In the early 1970s, simple rodent models of Parkinson's disease (e.g., the unilateral lesion model) were developed by Urban Ungerstedt and others, as discussed later in this chapter.

Parkinson's Disease

Parkinson's disease, which was initially described as "shaking palsy" by James Parkinson in 1817, is a progressive degenerative disorder of the brain that is manifested mainly as impairment of motor function. The original name, "shaking palsy," refers to a low-frequency tremor that is usually most prominent in the arms and hands but is also seen in the legs, mouth, and jaw. In addition to tremor, there are three other cardinal symptoms of Parkinson's disease: rigidity, postural instability, and bradykinesia, a loss and slowing of movements. Although the tremor is the most apparent symptom, the bradykinesia is usually the most disabling manifestation of the disease.

Bradykinesia involves a loss of movements, inability to initiate movements, and slowness of movements. Muscular rigidity can be detected by moving the limbs passively, upon which an unevenness or racheting effect is seen; this is known as cogwheel rigidity. The postural instability is seen as an inability to make postural corrections that are normally automatic; patients fall frequently or can maintain their posture only with a conscious effort. In addition to the four cardinal symptoms (bradykinesia, rigidity, tremor, and postural instability), many other signs and symptoms occur; these may include abnormal gait, a loss of facial expression, drooling and difficulty in swallowing, sensory abnormalities, and even skin problems (seborrhea of the scalp). There are also often psychiatric manifestations, mainly dementia and depression. The disease is progressive, usually beginning with mild symptoms, such as unilateral tremor, and progressing over 5–20 years. Untreated, the disease progresses to a state of severe and almost complete disability. Patients may ultimately become bedridden and unable to eat, dress themselves, or perform even the simplest activities.

Postmortem examination of the brains of patients with Parkinson's disease has revealed a loss of neurons in a part of the brain called the substantia nigra pars compacta, which will hereafter mainly be referred to as the SN. The SN is located in a region of the brain called the ventral mesencephalon, that is, the lower midbrain. Since these cells in humans (although *not* in lower animals) contain a dark pigment called neuromelanin, or melanin, this degeneration is seen as depigmentation when the appropriate part of the brain is casually examined. More detailed studies show a loss of neurons in the SN. In addition, surviving neurons in the SN of patients with Parkinson's disease show a characteristic abnormality called Lewy bodies, named after their discoverer. They are circular structures inside the neurons that appear to have a dense central core and a lighter-staining outer region, and are at least partly composed of neurofilaments. In patients with Parkinson's disease, Lewy bodies are seen not only in the SN but in other brain regions as well, including the locus ceruleus, raphe nuclei, hippocampus, amygdala, and cortex. Thus Parkinson's disease involves degeneration in a number of brain areas in addition to the SN, though the extent of degeneration in the SN is much greater than is seen in other brain regions. Also, the degree of motor impairment is correlated with the degree of SN degeneration. Thus, it is generally acknowledged that Parkinson's disease is primarily a disease of SN neuronal degeneration.

Neural Systems

Research in neuroscience, in general, tends to focus on collections of neurons with similar properties rather than on individual cells. Groups of similar neurons are often located together in certain brain regions (or nuclei). A group of similar neurons having similar biochemical properties and utilizing the same chemical substance as a neurotransmitter, together with the axonal and dendritic extensions of these cells and their connections with other cells, is often referred to as a system (figure 8.1). A great deal of research interest is focused on certain of these systems because of their importance in the control of behavior or other functions, or because they are thought to be responsible for particular diseases.

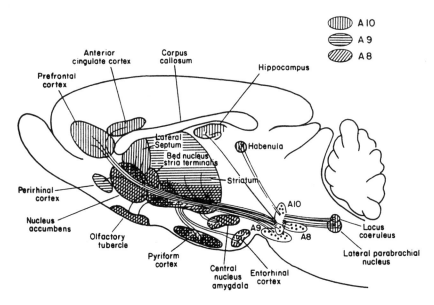

Figure 8.1
Distribution of systems of dopaminergic neurons in the brain. A8, and A9, and A10 are the three major collections of dopaminergic cell bodies. The brain regions shown are those identified as receiving dopaminergic afferents. Additional groups of dopamine neurons, not shown in the picture, are located in the hypothalamus, retina, and olfactory bulb. (From Cooper et al. 1996, with permission.)

Several neurochemical systems of particular importance involve neurons with cell bodies in the brain stem or mesencephalon, and utilize several relatively simple biochemical substances (monoamines) as neurotransmitters forming their primary connections with higher centers. These monoaminergic neurotransmitters mainly include norepinephrine, dopamine, and serotonin. The output from the cell bodies of this group of systems largely passes from caudal ("tail" end), to rostral (in the direction of the head) through the hypothalamus or diencephalon.

In the 1950s and early 1960s, it was noted that the hypothalamus appeared to play an important role in the control of behavior, especially motivational and physiological homeostatic mechanisms. For example, electrical stimulation of the brain was found to be rewarding in humans (Heath 1963; Monroe and Heath 1954). Animals were found to press levers vigorously at very high rates in order in initiate electrical stimulation of parts of the hypothalamus (Olds and Milner 1954). This phenomenon was termed "self-stimulation of the brain" or "electrical brain self-stimulation." Animals could be induced to eat or drink by similar electrical stimulation, or by injections of small amounts of certain drugs into the hypothalamus. Animals with hypothalamic lesions exhibited a profound lack of eating and drinking behavior, and loss of weight, with gradual recovery over a period of time. This pattern was called the lateral hypothalamic syndrome (see Teitelbaum 1971; Grossman 1979).

Considerable research was devoted to understanding the particular properties of these behavioral patterns related to hypothalamic stimulation or damage during the 1960s and early 1970s. In particular, the lateral hypothalamus appeared to be an important center for motivational control, since (a) lesions of this area produced a lateral hypothalamic syndrome of weight loss, as described above; (b) stimulation of this area produced eating, drinking, and general activation; and (c) animals would press bars at high rates to initiate electrical stimulation of this area.

The hypothalamus is close to the pituitary and contains several nuclei that are involved, through a variety of mechanisms, in the regulation of physiological functions. These functions include stimulation and inhibition of pituitary hormone release, sensing of blood glucose and blood pressure, control of sexual differentiation and sex hormones, and many other regulatory processes. In addition, as has been mentioned, the axons of dopaminergic, noradrenergic, and serotonergic systems pass through or near the hypothalamus. The techniques available in the early 1960s did not permit separate examination of the role of these various structural components in the control of behavior. Thus, electrical stimulation activates both neuronal fibers and cells of a variety of types that happen to lie close to the stimulating electrode. Lesions, at the time, were made electrically, using electrocoagulation, which essentially cooks the tissue, destroying all living components of the nearby brain tissue, including neurons, glial cells, neurites, and even blood vessels. Stimulation by administration of drugs was more specific, but the anatomical basis of the effects that these drugs were producing could not be discerned. Thus, until more specific methods were developed, it would not be possible to understand the specific circuits that were responsible for the behavioral effects evoked by manipulations in the hypothalamus.

During this same period, in 1963, Oleh Hornykiewicz and his coworkers discovered, on postmortem examination, that patients with Parkinson's disease showed a profound loss of the neurotransmitter dopamine (see Hornykiewicz 1966). The most useful direct result of this discovery was the development of L-DOPA treatment for Parkinson's disease. Since dopamine does not readily cross the blood-brain barrier, L-DOPA, the precursor for dopamine, was tried, and eventually this was found to be a highly effective treatment. Although the effectiveness of L-DOPA diminishes after long periods of treatment (on the order of 6–12 years) due to the development of various side effects and fluctuations in efficacy, it remains a major form of therapy for Parkinson's disease.

Several techniques were developed between 1962 and 1975 that have revolutionized neuroscience by making it possible to study specific neuronal systems in much greater detail. Some of these technical advances included methods for making lesions that destroy only neurons, or only certain types of neurons, without damaging other cells or nearby passing fibers, and staining techniques that have made it possible to identify specific types of neurons and their connections. Some of these techniques will be discussed in more detail in later chapters. Probably, however, the single technique that led to the most fundamental advance, at least in this particular area of research, was the Falck-Hillarp fluorescence histochemical technique (see Cooper, Bloom, and Roth 1996). This technique consists of a way of inducing cells that contain dopamine (as well as norephinephrine and serotonin) to become fluorescent, so that they can be identified microscopically. In essence, thin slices (or sections) that include the dopaminergic tissues are frozen, dried, and exposed to formaldehyde vapor. Dopamine reacts with formaldehyde to form a fluorescent molecule, so that when this procedure is performed under appropriate conditions, and the section is illuminated in the appropriate manner, the locations of dopamine in the tissue sections can be seen as areas of bright green or blue-green fluorescence. There are now two available methods for producing this type of histochemical reaction, one that involves the use of formaldehyde and one that employs liquid, glyoxylic acid.

By employing the histochemical fluorescence method, the locations of the cell groups in the brain stem that contain dopamine, norepinephrine, and serotonin were described by in the 1960s (Dahlstrom and Fuxe 1964). Possibly the experiments that gave the greatest stimulus to research in this field, however, were those which mapped the terminal regions—that is, the areas where axons from the cell groups form their connections, and thus the brain regions where the effects of activity in these systems are exerted—as well as the areas through which these axons pass on the way to forming these connections (Ungerstedt 1971c). In these experiments, Ungerstedt also described behavioral changes that were seen as a result of damage in these pathways, thus developing both the anatomical and the behavioral studies of the dopaminergic neuronal systems—the neuronal systems that are important for Parkinson's disease. These experiments will be described in more detail below.

The particular system that is of interest for the present is the nigrostriatal dopamine system. Anatomically, this system follows the general pattern for the monaminergic cell groups as described above: a relatively small cluster of dopamine-containing neurons in the substantia nigra pars compacta sends projections that pass through the hypothalamus and terminate in the neostriatum or caudate putamen. The anatomy of this terminal area is slightly different in rodents, compared with humans and nonhuman primates. In rodents, the caudate putamen is a single brain region, while in humans it is divided into two separate areas (the caudate nucleus and the putamen) by the white matter of the internal capsule. For rodents, the terms neostriatum, caudate putamen, corpus striatum, and striatum are often used interchangeably. Technically, the striatum or corpus striatum includes an adjacent nucleus called the globus pallidus, which serves quite different functions. For the remainder of this book, it is sufficient to remember that we will employ the term "striatum" to refer to the caudate putamen in rodents, where numerous dopaminergic axons terminate and mediate functions related to motor control.

The collection of neurons in the substantia nigra pars compacta is not the only such group. For example, there is a group of dopamine-containing neurons located in the ventral tegmental area, more medial and ventral to the SN cells, that projects axons to other areas, including the nucleus accumbens and the prefontal cortex. This second system is known as the *mesolimbic system.* Largely from experiments in rodents, it has been determined that this latter system is important in controlling a number of important behavioral functions, including stimulant and rewarding effects of drugs, exploratory behaviors, emotion, and motivation.

It is rather remarkable that both of these dopaminergic systems, the nigrostriatal and the mesolimbic, although minuscule, play such prominent roles in the control of behavior. In general, the mesolimbic system is though of as being important for motivation and emotion, while the nigrostriatal system is thought of as being important for motor function. This is, however, a considerable oversimplification, and the two systems cannot be completely separated in these terms. It is also remarkable that both systems appear to be particularly susceptible to dysfunction. In varying degrees, they are thought to be important in Parkinson's disease, schizophrenia, drug abuse, Tourette's syndrome, and toxic brain injury induced by agents such as the synthetic opiate contaminant MPTP and manganese. A number of drugs of abuse, such as amphetamine, PCP, and cocaine, appear to exert their effects through these systems. Moreover, dysfunction of other classes of striatal neurons is thought to be related to Huntington's disease and perhaps to mood disorders.

Current Animal Behavioral Models

Studies in Rodents

A classic series of experiments, reported by Urban Ungerstedt in 1971 (Ungerstedt 1971a, 1971b, 1971c, 1971d), proved to be the cornerstone for the eventual application of neural transplantation to Parkinson's disease. These experiments exploited a toxin, 6-hydroxydopamine, which selectively destroys dopamine- and norepinephrine-containing neurons when injected into local areas of the brain in appropriate concentrations. In the first of Ungerstedt's experiments, he injected 6-hydroxydopamine in various locations along the pathways from which dopaminergic (and other) neurons project rostrally (i.e., toward the head). Normally—in contrast to the cells and terminals—these fibers are extremely fine and cannot be distinguished microscopically along much of their course. Injection of 6-hydroxydopamine damages the fibers wherever it is injected, resulting in a buildup of dopamine caudal to the injection site. This allowed the pathways through which these fibers reached their destinations to be mapped precisely.

One consequence of this precise mapping of the dopamine projection pathways was, as it developed, that the nigrostriatal dopaminergic projection passed through the lateral hypothalamus, precisely the region that, when lesioned, produces the lateral hypothalamic syndrome and, when stimulated, engenders electrical self-stimulation of the brain. In 1971 Ungerstedt showed, by using the specific neurotoxin 6-hydroxydopamine rather than electrical lesioning, that damage of the dopaminergic neurons in the substantia nigra pars compacta produces a syndrome resembling the lateral hypothalamic syndrome. Therefore, it appeared that damage of the dopaminergic projection pathways of these substantia nigra neurons was largely or entirely responsible for the lateral hypothalamic syndrome. Ungerstedt also observed that this bilateral substantia nigra syndrome included deficits not only in eating and drinking but in motor function as well. In general, animals with destruction of the dopaminergic neurons in both left and right substantia nigra showed a marked overall paucity of movements, including a lack of locomotion, grooming, and other behaviors. This syndrome is reminiscent of the movement difficulties experienced by human patients with Parkinson's disease.

In 1971 Ungerstedt (see also Ungerstedt and Arbuthnott 1970) also examined the consequences of destroying the substantia nigra dopaminergic neurons on only one side of the brain, and made a very interesting observation. The dopaminergic neurons in the substantia nigra are bilaterally symmetrical, and project mainly to targets only on the same side of the brain, with very little crossing of fibers over the midline. Thus,

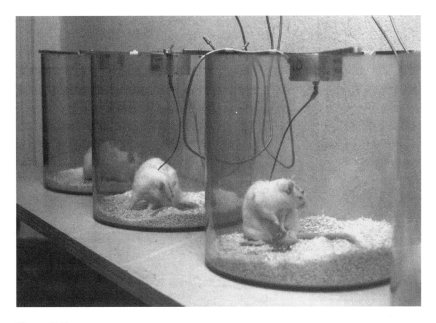

Figure 8.2
Rats being tested for rotational behavior. (Photograph courtesy of Roy Sundberg, National Institute of Mental Health.)

destruction of the dopaminergic neurons in one substantia nigra results in a loss of the dopamine-containing fibers that project to the striatum on only that side of the brain. When dopaminergic neurons on one side of the brain were destroyed in this manner, Ungerstedt observed that the animals initially became asymmetric. That is, their bodies were twisted and they tended to walk in circles away from the lesioned side. After a few days, however, the animals appeared to have compensated for the damage and were able to walk normally, without forced turning. After this period of recovery, when the animals were given a drug that stimulates dopaminergic systems, the asymmetric movement could be reinitiated. Apparently the recovery or compensatory mechanisms were disturbed by drug administration, and the animals began to show the forced circling again (figure 8.2).

Drugs that elicit this circling, or rotational, behavior are of two types. One category of drug (amphetamine is generally used) stimulates the release of dopamine from intact dopaminergic neurons. Since the

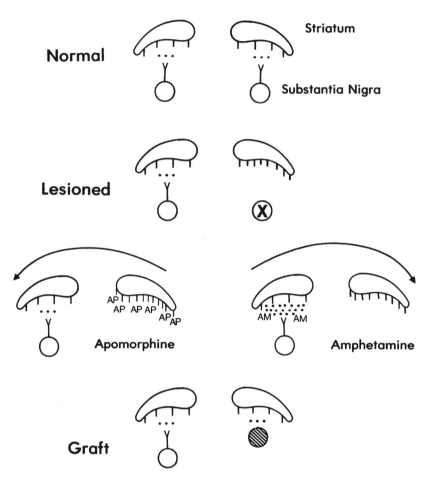

Figure 8.3
Diagram illustrating rotational behavior in the Parkinson's disease rodent model developed by Ungerstedt (1971c, 1971d) and Ungerstedt and Arbuthnott (1970). This model has frequently been used as a method for assessing effects of transplants in rats, although it is gradually being supplanted by more specific tests that measure motor function and motor coordination (see figure 10.5). The tear-shaped structure represents the neostriatum or caudate putamen; the circle represents the substantia nigra dopaminergic neurons; the dots indicate released dopamine; and the lines extending downward indicate dopamine receptors. Under normal conditions, the system is more or less symmetrical, so that there are similar amounts of dopamine released on both sides, and similar numbers of receptors on both sides of the brain. After the substantia nigra is destroyed on one side of the brain only, the animals are able to compensate so that they remain healthy

dopaminergic neurons remain intact only on the side of the brain that was *not* lesioned, amphetamine stimulates only the normal, nonlesioned side, causing the animals to turn toward the lesioned side. This behavior remains constant for many months after the injury. The rate at which the animals rotate can be used as a consistent indicator of the degree of, and thus as a measure of the severity of, the injury (figure 8.3).

The second category of drugs, of which apomorphine is the primary example, act by stimulating dopamine receptors directly. These receptors are located postsynaptically; that is, on neurons that receive inputs from dopaminergic neurons. Since this drug action does not require the neurons from which dopamine is released, apomorphine's activity is not eliminated by lesioning. For reasons that will be explained shortly, apomorphine and similar drugs cause animals to rotate in circles away from the side of the lesion.

Synapses operate by release of neurotransmitter that diffuses across the synaptic cleft and is sensed by receptor molecules located on the postsynaptic neuron. The postsynaptic neuron contains molecular mechanisms to, essentially, monitor the input of neurotransmitter to receptors and adjust the receptors accordingly. When neurotransmitter is no longer received, as is the case with the neurons having dopamine receptors (these neurons are called the medium spiny neurons, or spiny neurons), the receptors become *supersensitive*. In molecular terms, this means (usually) that more receptor molecules are produced.

Thus, after the nigrostriatal dopamine system is destroyed on one side of the brain, dopamine neurons in the striatum on the same side of the brain become supersensitive. When a drug such as apomorphine is

---

and show no obvious abnormality. However, the dopamine receptors on the injured side show an increased sensitivity (called supersensitivity) as a compensation for the injury. Drugs such as amphetamine and apomorphine challenge this compensation, so that the animals show an overt asymmetry and begin to rotate, that is, they turn in circles. Since amphetamine cannot cause dopamine release on the injured side of the brain, it causes release of dopamine only on the intact side, causing the animals to turn toward the side of the lesion. Apomorphine, on the other hand, causes a greater stimulation of dopamine receptors on the injured side, since the receptors there are supersensitive. Therefore, apomorphine causes rotation away from the side of the lesion.

administered to such an animal, it is distributed more or less equally to both sides of the brain. Since the dopamine receptors on the lesioned side (but not on the normal side) are supersensitive, the lesioned side is stimulated to a greater degree. This causes the animals to rotate away from the lesioned side.

Apomorphine-induced rotation is stable indefinitely, and can be used as a measure of lesion severity. Remember, however, that apomorphine-induced rotation indicates the effect of dopamine release on postsynaptic receptors, while amphetamine-induced rotation measures the asymmetry of dopamine release per se. Both testing methods are widely used to study effects of grafts in rat models of Parkinson's disease. It should also be noted that the rotational behavior testing methods have largely been supplanted by tests of motor coordination that do not rely on drug elicitation of behavior.

As a result of the work of Ungerstedt and other subsequent findings, it became possible to put together quite a neat model of the nigrostriatal dopaminergic system and its role in lesion-induced deficits and Parkinson's disease. The dopaminergic cell bodies located in the substantia nigra pars compacta give rise to a system of dopaminergic projections that, after passing rostrally through the diencephalon, produces a very widespread network of terminals in the caudate putamen in rodents, or the caudate nucleus and putamen in humans. In rats, degeneration of this system can be induced by the toxin 6-hydroxydopamine. In Parkinson's disease, degeneration of neurons in the substantia nigra pars compacta results in depletion of dopamine in targets in these terminal regions. In rodents, a syndrome of inactivity, aphagia, adipsia, lack of grooming behavior, and other deficits is seen. This syndrome appears to be analogous to the bradykinesia and at least a part of the movement disorders that are seen in Parkinson's disease in humans.

Studies in Monkeys

A second major Parkinson's disease model involves the use of the toxic drug MPTP (1-methyl–4-phenyl–1,2,3,6-tetrahydropyridine), which causes a Parkinson's-like syndrome when administered to monkeys. This drug was discovered as result of observations reported in 1979 and 1983. In 1982, William Langston and others observed a number of young drug addicts in San Jose and other areas in California who had developed a disorder very similar to Parkinson's disease; all of them had been injecting a synthetic heroin. Coincidentally, a report by Davis, Williams, and Markey (1979) described a subject who had been a graduate student and had developed a Parkinson's-like condition after injecting himself with a synthetic heroin that he had made himself, which had been contaminated with MPTP. On autopsy, this patient, who died from a subsequent cocaine overdose, showed a loss of SN cells. MPTP was later identified as the toxic agent, based on the observation that pure MPTP produced Parkinson's-like manifestations in monkeys.

MPTP is now widely used, in several ways, to produce model forms of Parkinson's disease in monkeys. It is, however, relatively nontoxic in lower animals. In mice, MPTP in very high doses causes minor and usually temporary dopamine depletion, and rats are almost completely resistant.

In monkeys, MPTP produces a severe Parkinson's-like syndrome, with loss of SN dopaminergic neurons (Burns et al. 1983). One difficulty is that animals tend to show spontaneous recovery from Parkinson's-like symptoms after MPTP administration (Kurlan et al. 1991). The recovery is probably less when severe damage is produced, but animals with very severe damage are extremely impaired and difficult to maintain in healthy condition. An alternative is the production of unilateral damage, which can be done by direct injection of MPTP into one carotid artery (Bankiewicz et al. 1986). Severe unilateral damage can be produced, and such animals are easily maintained but show little spontaneous recovery. These model forms of Parkinson's disease have frequently been employed to assess the efficacy of transplantation procedures in nonhuman primates.

Why Not Just Pump Dopamine into the Brain?

Since, in the following discussion, it will be seen that a primary goal of transplantation in Parkinson's disease (in many experiments) is simply to provide a new source of dopaminergic input to the striatum, the question naturally arose as to whether this goal might be accomplished more directly and predictably by simply pumping dopamine into the striatum. As it turns out, this is not quite so simple; nevertheless, it is a possibility.

There are actually two potentially attractive aspects to this idea, compared with the alternative of administering dopaminergic drugs (e.g., L-DOPA) by mouth. First, when drugs are administered orally, problems arise as a result of fluctuations in blood levels of the drugs that are related to drug absorption and metabolism. These are particularly severe in advanced stages of the disease, probably because the brain eventually loses its storage or buffering capacity for neurotransmitter (Mouradian et al. 1990). This problem can be circumvented to some extent by pumping appropriate drugs into the general circulation at a controlled rate, in order to stabilize the availability of drug to neurons in the striatum.

Second, there could be advantages associated with delivery of dopamine directly into the striatum rather than into the general circulation. There are some potential problems that arise as a result of administering drugs systemically rather than directly into the sites where they are needed. Drugs administered systemically may have peripheral effects or influence parts of the brain other than the striatum. For the most part, this problem does not appear to be as serious as one might expect. For one thing, the peripheral effects of L-DOPA administration are diminished by the concurrent administration of a DOPA decarboxylase inhibitor, which inhibits the formation of dopamine peripherally but cannot get into the brain. However, this problem is not simply or entirely overcome by administering a drug into the brain through a pump. Drugs administered in this way enter tissue at a single point or a few locations, and thus may not diffuse efficiently through the entire target organ, especially when the target is shaped somewhat irregularly, as is the striatum. In order to achieve the desired concentration of drug throughout the target organ, it may be necessary to deliver objectionably high concentrations at the point where the drug is being pumped into the brain. Biological systems may be more efficient than mechanical pumps in distributing dopamine throughout the target organ.

Beyond this, there are many reasons that mechanical pumps may be inferior to biological systems—that is, cells—in delivering chemical compounds. Cells have subtle mechanisms for regulating the release of compounds, and they often release several compounds, some of which may enhance effects of the primary compound. Cells may develop processes that deliver the compounds at some distance from the cell body, or the cells themselves may migrate or spread out to some degree, integrating themselves with the brain tissue. Thus, cells may become more widely distributed, resulting in more efficient delivery of chemical compounds. Cells can last longer than any foreseeable mechanical device. Moreover, cells are not generally sources of infection. They can be entirely compatible with host tissue, not inducing reactions that are eventually produced by most mechanical systems. The problem of immune system reaction to cells can also be controlled. Finally, cells make the compounds that need to be delivered themselves, from raw materials found at the site. No mechanical pump can perform this feat!

Further Reading

Cooper, J. R., Bloom, F. E., and Roth, R. H. (1996). *The Biochemical Basis of Neuropharmacology*. Seventh edition. Oxford University Press, New York.

9
Neural Transplantation in Parkinson's Disease: A Brief Synopsis

The discussion of neural transplantation in Parkinson's disease is a complex topic involving many lines of investigation with, in some cases, conflicting results. Superficially, it seems very simple: we just transplant dopamine-producing cells into the striatum of patients with Parkinson's disease, and they will get better. The topic is often presented more or less in those terms, especially to the general public. In reality, the issues are much more complex, and the details can be interesting. Rather than simply launching into a detailed discussion of the data, in this chapter I will give a brief synopsis of the basic information—that is, the fairly indisputable information—on the topic that is presently available. The following chapters will explore basic studies and human clinical trials in greater detail.

The essential information on transplantation in Parkinson's disease is presented in this chapter, so the following four chapters (chapters 10–13) are not essential for understanding the remainder of the book, and can be skipped if desired. Some readers may, however, be interested in more details on how this field has developed. In fact, some readers may be patients with Parkinson's disease, or their relatives, who would like to be better informed about the development of this field.

The basic principle of neural transplanation in Parkinson's disease, for the most part, is simply to replace the dopaminergic input to neurons in the neostriatum (figure 9.1). There are two neural transplantation procedures that have been explored fairly extensively, including trials in human patients with Parkinson's disease. These are (1) transplantation of chromaffin cells from the adrenal medulla, obtained from adult or relatively mature donors, and (2) transplantation of dopaminergic neurons obtained from the substantia nigra of fetal donors (figure 9.2).

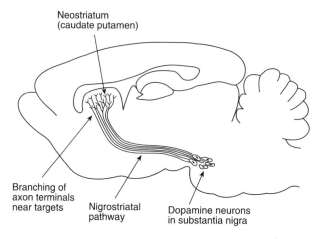

Neostriatum
(caudate putamen)

Branching of
axon terminals
near targets

Nigrostriatal
pathway

Dopamine neurons
in substantia nigra

Figure 9.1
Diagrammatical representation of a rat brain, showing the dopamine-containing neurons in the substantia nigra and the nigrostriatal pathway to the neostriatum. The goal of neural transplantation in Parkinson's disease, both in animal models and in human patients, is to replace this pathway.

In animals, transplants of fetal dopaminergic neurons can reverse some of the impairments that follow substantia nigra damage, especially fairly simple measures of motor function. Thus, measurements based on rotational behavior (see chapter 8) show that grafts produce fairly large improvements, but more sophisticated or complex measures of motor coordination usually indicate much less improvement. The deficits in eating, drinking, and general activity produced in rats by *bilateral* lesions of the substantia nigra are barely affected (chapter 10).

Transplanted dopaminergic neurons act like normal dopaminergic neurons in many respects: they are spontaneously active and produce new afferentation of the host brain, including the formation of synaptic connections with host neurons. Dopamine apparently is released into these synapses and also, apparently, in a more diffuse manner (Rose et al. 1985). The relative importance of dopamine released into synapses versus diffusion of dopamine from release sites into more remote locations of the host striatum is unclear.

Even though effects of fetal brain grafts can be substantial, there are significant limitations in the degree to which transplanted dopamine neu-

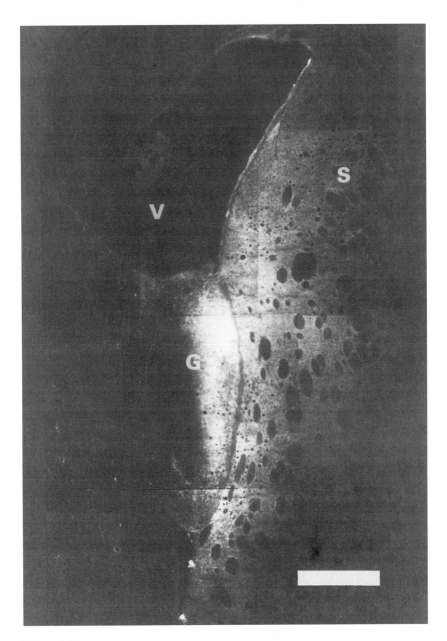

Figure 9.2
A substantia graft (G) in the lateral ventricle (V) of the rat brain, adjacent to the striatum (S). The section is stained by histochemical fluorescence to show catecholamine-containing fibers. The background is dark and the dopaminergic fibers are white. The graft contains both cell bodies and dopaminergic fibers (that cannot be distinguished in this section). The light areas in the striatum represent areas into which dopamine fibers from the graft have grown. The dark circles and oval shapes in the striatum are myelinated fiber bundles passing through it. (From Takashima et al. 1993.)

rons can improve behavioral deficits. As mentioned above, the effects of transplants can seem quite large if certain tests (e.g., measurements of amphetamine-induced rotation) are used. When more realistic tests are employed, however, such as spontaneous behaviors, tests of motor coordination, or even rotation induced by apomorphine, the effects are usually smaller. Correspondingly, there are also limits in the degree to which grafts reafferent the host brain. Thus, the integration of grafts with the host brain and behavioral efficacy roughly correspond, provided appropriate behavioral tests are employed. Both behavioral efficacy and anatomical integration are somewhat limited, in most circumstances.

In my view, there are two major and quite serious flaws in much of the rodent literature, especially earlier literature, on transplantation in Parkinson's disease models. The first is that many important experiments (which have, in some cases, formed the basis for human clinical trials) have not included appropriate controls. In many cases, in fact, rodent experiments that have provided a basis for further studies have made conclusions based on comparisons between animals that received transplants and animals that received neither control transplants nor any comparable surgery. Many of the effects that have been seen are, therefore, likely to be a combination of the actual effects of the transplants and nonspecific effects of surgery or damage that the surgery and the transplant itself produce. Although there have been a number of primate studies as well, it is generally difficult to include extensive control groups in these studies, and it is unrealistic to expect primate studies to make up for deficiencies in the rodent literature. Moreover, some programs have proceeded directly from rodent experiments to human clinical trials without any studies in primates. In the mid-1990s, however, a thorough and well-controlled experiment in monkeys demonstrated clearly that fetal substantia nigra transplantation can alleviate parkinsonian symptoms in higher animals (Taylor et al. 1995; see chapter 12 of this volume).

Second, a great deal of information has been based only on measurements of amphetamine-induced rotation. This is an excessively liberal measure of transplant efficacy, since amphetamine-induced rotation can often be eliminated completely by transplants that are only partially successful by any other measure (figure 9.3). An additional deficiency in the literature is that relatively little work has been performed in primates,

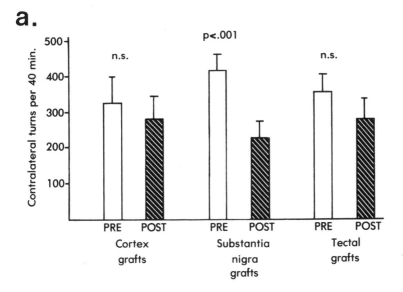

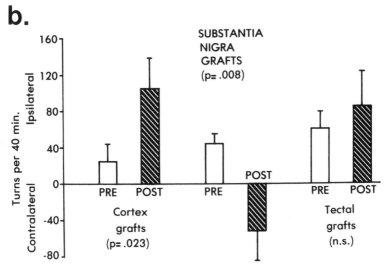

Figure 9.3
Decreases in amphetamine- and apomorphine-induced rotation produced by substantia nigra grafts in the lateral ventricles. "Pre" indicates prior to transplantation; "post" indicates after transplantation. a. Rotation induced by apomorphine. b. Rotation induced by amphetamine. Apomorphine-induced rotation was decreased by about 50 percent, and amphetamine-induced rotation was completely eliminated and actually reversed in direction. For both tests, statistically significant decreases were produced by the substantia nigra grafts, but not by control grafts of other fetal brain regions, tectum or cerebral cortex. (From W. J. Freed 1983.)

so that many variables relevant to transplantation in humans have been decided either on the basis of rodent experiments only or on conclusions reached from studies in human patients. Studies in humans have often preceded, rather than followed, appropriate primate experiments.

All available evidence is consistent with the idea that graft efficacy scales up with the size of the donor species (Brundin et al. 1986; Brundin, Strecker, Widner et al. 1988; Stromberg et al. 1988, 1989, 1991; van Horne et al. 1990). Thus, dopaminergic neurons from human donors are capable of extending axons for severalfold longer distances than similar grafts from rodent donors. The functional efficacy of grafts of tissue from human donors into rat hosts is also severalfold greater than similar grafts from rat donors. This suggests that effects of grafts in rodents (using rodent tissue) will be a reasonably accurate predictor of the efficacy that can be expected when similar transplantation procedures are performed in humans. Conversely, however, studies of human tissue grafts in rodent hosts are not accurate predictors of effects that will be seen in human patients, because such procedures are more effective than comparable experiments using the same species for donor and host. In other words, human grafts in rodent hosts work too well to be good predictors of the effects of same-species grafts.

It is not possible to precisely predict the donor age requirements for human tissue grafts simply by extrapolation from experiments in rodents. Thus, it has been necessary to conduct experiments on the transplantation of tissue from human donors of various ages, and for practical reasons, almost all of these experiments have involved transplantation of human tissue into rodent donors. Experiments along these lines have been reported by Stromberg and coworkers (1991), Brundin, Nilsson, et al. (1986), Brundin, Strecker, Widner et al. (1988), Freeman, Sanberg, et al. (1995), and van Horne et al. (1990), among others. The general conclusion is that for human donors, tissue of no more than nine weeks of gestational age is required. Thus, when one sees a clinical study in human patients in which fetal tissue from donors aged 11 to 14 gestational weeks was used, one might also expect that the dopaminergic neurons probably did not survive well.

The second procedure that has received a great deal of attention is transplantation of the adrenal medulla, the central mass of tissue in the

adrenal gland (it lies just above the kidney) into the neostriatum of patients with Parkinson's disease. The adrenal medulla is an endocrine
(hormone-producing) organ, and contains many thousands of chromaffin
cells, which can produce norepinephrine and epinephrine in great quantities. Since dopamine is a precursor of norepinephrine, they produce dopamine as well (although the chromaffin cells do not necessarily *secrete*
dopamine). Under normal circumstances, almost all of this dopamine is
converted to norepinephrine, but under some conditions, the relative
amount of dopamine contained in the adrenal medulla can be increased.

The original idea involved in transplanting adrenal medulla into the
brain was that the transplanted chromaffin cells would secrete dopamine,
and thereby substitute for fetal dopaminergic neurons. Although it appears that this (or something like it) may happen, effects produced in this
way by adrenal medulla grafts are very small—on the order of a 20 percent reduction in apomorphine-induced rotation, which is small indeed
(Takashima et al. 1992). Other nonspecific effects produced by adrenal
medulla grafts, related to general stress from the surgery and the minor
damage and stimulatory effects on the host brain caused by graft implantation, may add to the apparent magnitude of the grafts' effect slightly,
but the effects of adrenal medulla grafts are distinctly smaller than those
of fetal substantia nigra grafts. At present, the adrenal medulla transplantation procedure is of interest mainly in terms of being another procedure that can be compared with substantia nigra transplantation. It is not
a viable alternative to substantia nigra for transplantation in Parkinson's
disease.

A great deal of confusion in this area has been generated by the fact
that adrenal medulla grafts do not survive particularly well in the brain.
Some experiments in which adrenal medulla grafts produced behavioral
improvement observed survival of some, although only a minority, of
the transplanted chromaffin cells. In other experiments, adrenal medulla
grafts were found not to have survived (e.g., Bohn et al. 1987; Fiandaca
et al. 1988). Such experiments normally would receive little notice, except
for the fact that in some cases, effects were seen anyway. In particular,
adrenal medulla grafts (or the brain injury produced by them) appeared
to be capable of promoting recovery or sprouting of dopaminergic fibers.
These effects cannot exactly be considered effects of adrenal chromaffin

cell grafts, but are in some way associated with either the procedure or with the survival of other cell types (that is, cells other than chromaffin cells contained in the adrenal medulla) after transplantation.

Thus, there has been some confusion of (1) effects of adrenal medulla grafts per se and (2) effects that are seen when adrenal medulla grafts are implanted but do not survive. Many "effects" of adrenal medulla grafts that have been reported in humans, perhaps including the clinical improvement, are probably of the latter variety.

It would seem that there are a variety of nonspecific effects, such as damage to the host brain induced by surgery, which make it appear that adrenal medulla grafts can influence the host brain even when they do not survive, and thus have contributed to this confusion. This again underscores that it is essential to include controls which receive grafts of other tissues when examining any sort of "effects" of grafts in animals. Certainly, however, when adrenal medulla (or any other type of graft) is implanted into the brain, but on autopsy the grafts are consistently seen not to have survived, any changes that are observed are not "effects of the graft." Rather, changes observed under such circumstances are consequences of brain injury or other nonspecific effects, or in some cases may be semispecific effects produced by cells other than adrenal chromaffin cells that survive in the transplants.

Studies of adrenal medulla grafts are, therefore, really studies of adrenal medulla grafts only when the grafts (or at least some of the grafts) survive. Many human patients (several hundred) received adrenal medulla grafts between 1987 and 1990. In human studies, there have now been a number of autopsies, and there has been no example of good graft survival in any of these. Many of the published autopsies were from patients who did not show improvement, or for whom the improvement had disappeared by the time of death, although there is at least one example from a patient who did show some improvement. This graft also did not survive (chapter 11). Thus, it seems probable that the effects of adrenal chromaffin cell grafts in human patients were mainly nonspecific, related to injury or trophic effects of some type.

Even though, in all probability, the adrenal chromaffin cells did not survive in the human patients, clinical improvements were observed. There were improvements in rating scales and other measures of motor function. The most pronounced and long-lasting effects were in percent-ages of the day in "on" and "off" states. This requires a little explanation. In advanced stages of Parkinson's disease, when patients have received L-DOPA treatment for extended periods, they usually begin to experience periods of each day when they are "on." That is, the drug treatment is working and the patient can function fairly normally. "On" periods alternate with "off" periods during which the drug is ineffective and the patients are essentially as they would be without treatment. With pro-gression of the disease, the "on"–"off" alternation becomes more pro-nounced and the "off" periods become longer, so that more and more of the day is spent in the "off" state. This is the primary mode of drug treatment failure in Parkinson's disease. In advanced stages, parts of the "on" periods are accompanied by chorea (involuntary writhing move-ments). The changes between "on" and "off" states may be fairly abrupt, and there are usually several such alternations per day.

Although this is a complex issue, failure to recognize that a change in "on" and "off" states was the major change that occurs may have contributed to an early overestimation of the degree of improvement. The time course of the improvement is particularly interesting: clinical im-provements developed between three and six months after transplanta-tion, were fairly stable for up to one year, and declined afterward. By four years after adrenal medulla transplantation, the improvements had dissipated, with the exception of a small (but still significant) improve-ment in "on" and "off" times. This provides, if nothing else, an important backdrop for evaluating effects seen following fetal brain tissue grafts in humans: if fetal substantia nigra graft produces a clinical effect similar to that seen after adrenal medulla grafts, it probably is nothing to get very excited about. Since comparisons of the amount of improvement are often quite difficult (although sometimes possible), it is particularly useful to compare the time course of improvements that are seen with various procedures. When substantia nigra grafts produce clinical improvement over the same time course that was seen after adrenal medulla grafts, we have to suspect that they might be working in the same way.

One general problem with the entire idea of employing autologous ad-renal medulla transplants is the age of the donor tissue. The original idea behind employing adrenal medulla for transplantation was that one adrenal gland could be removed from the prospective graft recipient, as a source of tissue for transplantation. This was the method used in almost all of the human studies of adrenal medulla transplantation. In animal studies, however, the donor tissue was obtained from young animals. Later evidence confirmed that adrenal medulla grafts are effective only when obtained from relatively young donors (W. J. Freed 1983; Freed, Cannon-Spoor, and Krauthamer 1985; Date et al. 1993). Grafts were entirely ineffective when obtained from aging donors, or even from the equivalent of "middle-aged" rats. Since patients with Parkinson's disease are generally older, this procedure was essentially doomed from the start on that basis alone.

Another very serious problem with adrenal medulla transplantation, in addition to the small effects seen, is the high frequency of side effects, including a fairly large number of deaths. Some of these side effects are related to the surgery. Other side effects, however, appear to be psychological in nature, including psychosis, depression, and unusual dissociative states. In retrospect, it is not surprising that a foreign cell type, which is capable of secreting a number of substances other than dopamine—substances that are not normally produced by dopaminergic neurons—would produce unexpected effects when used, basically, as a replacement for dopaminergic neurons. This is probably an important lesson that should be remembered for the future, especially when substitute cells of any type are used: ectopic transplantation of cells may produce unexpected effects.

An interesting comparison involves studies in which dopaminergic neurons were transplanted into neonatal animals. The immature brain is a relatively hospitable environment for graft development. In these experiments, substantia nigra was transplanted into normal newborn host animals (Schwarz and Freed 1987). The animals were then allowed to grow to maturity, all the while bearing the additional graft tissue in their brains. The animals then received complete bilateral lesions of the dopaminergic neurons in their substantia nigra. These lesions normally produce profound behavioral deficits, including aphagia (not eating), adipsia (not drinking), loss of weight, motor inactivity, loss of grooming, general malaise, and death within a few weeks unless the animals are artificially kept alive with intensive feeding by intubation. Under these neonatal transplantation conditions, substantia nigra grafts produced a very complete prevention of behavioral deficits, including alleviation of motor impairment, retention of grooming behavior, and prevention of weight loss and general malaise. Recent studies have shown that grafts of dopaminergic neurons in neonatal animals become more completely integrated into the host brain circuitry (Nikkhah et al. 1995). Since the behavioral recovery and integration of the grafts into host brain are less complete in adult hosts, it appears that conditions in the neonatal brain are more favorable for graft development.

There have now been a number of studies of fetal brain grafts in human patients with Parkinson's disease, and for the most part some improvements in the clinical state of these patients has been observed. Often, however, improvements were reported over a time course of two to six months, similar to the time course observed for adrenal medulla grafts in human patients. In addition, many of the initial experiments used tissue that was probably too mature for optimal graft survival. However, there also have been several studies that used tissue and transplantation conditions which are likely to have resulted in the survival of the transplanted dopaminergic neurons. In these experiments, there have been indications that some specific clinical improvement, possibly related to physiological integration of the grafts with host brain, has occurred. Particularly encouraging has been the protracted time course of improvement that has been seen in some studies, in which patients have improved gradually, with significant improvement continuing more than one year after transplantation. In particular, clinical studies by C. R. Freed and coworkers (1992) and by O. Lindvall and coworkers and H. Widner and coworkers (Lindvall et al. 1992; Widner et al. 1992) have observed improvements that have progressed substantially, starting approximately one year after transplantation (see chapter 13 for more details), as well as some improvements that were seen earlier.

More recently, excellent graft survival was observed in two patients with Parkinson's disease who died 18 months following transplantation of fetal mesencephalic tissue to the putamen. These patients were subjects in a clinical trial at the University of South Florida that included a larger number of subjects. Some early clinical improvements were seen, although these were not especially remarkable (figure 9.4; compare with

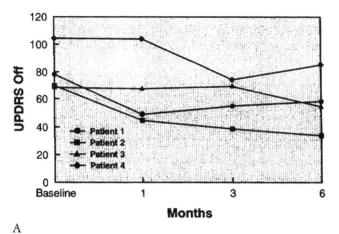

A

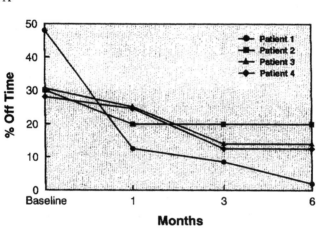

B

Figure 9.4
Improvement after fetal substantia nigra grafts in four human patients. These are clinical results for the study in which two patients died (of causes unrelated to transplantation) and were found to have grafts with numerous surviving dopaminergic neurons (figure 9.5). The upper graph shows ratings by the Unified Parkinson's Disease Rating Scale (UPDRS) taken during the "off" state for four patients. There was some improvement in three of the patients; for two patients, most of the improvement developed within one month, and the third showed improvement by two months after transplantation. The lower graph shows the percent of the day in the "off" state. Again, most of the improvement was seen within three months after transplantation. (From Freeman, Olanow et al. 1995; reproduced with permission.)

figures 11.3, 13.1, 13.4, and 13.5), as well as some longer-lasting effects. In the first patient who died, tissue from seven embryos, aged 6.5 to 9 weeks, was used (results for the two patients were similar). Transplants were made into 24–32 sites on each side of the brain, so that the grafts were spaced no more than 5 mm apart throughout the target area. The patient improved markedly, and the improvement was sustained until the patient died 18 months after surgery, of a pulmonary embolism. Examination of the brain revealed surviving dopaminergic neurons at multiple sites, with virtually no evidence of an adverse reaction of the host brain (e.g., scarring or inflammation). In the words of the author, "each graft displayed seamless integration within the host striatum" (Kordower et al. 1995, 1121). Innumerable tyrosine hydroxylase-containing fibers had grown out of the grafts, entering into the host brain (figure 9.5).

These data essentially demonstrate that what works in the rodent and primate also works in humans. Our confidence that neural transplantation can be used as a therapy for at least a few selected diseases should be greatly bolstered by this finding.

In the following chapters, some of the experiments that led to the above conclusions will be described, in some cases in detail. Since the literature on this topic is large, many studies are necessarily omitted. Additional references can be found in the general reading sources provided. The goal in the following chapters has been to attain brevity by selection of the most important studies rather than through simplification. The important details for understanding exactly what has been done, what is known, and what is not known are included.

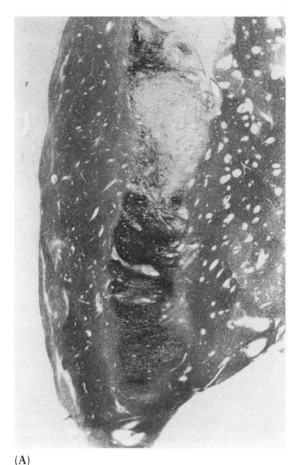

(A)

Figure 9.5
Illustration of surviving transplanted fetal dopamine neurons in a human patient with Parkinson's disease. The patient died of unrelated causes 18 months after surgery, and excellent graft survival was observed, corresponding to continued clinical improvement. The photos show dopamine neurons stained to reveal the enzyme tyrosine hydroxylase. (A) A graft shown at low magnification. The graft is in the center, and the dark areas on either side represent reafferented parts of the host brain. (B) A higher magnification picture, showing numerous surviving transplanted dopamine neurons. Neurites extend from the graft into the host brain. (C) Two transplanted neurons, with extensive networks of neurites. (Photographs courtesy of Jeffrey Kordower, Rush-Presbyterian-St. Luke's Medical Center, Chicago. Kordower et al. 1995, 1996.)

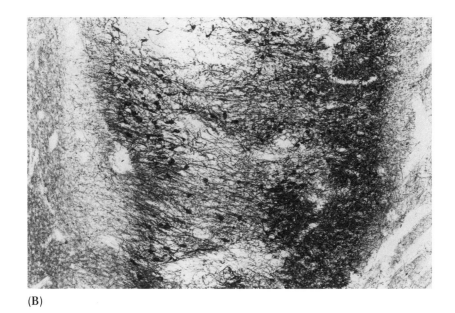

(B)

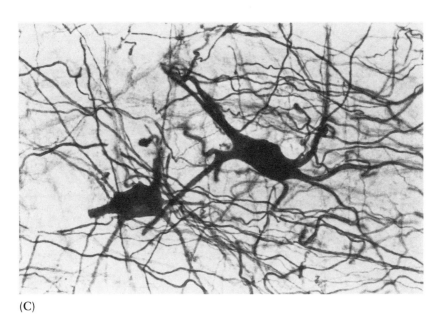

(C)

10

Fetal Brain Tissue Transplantation in Parkinson's Disease: Experiments in Animals

Initial studies of neural transplantation in Parkinson's disease models employed rats with unilateral destruction of dopaminergic neurons induced by the neurotoxin 6-hydroxydopamine, a technique that was discussed in chapter 8. A number of experiments have also employed primates as a model, and the majority of these experiments have used the MPTP model of Parkinson's disease, also described in chapter 8. The MPTP model, in some respects, is very closely analogous to Parkinson's disease and is an almost ideal model, or at least it is as close to ideal as one might reasonably expect of a model in animals. Because of the much greater difficulty, and cost in time and money, associated with studies in primates, however, a much greater amount of data has been obtained for rodents than for primates, and development of neural transplantation in Parkinson's disease has relied largely on rodent models.

Basic Studies in Rodents

The use of rodents permits the use of large numbers of animals, which is essential for basic research on mechanisms and properties of grafts, because it allows for controlled studies and for comparisons of various techniques. Thus, most of what is known about the basic properties of brain grafts is derived from experiments in rats. The body of information available on this topic is huge and growing, and some of it is arcane and of interest only to specialists. I will limit the discussion here to topics that are relevant to human application. In addition, there is a substantial literature on techniques that might be used to enhance the effects or survival of grafts, such as cografting with other tissues and treatment with various drugs and trophic factors. Not all of this literature will be described. Details of some of the other studies may be obtained from the list for further reading.

Most studies in rodents have employed the 6-hydroxydopamine model of Parkinson's disease developed by Ungerstedt, which was described in chapter 8. Several aspects of these experiments are virtually universal: (1) small fragments, or suspensions made from small fragments, of tissue are implanted and allowed to form new connections with the host brain, as was discussed in chapter 4; (2) fetal tissue is used; and (3) the tissue is usually (but not always) transplanted into the site where dopaminergic fibers terminate, not into the substantia nigra, where the cell bodies are located.

The earliest experiments on transplantation of fetal substantia nigra were not attempts to repair damage of the host's brain, but instead examined the survival and growth of transplanted dopaminergic neurons. Seiger and Olson (1997) obtained important information regarding the use of dopaminergic neurons for transplantation through studies of grafting into the anterior chamber of the eye. In 1976, Stenevi and coworkers reported on attempts to transplant dopaminergic neurons into the brain, but with very little success. Almost none of the transplanted dopamine neurons survived, probably because the transplantation technique was not optimal. In 1979, Bischoff et al. reported on studies of transplanted dopaminergic neurons in the hippocampus.

In order to start the discussion of this topic, the first few experiments which found that fetal substantia nigra (SN) transplantation could produce functional improvements in animal models of Parkinson's disease, reported in the literature in 1979 and 1980, will be described. In the first experiment, published in *Science* in 1979, the dopaminergic neurons in the substantia nigra were destroyed on one side of the brain (unilaterally) in a group of 29 rats. The animals were then tested repeatedly for apomorphine-induced rotational behavior (Perlow et al. 1979). The rotational behavior was measured by attaching the animals to rubber-band harnesses, using automated devices. The animals then received grafts of fetal ventral mesencephalon, which contains the dopaminergic SN neurons, obtained from pregnant donor rats of 17 days' gestational age. These tissue fragments were transplanted into the lateral ventricle on the same side of the brain as the lesions, by injecting the tissue through a large (approximately 1 mm in diameter) needle. A smaller number of animals (n = 7) received similar-sized grafts of pieces of sciatic nerve, obtained from the pregnant tissue donors; these latter animals were the control group.

Beginning four weeks after transplantation, the animals were tested for apomorphine-induced rotational behavior a number of times over a period of approximately one month. The surgery and testing were performed at the National Institute of Mental Health Neuroscience Center at St. Elizabeths, in Washington, D.C. When the testing had been completed, the animals were sent to our collaborators Lars Olson and Ake Seiger in Stockholm, and their brains were examined for the presence of grafts using the Falck-Hillarp fluorescence histochemical technique.

In this experiment, animals that received substantia nigra grafts showed reductions in apomorphine-induced rotational behavior of approximately 50 percent, while the control animals, which received sciatic nerve, showed only slight reductions (about 10 percent). Histochemical examination of the brain performed on some animals that showed large reductions in rotation. All of the animals had surviving grafts with catecholaminergic neurons and reafferentation of the brain, regardless of whether the grafts were effective. It appeared that the grafts were more effective if located in more anterior parts of the ventricle; grafts with a more posterior location may not have effectively contacted crucial regions of the striatum. The location of some of the grafts in more posterior parts of the ventricular system probably reflected errors in the transplantation technique. In later experiments, the location of the grafts was more consistent, so that they were almost always in contact with the relevant areas of the brain.

The second experiment (Freed et al. 1980) involved examination of the long-term effects of SN grafts in another series of animals. Testing and transplantation were performed in the same manner, and the animals were repeatedly tested for changes in apomorphine-induced rotation over a period of six months. There was no loss in the efficacy of the grafts during the six months; in fact, it increased slightly. The grafts appeared to reafferent the medial one-third of the striatum, the section closest to the grafts and to the ventricle, to a substantial degree. In addition to histochemical evaluation of the grafts, the ability of these grafts to influence the host brain was confirmed by increased dopamine concentrations in small tissue punches taken from the striatum. Dopamine, which had been almost completely depleted by the lesions, was increased to about one-third of normal values in parts of striatum where new afferents had grown from the grafts. In control animals that received sciatic nerve grafts, and in parts of the host striatum that were not adjacent to the graft, dopamine concentrations remained very much depleted, less than 10 percent of normal values. These experiments thus showed that substantia nigra grafts could induce some amelioration of the behavioral deficits subsequent to substantia nigra lesions, and that this amelioration is associated with the development of new dopaminergic striatal afferentation (figure 10.1).

Another group of researchers, located in Lund, Sweden, performed a related series of experiments at around the same time or shortly afterward (Bjorklund and Stenevi 1979; Bjorklund, Dunnett, et al. 1980; Bjorklund, Schmidt, and Stenevi 1980). Rather than transplanting tissue into the lateral ventricles, this group initially employed a technique for transplanting the tissue into the cerebral cortex. Their method involved removing a small area of cerebral cortex, waiting for a period of time, and then transplanting the tissue into the lesion site. This allowed the transplanted tissue to come into contact with new blood vessels that had formed at the edges of the area of removed tissue, which presumably promoted graft survival. In the earlier experiments by this group, reported by Stenevi and coworkers in 1976, simple injection of fetal brain tissue into the brain had resulted in poor graft survival.

In their first experiment (Bjorklund and Stenevi 1979), animals were tested for amphetamine-induced rotation, and three of the four animals tested showed decreases. There were no control animals. In a more complete experiment (Bjorklund, Dunnett et al. 1980), a larger number of animals was tested for changes in amphetamine-induced rotation. Although again there were no controls, this experiment included a manipulation in which the grafts were surgically removed from some of the animals. Removal of the grafts was shown to restore the amphetamine-induced rotation to pretransplantation levels, whereas rotation remained decreased in animals from which the grafts were not removed. As in our

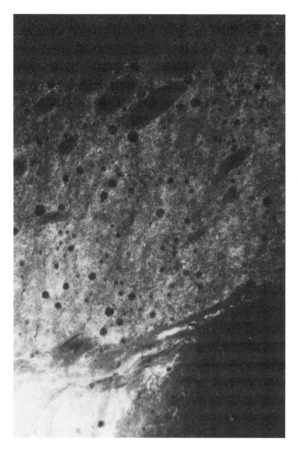

Figure 10.1
Illustration of growth of dopaminergic fibers from a fetal substantia nigra graft, stained with histochemical fluorescence, into the host rat brain. The graft is the brightly stained white structure in the upper left of the picture. Fibers growing into the host brain appear as fine, brightly stained white patches, gradually diminishing in intensity from left to right, as they extend into the host neostriatum over approximately 2 mm from left to right.

experiments, the grafts produced new afferents to parts of the striatum adjacent to the grafts. These experiments, however, employed only amphetamine-induced rotation as a functional measure—it measures the ability of the grafts to release dopamine rather than an enduring effect of the grafts upon the host brain per se.

An important innovation, reported by this same group, was the development of methods for transplantation of dissociated cell preparations rather than intact tissue fragments. (This technique was mentioned in chapter 4.) This technique involves mechanical disruption of tissue fragments, sometimes with the aid of enzymes, to form suspensions of dissociated cells, which can then be injected directly into brain tissue. While earlier studies of transplantation by injection of tissue fragments directly into the striatum (Stenevi et al. 1976) had not been very successful, this dissociated cell transplantation technique facilitated improved survival of dopaminergic cells following transplantation directly into the brain parenchyma by simple injection (Bjorklund, Schmidt and Stenevi 1980). In this first experiment using the technique, dissociated cell preparations from the SN were shown to decrease amphetamine-induced rotation when transplanted into the rat striatum (figure 10.2). A further refinement of this technique involves the microinjection of small numbers of cells, using fine needles (Nikkhah et al. 1995).

For dissociated cell transplants, it appeared that cells from a slightly earlier stage of fetal development were required; transplants obtained from donors of 15 days' gestation survived and decreased amphetamine-induced rotation, whereas transplants from 17-day gestational donors did not survive well and produced only slight behavioral changes (Bjorklund, Schmitt, and Stenevi 1980). In contrast, 17-day gestational rat tissue is efficacious when using techniques that employ solid tissue fragments, including intraventricular transplantation and transplantation to lesion cavities.

Since those early studies there have, of course, been numerous experiments to which refinements and additional details have been added. For example, several studies have shown that grafts can produce improvements in behaviors other than simple rotation (e.g., Mandel et al. 1990; see also section "Behavioral Tests," below) can produce changes in host brain neurotransmitter receptors (W. J. Freed, Ko et al. 1983; W. Freed,

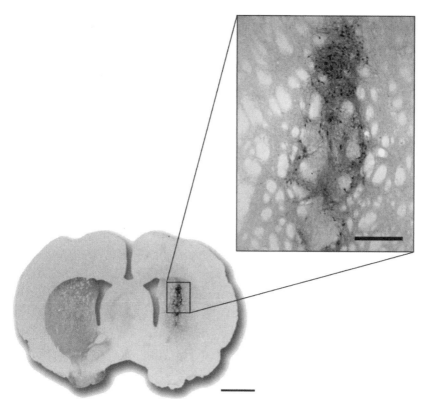

Figure 10.2
Dissociated fetal dopaminergic neurons transplanted into the rat striatum. The graft in the rat's brain is on the lower left (scale bar: 2 mm). The numerous dopaminergic neurons in the graft are in the upper right at higher magnification (scale bar: 0.25 mm). (Courtesy of Patrick Brundin and Gabriele Schierle, Wallenberg Neuroscience Center, Lund University, Lund, Sweden.)

Olson et al. 1985), and that grafts can form synapses with host neurons (Bolam et al. 1987; Freund et al. 1985; Mahalik et al. 1985).

Donor Tissue Age: Experiments in Rats

The use of fetal tissue is a general axiom of neural transplantation, for several related reasons. In essence, fetal tissue has the capacity to survive transplantation to a new location and to develop connections with the host brain. Some of this resilience is the result of fetal tissue's having a greater ability to resist anoxia, and therefore to more readily survive the stress and disruptive events associated with transplantation. The major reason, however, is that fetal neurons have not yet extended neurites. Thus, neurites are not severed when the cells are removed from the brain and fetal neurons retain the capacity to extend neurites. In addition, the trauma of removal is minimized.

Adult neurons have developed extensive processes, both axons and dendrites, that connect them to other cells of the CNS. Fetal neurons, once differentiated, begin the process of developing these connections. Removal of neurons from the brain entails varying degrees of disruption, which can be lethal to differentiated neurons. When fetal neurons are used for transplantation, it appears that tissue in a slightly more mature stage of development can be used if solid fragments of tissue are used, while younger tissue is needed if the tissue is disrupted into individual cells.

Within the general limitation that fetal tissue must be used, there remains the question of gestational age of the tissue. Can any fetus be used, or is it necessary to employ tissue from very early stages of development? Furthermore, are larger effects seen if tissue at a very early stage of development is employed? There is a great deal of data on this topic in rats, and the data are of two types. First, there are experiments on transplantation of rat tissue into rats, and more recently there have been a number of experiments on transplantation of human tissue into rat brains. In these human-to-rat transplantation experiments, some form of immunosuppression must be used to prevent graft rejection.

The human is born after a gestational period of nine months, while the gestation in the rat is 21 days. The rat is born in a much less mature state than the human. In comparing rat and human development, a rough approximation would be that one day of rat development equals five days of human development, and that the rat is born at a stage of development equivalent to about five months of human gestation. Very approximate equivalent ages for development of the dopaminergic system in rodents and humans are shown in table 10.1.

The first experiment on brain tissue transplantation in rats that looked at this issue directly was the study by Bjorklund, Schmitt, and Stenevi

Table 10.1
Development of the nigrostriatal dopaminergic system

Rat	Human		
Days	Weeks	Trimester	Landmarks of Brain Development
10–11	3–4	1	Neural tube closure
12	6	1	Formation of cerebral hemispheres
12–13	7–8	1	Appearance of dopamine neurons
14–15	10–11	1	Aggregation of dopamine neuroblasts Beginning of development of projections of dopamine neuroblasts to striatum
17–19	12–14	1–2	Increasing dopaminergic afferentation of striatum Segregation of dopaminergic cells into groups
19–21	14–16	2	Further segregation of dopaminegic cells into groups Start of patchy dopaminergic afferentation of striatum
(birth) P 1–28	16–18	2	Distinctly patchy afferentation of striatum
P 8–22	18–24	2	Development of dopaminergic projections in mature form
———	40	(birth)	

P, postnatal.

(1980), in which effects of dissociated cell grafts were examined. In this experiment, grafts from 15-day gestational donors were effective, while tissue from 17-day gestational donors was not. A later experiment, by Brundin and coworkers (1986), found that dissociated cell grafts from 15- and 16-day gestational donors were effective, but there was better survival of cells from the 15-day donors. It appeared that the younger donor tissue was less vulnerable to damage directly associated with the dissociation procedure. Therefore, although grafts of dissociated cells from 16-day gestational donors can be effective (Bjorklund, Schmitt, and Stenevi 1980; Brundin, Barbin, et al. 1988), dopaminergic neurons appear to survive somewhat better when slightly younger donors are used. Another study that obtained larger numbers of surviving dopaminergic cells (Sauer and Brundin 1991) used grafts from 14–15 days' gestational donors. Thus, from the data available for rats, it seems that dissociated cell grafts from donor rats of up to about 15 days' gestation are optimally effective. There is still a definite possibility that there are advantages to using slightly younger donors, of perhaps 14 days' gestation.

For transplantation of solid tissue fragments into the ventricles, there are also data on donor tissue ages. Grafts from 11, 13, 15, 17, and 19 days' gestation were compared in one experiment (Simonds and Freed 1990). The largest effects were produced by grafts from 15-day gestational donors, with slightly smaller effects being produced by tissue from 11-, 13-, and 17-day donors. Interestingly, grafts from the younger donors required a longer time interval for the development of maximal efficacy. While the grafts from 15- and 17-day donors were maximally effective by 6 weeks after transplantation, grafts from 11-, and 13-day donors did not produce their maximum effects until 12 weeks after transplantation. Thus, it seems that grafts from very young donors may require extended time intervals for the development of maximal efficacy. Whether further increases in efficacy would have developed beyond 12 weeks was not investigated.

In general, therefore, it seems that 14–15-day gestational tissue produces optimal results in rats for both solid and dissociated tissue transplantation methods. Sixteen days of gestation in rats is the point at which decrements in graft efficacy begin to be seen. Although it is probably possible to obtain good effects with tissue one day or so older in solid tissue transplantation methods, in rats the difference in donor ages required for the two different techniques is no more than about one day.

Donor Age Requirement: Data from Human-to-Rat Transplants

Ultimately, the major reason for examining the issue of donor age is to learn what ages of tissue would be required for transplantation in human patients. There are several potential means for obtaining this kind of data. One might examine the survival of dopamine neurons in culture, when transplanted into rats, or when transplanted into monkeys or even humans. The use of rats as a host species has generally been considered to be the best method. Experiments in culture do not sufficiently mimic the situation that is present in transplantation, and performing initial experiments in monkey hosts would provide relatively little additional information as well as being extraordinarily expensive and time-consuming. Grafts of human tissue into rodent hosts would normally be rejected, but graft survival can be obtained by using immunosuppressant drugs or immunodeficient rat host animals. Interestingly, grafts of human fetal brain tissue become quite well integrated with the rat host brain, even forming synapses with rat neurons (Clarke et al. 1988; Mahalik et al. 1989).

Stromberg, van Horne, and associates have reported on several experiments involving the transplantation of human tissue into rodents, using both animals immunosuppressed with cyclosporine and genetically immunodeficient rats (Stromberg et al. 1986, 1988, 1989; van Horne et al. 1990). The use of the two models is important because of the possibility that either cyclosporine or the immunodeficiency state would itself have an effect on the transplanted tissue. In these experiments, grafts of human fetal dopaminergic neurons were found to produce large behavioral effects in rodent host animals when donor tissue of 8.5–10 weeks' gestational age was used (Stromberg et al. 1988; van Horne et al. 1990). Similar effects were found using athymic immunodeficient rats (i.e., animals lacking the thymus gland, an immunologically important organ).

Another series of experiments, by Brundin, Nilsson et al. (1986) and Brundin, Strecker, Widner, et al. (1988), employed transplantation of human tissue into rat hosts, in the form of grafts of dissociated cells. Grafts from donors of 6. 5 to 9 weeks of gestation were effective in reducing amphetamine-induced rotation, whereas grafts from donors of 11 to 19 weeks of gestation were ineffective. Grafts from a donor of 8 weeks' gestation were also tested for effects on apomorphine-induced rotation and spontaneous rotation, and were found to be effective; however, the other donor age groups were tested only for effects on amphetamine-induced rotational behavior. This series of experiments therefore also suggests that for human donors, tissue younger than 11 weeks is required.

A third series of experiments on this topic was performed by Freeman, Spence, et al. (1991) and Freeman, Sanberg, et al. (1995). Their first study involved an examination of the development of human dopaminergic neurons in vivo, in fetal tissue samples. It was found that the dopaminergic neurons began to develop neurites at about 8 weeks of gestation; by 10–11 weeks the dopaminergic neurons had migrated to their final positions, and most had developed neurites. In the second study, Freeman and coworkers (1995a) examined the survival of human dopaminergic neurons of different gestational ages, when transplanted into the rat brain in either solid or dissociated forms. This is the only experiment that has directly compared donor ages for solid and dissociated grafts, and is therefore of considerable importance for human clinical trials.

For both solid and dissociated grafts, donors younger than 56 days resulted in good graft survival. Virtually no surviving dopaminergic neurons were found in grafts from 72-day gestational donors, for both transplantation procedures. There did appear to be a developmental period around 65 days for which solid grafts showed good survival but dissociated cell grafts survived poorly.

The three series of experiments described above are in general agreement. Thus, for human clinical transplantation it appears that the following conclusions can be made. First, fetal donor tissue of more than 10 weeks' gestational age is too mature, whereas tissue from donors of 8 weeks' gestational age or younger is likely to be viable, whether dissociated cell or solid tissue transplantation techniques are used. There is a stage of development, of about 9 weeks' gestation, that may yield good graft survival for solid tissue grafts but not for dissociated cells.

Time Course for Improvement

There appear to be several factors that interact to determine the time course over which improvement occurs. These are the donor and recipient species, as well as the age of the donor and possibly other factors, such as transplantation site. It would be useful if we were able to predict, from animal data, the expected time course for improvement in humans. The data available on this topic are, however, very limited, and conclusions about the expected time course for improvement in humans can be made mainly only by inference, and are therefore speculative.

In most of our studies in rats, the major improvement that is seen has appeared to occur during the first six weeks. When animals were followed over longer time periods—for six months in one experiment and one year in another—it appeared that progressive increases in graft efficacy continued to develop quite slowly. In one experiment, the grafts gradually became more effective over the course of one year, culminating in decreases in apomorphine-induced rotation of more than 80 percent (W. J. Freed and Cannon-Spoor 1989). Studies by Dunnett and coworkers (1983a) observed a similar time course for development of effects of dissociated cell grafts: decreases in amphetamine-induced rotation developed within 3 to 6 weeks after transplantation, with some continued increase in efficacy thereafter up to about 25 weeks. Apomorphine-induced rotation also improved (but only slightly) during the three to six weeks, but there was no progressive improvement after six weeks. Thus, in rats it seems that most of the efficacy develops over about three to six weeks, with a slow and modest continued improvement thereafter.

The time course of improvement also seems to depend on donor age. In an experiment by Simonds and Freed (1990), for example, the efficacy of 15- or 17-day gestational fetal substantia nigra grafts was maximal by 6 weeks after transplantion, whereas the effects of 11- or 13-day gestational grafts continued to increase between 6 and 12 weeks.

In primates, improvement seems to develop more slowly. In a study by Taylor and associates (1990), parkinsonian signs decreased gradually over the course of 2–8 months after transplantation. Annett et al. (1990) observed improvement in spontaneous rotation in marmosets, a smaller monkey species, over the course of 12–24 weeks.

A third type of animal data on the time course for development of improvement involves studies of transplantation of human fetal tissue into rat hosts. In general, it appears that human fetal tissue develops more slowly than does rat tissue, in accordance with intrinsic developmental mechanisms (Seiger et al. 1988). The maturation of substantia nigra dopaminergic cells appears to progress gradually over two to six months (Seiger et al. 1988), with behavioral improvement gradually developing over the course of about five months after transplantation (van Horne et al. 1990; see also figure 10.3). Experiments by Brundin et al. on the transplantation of human fetal tissue into rat hosts showed that tissue from a 9-week gestational human donor progressively decreased amphetamine-induced rotation over 15–20 weeks after transplantation, with the decreases becoming statistically significant only at 19–20 weeks. Amphetamine-induced rotation was decreased by about 60 percent after 15.5 weeks, and about 80 percent after 19–20 weeks. In contrast, mouse

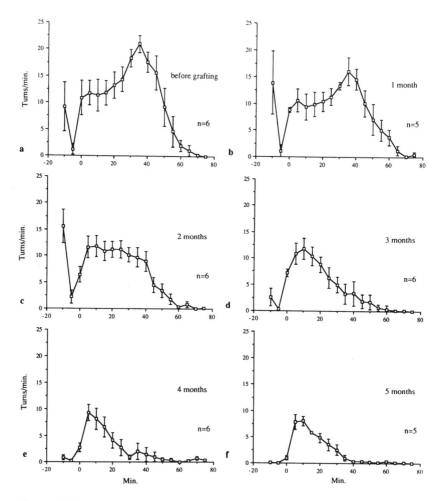

Figure 10.3
Data showing the time course of decreases in rotational behavior produced by grafts of human substantia nigra in the rat brain. Each graph displays data from one time period after transplantation. The curves indicate the profile of rotations over the course of 80 minutes following injection of apomorphine. The rotation induced by apomorphine gradually decreases over the course of five months following transplantation. (From van Horne et al. 1990, with permission.)

donor tissue decreased amphetamine-induced rotation by nearly 100 percent after six weeks. Thus, the effects of human donor tissue clearly seem to develop considerably more slowly than effects of rodent donor tissue.

Based on these limited data, I would like to try to speculate on the time course over which improvement would be expected in human subjects. It would appear that rat donor tissue requires—very roughly—about three weeks (plus or minus 7 to 10 days) to develop half of its maximal efficacy. Human donor tissue reaches half of its maximal efficacy in about 15 weeks (plus or minus 2–3 weeks) when transplanted into rats. Thus, human tissue develops about five times more slowly than rat tissue. This estimate is consistent with the earlier estimation that one day of rat development is equivalent to about five days of human development.

There are no comparable data for the contribution of the host species. That is, would it take longer for rat donor tissue to produce an effect in humans as compared with rats? It would seem likely that this would be the case, since larger areas must be reafferented. Lacking these data, however, it is impossible to make any reasonable prediction regarding the time course for improvement following transplantation of human tissue into humans. Nonetheless, it is probably safe to conclude that it should require at least as long for effects of fetal grafts of human tissue to become manifest when transplanted into humans as when transplanted into rats.

What would we therefore expect in humans? Probably, effects that occur earlier than four months after transplantation should be suspect. That is, we have to be especially cautious about effects seen one to three months after surgery, as possibly being related to surgical trauma, or simply a placebo effect. It would not, in my opinion, be at all surprising if brain grafts in human patients required more than one year for maximal effects to develop. Remember this for the following chapters.

Behavioral Tests

The studies that we have talked about thus far have mainly employed rotational behavior to assess effects of grafted fetal dopaminergic neurons. In many ways, this test does not tell us much about the ability of transplants to restore coordinated motor function, since anything that would decrease the rotational behavior (such as anesthetizing the animals, or completely destroying their neostriatum) would appear to produce improvement. There are, however, much better tests for efficacy of transplants, and when these tests are employed, effects of transplants are much less robust. (A detailed discussion of this issue can be found in Brundin, Duan, and Saver (1994) see also "Further Reading" at the end of this chapter.)

One test that has been used involves stimulating the animals' skin with a small hair or other flexible probe, or some variation of this test. Animals with lesions of the substantia nigra show deficits in their ability to orient toward this kind of stimuli, and grafts of fetal dopaminergic neurons are effective in reversing this deficit (Dunnett et al. 1981b, 1983b; Dunnett, Whishaw et al. 1987; Mandel et al. 1990; Nikkhah et al. 1993; see also figure 10.4). A modification of this test, called "disengage behavior," in which the animals are given a similar sensory stimulus while they are eating, did not show positive effects of transplants (Mandel et al. 1990).

When transplants have been tested using measures of skilled motor function—specifically, reaching though a small opening to retrieve food pellets (figure 10.5)—positive effects were not found (Dunnett et al. 1987; Montoya et al. 1988), even though recovery on this test was produced by striatal grafts in animals with striatal lesions (Dunnett, Isacson et al. 1988; see chapter 17 in this volume and figure 10.6). The deficit measured in this test is probably the best parallel with the motor function deficits seen in Parkinson's disease, and the failure of grafts to produce improvement is therefore not encouraging; the implications of this will be discussed in the conclusions of chapter 13. More recently, it has been found that some improvement in both the disengage behavior test and the skilled paw-reaching test can be produced by the microtransplantation technique, in which small grafts are placed into a relatively large number of locations through very fine glass pipettes (Nikkhah et al. 1993); this method probably could not, however, be used in human patients.

Method of Transplantation and Transplantation Sites

Fetal substantia nigra and other tissues (e.g., adrenal medulla) are usually transplanted into or near the striatum rather than in the substantia nigra, where it "belongs" (figure 10.7). This is because the goal of

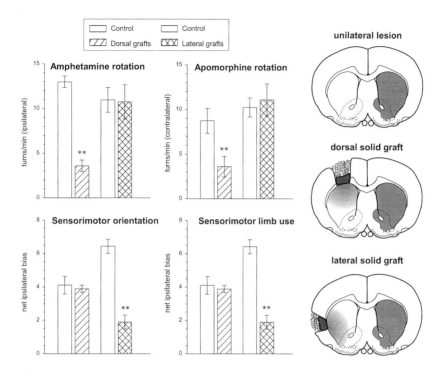

Figure 10.4
Effects of substantia nigra grafts on contralateral sensory neglect. Animals with lesions of the substantia nigra ignore sensory stimuli on the side of the body opposite the lesion. This sensory neglect is tested by stimulating the animals' skin with a flexible fiber. Normal animals turn toward the stimulus, while animals with substantia nigra injury ignore it. In this experiment, animals received grafts either dorsal or lateral to the striatum, as indicated on the right of the figure. Four behavioral tests were used: rotation induced by (i) amphetamine or, (ii) apomorphine, (iii) sensorimotor orientation or contralateral sensorimotor neglect (lower left), and (iv) limb used. The dorsal grafts produced improvements in rotation, and the lateral grafts improved sensorimotor orientation and limb use bias. (From Dunnett and Bjorklund 1984, with permission; courtesy of Steven B. Dunnett, Cambridge University.)

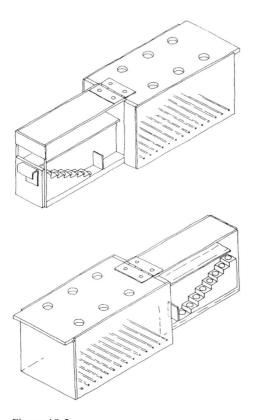

Figure 10.5
The "staircase" apparatus, employed for testing the motor coordination of rats. In order to get food pellets, animals must reach through either of two openings on the side of the enclosure. The animal can reach food through the left opening only by using the left paw, and through the right opening using the right paw. There are two staircases, one on each side, and in each of the seven steps there is a small well that contains two food pellets. The pellets located in lower steps are progressively more difficult for the animals to retrieve. The number of food pellets that the animal is able to retrieve during 15 minutes is determined. (Reproduced from Abrous and Dunnett (1994), by permission; courtesy of Steven B. Dunnett, Cambridge University.)

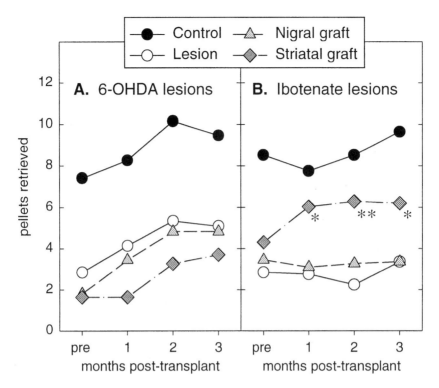

Figure 10.6

Effects of lesions and transplants on performance in the staircase apparatus. The data show the numbers of pellets retrieved by the animals at various times after lesioning and transplantation. The two graphs on the left show effects of lesions of the substantia nigra with the neurotoxic substance 6-hydroxydopamine, or 6-OHDA, and the graphs on the right show effects related to lesions of the striatum produced by ibolenic acid (see chapter 17). The upper graph of each pair shows the side ipsilateral (i.e., the same side) to the lesion, and the lower graph shows performance on the side contralateral (the opposite side) to the lesion, where effects would mainly be expected.

First, look at the data for the "controls," which in this case means animals with no lesions, shown by black circles with dotted lines. The performance of these animals improved over time, as a result of practice. Next, compare the black circles with dotted lines with the white circles with dotted lines. The white circles show animals with substantia nigra lesions only (left graphs) or striatal lesions only (right graphs). The lesions caused the animals to perform more poorly (collect fewer food pellets).

For both cases, the animals received both fetal substantia nigra and striatal grafts. Note that in the [lower] right panel, the striatal grafts (diamonds) improved the animals' performance, while the substantia nigra grafts (triangles) did not. In the [lower] left panel, however, neither type of graft improved the performance of the animals with substantia nigra lesions produced by 6-OHDA. Data from Montoya et al. (1990), with permission, provided courtesy of Steven B. Dunnett, Cambridge University.

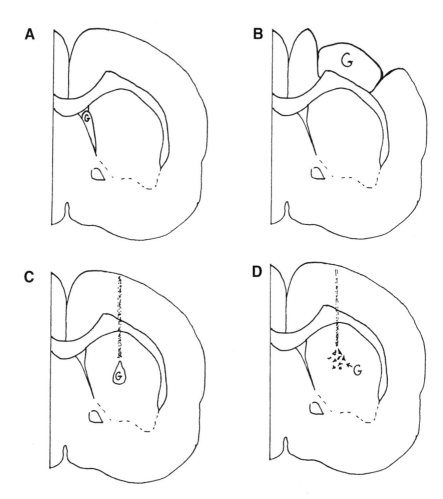

Figure 10.7
Methods that have been used for transplanting fetal substantia nigra into or near the neostriatum in rat studies. G, graft. Locations used include the lateral ventricle (a) and cavities created by removing a part of the cerebral cortex (b); and the neostriatum (c); in the latter, both solid tissue fragments and dissociated cells (d) are injected.

transplantation experiments is to replace the inputs from the substantia nigra dopaminergic neurons to neurons in the striatum, and these are likely to develop more easily if the axons of dopaminergic neurons are required to grow only a short distance.

The nigrostriatal dopamine system, which consists of dopaminergic cell bodies in the substantia nigra pars compacta and the projections from these axons to form synapses in the neostriatum, develops before birth and depends upon the presence of appropriate soluble growth factors as well as an appropriate substrate, or scaffolding, for the extension of axons from the dopaminergic cell bodies to targets in the striatum. These conditions are not present, or are present in suboptimal amounts, in the adult.

The method that is used for transplanting tissue into the brain has some influence on interpretation of results and the types of control groups that are required. In testing effects of grafts on behavior of animals, transplantation into prepared cavities in the cerebral cortex, for example, in theory requires that control animals which receive similar cavities (but no grafts, or control grafts) be tested, in the event that the cortical lesion alone influences the behavior. Grafts of solid or dissociated tissue into the brain parenchyma can influence the brain in two ways: (1) through injuring the brain directly and (2) through cellular reactions to the presence of foreign tissue. Grafts in the lateral ventricle seem to be somewhat less likely to injure the surrounding brain, although some degree of brain injury is inevitably produced even by this procedure (and control animals that receive inactive grafts are still needed). In human patients, procedures for transplantation into the ventricles have included the production of cavities in the ventricular wall, so that brain injury is also associated with these grafts (Madrazo et al. 1987). In general, transplantation into the ventricles is also not a practical procedure for human use because of the relatively poor contact between the graft and the host brain.

The relevance of brain injury to graft survival and efficacy is highlighted by recent findings that the size of the needle used for implantation of tissue into the human brain appears to be an important factor. Since the human brain is larger, there is a tendency to employ larger needles for injection of tissue, in part because larger needles are more rigid and less likely to be deflected while being lowered into the brain. Apparently the use of relatively large needles impairs the survival of grafted cells after transplantation (Brundin, Strecker, Clark, et al. 1988). Thus, the use of smaller needles, about 1 mm in diameter or less, is currently favored. One strategy employed in order to make the injection needles smaller is to taper them, so that rigidity is maintained throughout most of the needle's length but the tip is smaller, and therefore damages less tissue at the injection site. Thus, even the minor injury that is induced by a relatively small injection needle appears to induce a sufficient degree of brain injury that graft survival is adversely affected.

One technique that has received some attention recently is the microinjection of small numbers of dissociated cells into a relatively large number of locations (Nikkhah, Cunningham et al. 1993, 1994). Fine glass pipettes can be used for delivery of cells in this method, which minimizes disruption of the host brain. Greater survival of the transplanted cells and improved behavioral recovery are seen with this technique, compared with transplantation of cells through metal needles. Although it is relatively straightforward to do this in rats, making transplants in this manner in human patients, through fine glass needles, presents some considerable difficulties. The principle seems important, nevertheless: it is best to minimize disturbance of the host brain tissue and to maximize dispersion of the transplanted cells.

Increasing Graft Efficacy: Growth Factors and Transplants in the Substantia Nigra

There have been many studies of methods to enhance the survival or effectiveness of grafts of dopaminergic neurons. Because of the limited survival of transplanted neurons in animals and in human patients, this is a very active area of study. Possible methods to enhance graft survival have involved the use of growth factors, antioxidants, or other agents to block cell damage and injury; microtransplantation to obtain improved distribution of grafts throughout the target region; and improvements in tissue handling and dissection. A potent substance that enhances the survival and maturation of dopaminergic neurons, glial cell line–derived neurotrophic factor (GDNF), has been discovered and may eventually be used in treating Parkinson's disease, either to enhance effects of grafts or possibly even alone, to protect neurons from disease-related injury.

Neurons may be stimulated by chemicals called growth factors or trophic factors, which increase their capacity to extend neurites. These are peptide molecules (with abbreviations such as NGF, NT–3, BDNF, bFGF, and GDNF). It has long been recognized that each trophic factor is effective only for certain types of neurons. NGF, the classical example, acts on peripheral sympathetic neurons, immature peripheral sensory neurons, and CNS cholinergic neurons. Recently, certain of these substances have been shown to have activity for central dopaminergic neurons, especially glia cell line–derived neurotrophic factor (GDNF). GDNF has the ability to dramatically and potently stimulate the survival and growth of dopaminergic neurons, both in culture and after transplantation (Apostolides et al. 1998; Gash et al. 1995; Gash et al. 1996; Rosenblad et al. 1996; Tomac et al. 1995).

When a neuron is appropriately stimulated with such factors, internal mechanisms that control neurite extension are activated. This increases the capacity of the cell to extend neurites. In the absence of any other influence, such as a growth factor being added to a tissue culture medium, the neuron will indiscriminately extend neurites in all directions. For example, adrenal chromaffin cells stimulated with NGF, or dopaminergic cells stimulated with glia cell line–derived neurotrophic factor, in tissue culture produce a halo of neurites surrounding the cell. Instead of simply being added to the entire medium if the growth factor is added in such a way that there is a gradient of concentration, the growing neurites will follow the concentration gradient. Neurite extension may also be augmented and guided by the presence of appropriate substrates; neurites that are otherwise stimulated (i.e., by growth factors) may preferentially extend where appropriate substrate is present. In normal development, substrates and growth factors interact in a complex manner to guide axonal development and target-finding.

Although the possibility of using GDNF is promising, it is a little more complex than simply adding GDNF to transplanted dopaminergic neurons. There remains the problem of delivery, as well as the related issue of whether a short period of trophic factor administration is sufficient over the long term, or whether administration has to be continuous.

Perhaps, if a single application is sufficient (current evidence suggests that this may be the case), the implanted graft could be mixed with a fluid containing the appropriate growth factor. Even if application over a few weeks, or a month or two, is needed, administration via a mechanical pump would not pose an insurmountable obstacle. If, on the other hand, the beneficial effect of a growth factor requires long-term administration, methods such as cotransplantation of growth factor-secreting cells would be required. This latter is also a possibility. Several experiments have examined the possibility of using GDNF to enhance grafts of dopaminergic neurons, and have reported beneficial effects even with short-term administration (Apostolides et al. 1998; Rosenblad et al. 1996).

As mentioned earlier, one dream of neural transplantation is to reconstruct a complete pathway rather than simply provide an un-modulated input to a target region. In order for this to occur in the Parkinson's disease model, grafts of dopaminergic neurons would have to be placed into the substantia nigra itself rather than into the striatal target area. This is because some of the inputs to the dopaminergic neurons normally originate in the substantia nigra, and these inputs would not be able to reach transplanted neurons in other locations. In some recent experiments, it has been found that dopaminergic neurons transplanted into the substantia nigra do produce some functional improvements, even though their axons do not extend to their primary targets in the striatum (Robertson et al. 1991; Nikkhah, Bentlage et al. 1994; Johnston and Becker 1997). In order for grafts located in the substantia nigra to be fully effective, however, connections with the striatum as well as the substantia nigra have to be established. The first experiment that attempted to accomplish this was reported by Dunnett and coworkers in 1989. Since then, several experiments have focused on techniques to allow dopaminergic neurons to reconstruct a nigrostriatal pathway after transplantation into the substantia nigra.

In one experiment, Zhou and coworkers (1996) transplanted dopaminergic neurons into the substantia nigra and employed injections of kainic acid to create a pathway allowing the dopaminergic axons to reach the striatum. It had been observed previously that the growth of dopaminergic axons into the striatum was enhanced by local injections of kainic acid, a neurotoxic substance (Takashima et al. 1993). Zhou and cowork-

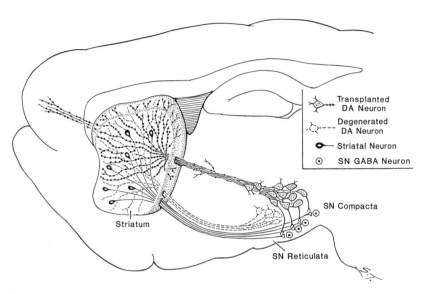

Figure 10.8
The method employed by Zhou and coworkers (1996) to obtain growth of dopaminergic axons into the striatum after transplantation into the substantia nigra. Injections of kainic acid, made along a pathway extending from the substantia nigra to the striatum, apparently created an environment favorable to long-distance growth of dopaminergic neurites. (From Zhou et al., 1996, with permission; courtesy of Feng Zhou, Department of Anatomy, Indiana University.)

ers injected kainic acid, in small doses, along a tract extending from the substantia nigra to the striatum, in such a manner that neurites growing from the transplants could grow along the tract. To accomplish this, the transplants were injected into the brain, followed by injections of kainic acid along a pathway extending to the striatum (figure 10.8). Although kainic acid is neurotoxic, small amounts were used so that there was little injury to the brain or to the transplanted cells.

It was found, by tracing experiments, that axons of the transplanted neurons grew along the kainic acid injection tract, following this pathway to reach the striatum. These axons remained in tightly grouped bundles until reaching the striatum, whereupon the fibers spread out considerably, growing into large parts of the striatum. In addition, the grafts sent fibers into the substantia nigra. This technique was also found to be effective in reliably decreasing amphetamine-induced rotation. We do not know, however, whether this method is more effective (behaviorally speaking) than simple transplantation into the striatum, since it has not been evaluated using other kinds of behavioral tests. Nonetheless, it does allow for the possibility of restoring more complete nigrostriatal neural circuitry.

Another strategy, investigated by Wang et al. (1996), involves injections of GDNF rather than kainic acid between the substantia nigra and striatum to promote the growth of dopaminergic fibers. This approach was found to produce results similar to those seen after injections of kainic acid, with processes extending from the substantia nigra into the striatum. This technique to promote the growth of dopaminergic neurites along their normal growth pathway employed GDNF infusions at a single point in time, when the grafts were implanted, and thus did not seem to require continuous infusions.

A third series of experiments, by Mendez and coworkers (Mendez and Hong 1997; Mendez et al. 1996) showed that the nigrostriatal pathway apparently could be reconstructed by placing grafts into *both* the substantia nigra and striatum. When grafts of dopaminergic neurons were placed into both locations, dopaminergic axons were found to extend along the original course of the nigrostriatal pathway, producing a more complete reafferentation of the striatum, behavioral recovery in terms of measures of rotation, and connections between substantia nigra and striatum. A fourth experiment employed cells that produce a growth factor (FGF–4) to form a bridge between the SN and striatum (Brecknell et al. 1996). It is likely that further developments along these lines will lead to transplantation techniques that more accurately reflect normal brain circuitry.

It has been estimated that 5–10 percent of rat dopaminergic cells survive transplantation. Typically, therefore, 1,000–3,000 dopamine cells survive in rat transplant recipients. Assuming that a similar percentage of cells survive in humans, 10,000–30,000 surviving cells might be expected. In the best cases, based on postmortem examination of graft recipients, more than 200,000 dopaminergic neurons have been found—only about 6 percent of the total number initially implanted (Kordower et al. 1995). A likely route to improving graft efficacy, or at least decreasing the number of human fetuses needed for transplantation, would be to improve the survival rate for transplanted dopamine neurons. Considerable effort has been devoted to that topic, looking at possibilities such as improving tissue preparation and storage techniques, using compounds to prevent toxic injury, and treatment with growth and trophic factors.

One possible means of increasing the effectiveness of SN grafts, which has hardly been explored, would be to improve the properties of the striatum as a target for the growth of dopaminergic axons. Certain molecules that are present on cell surfaces or extracellular matrix, such as laminin and L1, are known to promote the growth of dopaminergic axons. There are also certain manipulations that appear to improve the properties of the striatum as a substrate for extension of dopaminergic axons, including damaging the cerebral cortex (W.J. Freed and Cannon-Spoor 1988) and administering the neurotoxin kainic acid (Takashima et al. 1993; Zhou et al. 1996). Although these methods damage the brain, and thus obviously could not be used in humans, there may be nontoxic means of producing a similar result.

Conclusions

Briefly, it should also be mentioned that in addition to limited cell survival and neurite extension, SN grafts are subject to other potential limitations. One is the availability of synaptic sites. Neurites not only must grow from grafts into target areas in the striatum, they also must find appropriate sites and establish synapses once they get there. After the original dopaminergic afferentation degenerates in Parkinson's disease, synaptic sites also may degenerate, become blocked by astrocytes, or become occupied by abnormal synaptic inputs. There also may be permanent degenerative changes in host target cells that unavoidably limit graft efficacy. Dopaminergic synapses occur largely on the dendritic spines of neurons in the striatum, and if these spines degenerate, growing dopaminergic axons may not find appropriate targets. Also, the circuits involved are more complex than simple dopaminergic inputs to the striatum, and complete restoration of these circuits to precisely their original form is improbable.

It should also be emphasized that much of the work on neural transplantation animal models of Parkinson's disease has been based on the use of very simple models of behavior, especially rotational behavior. In some studies, grafts have been found to be partially effective with more complex behavioral tests, such as orienting toward sensory stimuli or tests of motor coordination involving reaching to obtain food pellets (see section "Behavioral Tests," above). In general, however, fetal substantia nigra grafts are much less effective when their effects are measured using tests of more complex behavioral functions or when they are compared with simple tests of drug-induced rotation. This leads to some concern that there could be fundamental limitations on transplantation of dopaminergic neurons in Parkinson's disease, an issue that will be mentioned again in the conclusion of chapter 13.

Thus, there is a great deal of experimental work that can potentially be done in this area to improve the properties of SN grafts. One might imagine, without a great deal of technological innovation, the following conditions: 90 percent of transplanted dopaminergic neurons would survive. They would be healthy and metabolically highly active. They would have the capacity to extend neurites robustly, perhaps stimulated to do so by GDNF. The striatum of the host would be modified, perhaps by a drug or, only slightly more fancifully, by an attenuated virus that targets striatal cells, inducing them to produce a molecule favorable for neurite extension. Thus, the host mature striatum might be made as favorable for growth of dopamine axons as the immature fetal striatum. Under such conditions, transplants of fetal dopaminergic neurons might, indeed, be very effective.

Further Reading

Bjorklund, A., Lindvall, O., Isacson, O., Brundin, P., Wictorin, K., Strecker, R. E., Clarke, D. J., and Dunnett, S. B. (1987). Mechanisms of action of intracerebral neural implants: Studies on nigral and striatal grafts to the lesioned striatum. *Trends Neurosci.* 10: 509–516.

Brundin, P., Duan, W.-M., and Sauer, H. (1994). Functional effects of mesencephalic dopamine neurons and adrenal chromaffin cells grafted to the rodent striatum. In: *Functional Neural Transplantation,* S. B. Dunnett and A. Bjorklund (eds.), pp. 9–46. Raven Press, New York.

Freed, W. J. (1991). Substantia nigra grafts and Parkinson's disease: From animal experiments to human therapeutic trials. *Rest. Neurol. Neurosci.* 3: 109–134.

11

Adrenal Medulla Transplantation

In the world of neural tissue transplantation, the topic of adrenal medulla transplantation is the most unusual story of all. Experiments on this topic comprise a very messy, confusing, and convoluted body of literature. It should be emphasized that, as a potential treatment for Parkinson's disease, adrenal medulla transplantation is no longer a promising therapeutic technique. At present, it is mostly of historical interest—but it makes an interesting story.

The clinical studies of adrenal medulla grafts can be summarized as having produced clinical improvements, but these improvements gradually dissipated, starting after about nine months. Substantia nigra transplantation appears to have major advantages: it seems to be more effective, and for much longer periods of time. It probably produces fewer side effects, and suffers only from the drawback of requiring a fetal donor. Adrenal medulla transplantation for Parkinson's disease remains of interest mainly because of what it can show us about effects of transplants on the brain and development of clinical transplantation techniques.

Adrenal medulla transplantation has been performed in a substantial number of human patients; fetal tissue transplantation has only recently caught up in terms of numbers of patients operated on. It was initiated in human patients as an experimental procedure on the basis of the sketchiest imaginable animal data. Even in animals, the procedure is only moderately effective, and all of the things that adrenal medulla grafts do to the brain are not entirely understood even now, more than ten years after the first human study. Adrenal medulla transplantation has been used for Huntington's chorea and progressive supranuclear palsy (Koller et al. 1989) in addition to Parkinson's disease, based simply on the hope that it might produce some benefit. In contrast, a fourth application, the use of adrenal medulla transplantation for chronic pain, has been developed systematically from a series of animal studies, and is the subject of chapter 14. Many researchers are of the opinion that, in the long run, adrenal medulla transplantation might be most useful for chronic pain.

For the moment, I will postpone the discussion of whether the procedure does or doesn't work: it is the logistical simplicity of the procedure that is, in part, responsible for its popularity—no separate donor is required. The subject who is to receive an adrenal medulla transplant into the brain simply has one adrenal gland removed (each person has two, and usually can get along quite well with only one), and the central part of the gland (the adrenal medulla) is transplanted into the brain. There are data which suggest that some of the beneficial effects may be related to trophic influences on the brain, promoting circuit remodeling in response to injury. When viewed in this manner, it is understandable, and perhaps not so objectionable, that adrenal medulla transplantation would be tried in serious degenerative diseases for which there is no other hope.

On the other hand, it should be mentioned that the use of this "simple" autotransplantation method, requiring no separate donor, may have contributed to the relative clinical failure of the procedure; several rodent studies suggest that adrenal medulla tissue from aging donors is relatively ineffective. This may be either because aging adrenal medulla is less plastic or because it is less able to stimulate plasticity in the host brain. When it is used for Parkinson's disease, the patient (who also serves as donor) may to be too old for adrenal medulla transplantation to be effective (W. J. Freed 1983; W. J. Freed, Cannon-Spoor, and Krauthamer 1985; Date et al. 1993; also see Stromberg et al. 1990). Thus, the autotransplantation technique is seductively simple, but most animal experiments, when examined carefully, suggest that adrenal medulla transplantation done in this way is not effective in animal models of Parkinson's disease. Also, most of the animals studies measured only a very simple motor behavior (rotational behavior), which does not necessarily provide a good predictor of clinical improvement in Parkinson's disease.

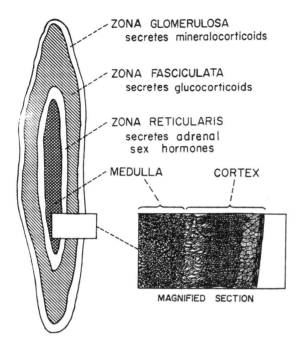

Figure 11.1
Anatomy of the adrenal gland. The two major divisions are the adrenal medulla (center) and adrenal cortex (outer layer). There is also a capsule, consisting of an outer membrane and an intermediate zone, the zona reticularis, that may contain both adrenal cortical and medullary cells. The adrenal glands are located just superior to (above) the kidneys.

Anatomy

The adrenal gland, also called the suprarenal gland, is located just above (superior to, or toward the head) the kidney. It is embedded in the fatty tissue surrounding the kidney.

The adrenal gland is comprised mainly of an outer layer, called the adrenal cortex, and a core called the medulla (figure 11.1). Additional anatomical regions include an outer capsule and an intermediate transition zone located between the medulla and the cortex (zona reticularis), which is considered part of the cortex. In some species adrenal medulla- and cortex-type cells are intermixed in the zona reticularis. The sharpness of the anatomical separation between adrenal medulla and cortex varies between mammalian species; for example, in the rat the medulla and cortex are not sharply separated, and there is a substantial transition zone where cortical and medulla cells are intermeshed. In monkeys, the transition is quite sharp, and the medulla and cortex can simply be pulled apart. In humans, the adrenal gland has a relatively complex structure, with the medulla being separated in many lobules, which makes dissection quite difficult.

Cell Types and Functions of the Adrenal Gland

When the adrenal gland is used as a source of tissue for transplantation into the brain, it is the adrenal medulla, the core area of the gland, that is employed (figure 11.1). Chromaffin cells, found in the medulla, share many of the properties of neurons (sometimes they are called "paraneuronal") and contain catecholamines. Normally, the purpose of these cells is to secrete catecholamines (epinephrine and norepinephrine), which produce a state of arousal in response to stress, into the blood. This arousal state is thought of as preparing the body to deal with emergencies. Changes that are produced include increases in heart rate and blood flow to skeletal muscles, and in metabolism.

The chromaffin cells are derived embryologically from the neural crest, which is also the source of neurons of the peripheral autonomic, spinal, and cranial ganglia. Chromaffin cells consequently retain the capacity to differentiate into neuronlike cells when exposed to certain trophic factors, especially NGF. Unlike neurons, chromaffin cells can survive removal, culturing, and transplantation even when taken from adult donors. Occasionally, chromaffin cells divide in adult animals.

Most of the chromaffin cells (especially the ones that produce epinephrine) are squarish in shape, sometimes being described as "cuboidal," and do not have extensive processes. Throughout the following discussion, however, it should be remembered that the adrenal medulla does not contain only chromaffin cells; other cell types, including endothelial cells (which line blood vessels), Schwann cells (which cover the axons of peripheral nerves with myelin), and fibroblasts are also present.

The normal physiological functions of the adrenal medulla and cortex are also quite different, although related. Cells of the adrenal cortex produce hormones (corticosteroids) that regulate various metabolic functions, whereas the chromaffin cells of the adrenal medulla produce the catecholamine hormones epinephrine and norepinephrine. Corticosteroids also regulate the form of adrenal chromaffin cells in the adrenal medulla. The blood supply of the adrenal medulla passes through adrenal cortex, so that cells of the adrenal medulla that are near blood vessels are exposed to high concentrations of corticosteroids. Corticosteroids induce the activity of the enzyme PNMT (phenethanolamine N-methyltransferase), and induce other changes in chromaffin cells so that those near blood vessels tend to be of the epinephrine-producing type. Norepinephrine cells are not adjacent to blood vessels, and thus are not exposed to high corticosteroid concentrations.

Transplantation

In 1970 Olson studied the properties of adrenal chromaffin cells transplanted to the anterior chamber of the eye. He found that under these conditions, these cells developed extensive processes, generally with neuronlike properties. Later, Unsicker and coworkers (1978; Grothe et al. 1985) determined that chromaffin cells are maintained in a endocrine phenotype by the presence of corticosteroids from the adrenal cortex, and that when they are removed from the influence of corticosteroids (e.g., by maintaining them in culture), they develop a noradrenergic phenotype and produce some processes or cytoplasmic extensions. A much greater degree of process formation can be induced when these chromaffin cells are exposed to nerve growth factor (NGF). Under these conditions, they can be induced to develop processes and adopt a more neuronal phenotype. Thus, corticosteroids and nerve growth factor play reciprocal roles in controlling chromaffin cell phenotypic expression of neuronal vs. endocrine properties. Corticosteroids promote epinephrine production and a rounded-squarish shape; NGF promotes decreased synthesis of epinephrine in favor of norepinephrine production, and process formation.

NGF treatment cannot, however, induce chromaffin cells to become dopaminergic neurons per se; if anything, the differentiation induced by NGF induces these cells to become similar to sympathetic noradrenergic neurons. Still, these cells may produce and perhaps release considerable amounts of dopamine. Some dopamine is present in adrenal chromaffin cells even when they are differentiated in an entirely endocrine phenotype.

Because the chromaffin cells of the adrenal medulla produce dopamine and can develop neurites, they were transplanted into animals with unilateral lesions of the substantia nigra, in the same manner as fetal dopaminergic neurons (W.J. Freed et al. 1981; W.J. Freed, Karoum et al. 1983; W.J. Freed 1983). The rationale for this experiment was that the chromaffin cells might be able to differentiate into a phenotypic form (in other words, change their properties after transplantation) that would permit them to substitute for dopaminergic neurons to some degree. Fragments of adrenal medulla were transplanted into the lateral ventricles of rats with unilateral lesions of their dopaminergic neurons (figure 11.2). Like dopaminergic neurons, these adrenal medulla grafts caused decreases in rotational behavior. Surviving chromaffin cells were found, and they produced catecholamines. However, no new connections between the transplanted chromaffin cells and the host brain were formed. At this point, explanation of the effect of adrenal medulla grafts seemed relatively simple; they were suspected to produce catecholamines that reached the host brain by diffusion rather than by release at synapses.

How Do Adrenal Medulla Grafts Work?

The subsequent literature on effects of adrenal medulla grafts, however, suggested that the situation was considerably more complex (to say the least!). It appears that several additional effects can be attributed to these grafts. The entire literature on this topic will not be reviewed here, and details can be obtained from the list for further reading (e.g., Freed et al. 1990). Without discussing every detail, what is the bottom line? It appears that the effects of adrenal medulla grafts on the host brain depend partly on the particular model that is used. When rats with complete lesions of the substantia nigra, induced by administration of 6-OHDA directly into the brain, are used, adrenal medulla grafts may work at least

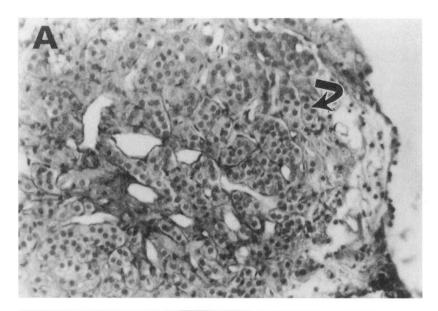

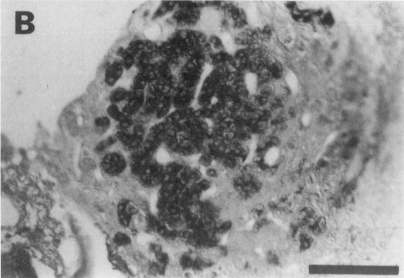

Figure 11.2
An adrenal medulla graft in the lateral ventricle of the rat brain. The upper panel (A) shows a section stained with cresyl violet, a tinctorial stain that shows all cells. The clusters of cells in the center of the graft (e.g., those indicated by the curved arrow) are chromaffin cells. The empty spaces are blood vessels. The lower panel (B) shows a section stained immunohistochemically for tyrosine hydroxylase. The darkly stained cells in (B) are chromaffin cells that are positive for tyrosine hydroxylase. The bar at the bottom of the picture is 0.1 mm long. (From W.J. Freed, Poltorak, and Becker 1990.)

partly as initially thought: they produce catecholamines which diffuse into the host brain. At best, however, this effect is very small, and requires that substantial numbers of the transplanted chromaffin cells survive (Takashima et al. 1992). When the grafts do not survive, some effects may be seen, but these are apparently nonspecific effects related to the surgery or associated damage of the host brain. Moreover, the specific effects are *very* small; in fact, they can be detected only under the most carefully controlled conditions. In many experiments, the specific effects may have seemed much larger than they actually are because they have been magnified by the presence of the nonspecific effects related to host brain injury.

Trophic Effects of Adrenal Medulla Grafts

When other models are used, especially MPTP lesions under conditions that produce only a partial destruction of the dopaminergic neurons, additional effects may be seen. In these cases, it appears that effects of adrenal medulla grafts primarily involve trophic effects on the host brain. Thus, adrenal medulla grafts may stimulate recovery of dopaminergic neurons that were not killed by the MPTP lesion, or sprouting of residual neurons that were not initially injured (Bohn et al. 1987). This effect appears to be due in part to the production of the trophic molecules by these grafts, including basic FGF and GDNF (Otto and Unsicker 1990; Unsicker 1993; Unsicker and Krieglstein 1996; Krieglstein et al. 1996), and perhaps also the cell surface molecule L1, which can stimulate growth of dopaminergic fibers (Poltorak and Freed 1990; Poltorak et al. 1990, 1992, 1993).

This trophic effect was first described by Bohn and coworkers in 1987 (see also Bing et al. 1988), and has been confirmed in several subsequent studies of animals with MPTP-induced injury. It still is not entirely clear, however, whether these trophic effects (1) require the survival of chromaffin cells, being induced by substances that chromaffin cells manufacture (e.g., basic FGF); (2) depend on survival of other cells of the adrenal medulla (e.g., fibroblasts, Schwann cells, or endothelial cells); or (3) are due to implantation-associated brain injury. Carefully controlled studies to address this question have not been completed. It appears likely, however, that the trophic effects may involve some combination of all three possibilities. There are animal experiments which suggest that each of the three mechanisms can occur.

Transplantation Site

The initial experiments on adrenal medulla grafts employed transplantation into the lateral ventricle. In this location, the chromaffin cells survive reasonably well, but the vast majority do not survive. In some animals, none of the grafted chromaffin cells survive, and in others only small numbers of surviving cells are found.

Since the original intent of adrenal medulla transplantation was to obtain secretion of catecholamines into the surrounding medium, the ventricle is in some respects a poor place to put adrenal medulla grafts. Catecholamines released into the ventricle would be diluted by the cerebrospinal fluid (CSF), and largely washed away into the ventricular system rather than reaching receptor sites in the striatum where they can influence the host brain. It seems that it would be better to transplant adrenal medulla grafts into the striatum, so that catecholamines released from the grafts can interact with postsynaptic receptors directly. Unfortunately, the survival of adrenal chromaffin cells in the striatal parenchyma is very poor. The vast majority die within a few hours after transplantation (Stromberg et al. 1984).

It is well known that nearly all kinds of primary cells require the presence of certain chemical factors for survival. Each cell type requires a certain set of trophic factors for survival. Adrenal chromaffin cells are no exception, and one of the factors that can increase their survival is NGF (Unsicker et al. 1978). Concentrations of NGF in the striatum are very low (Korsching et al. 1985). Thus, it may be that adrenal chromaffin cells do not survive well in the striatum because insufficient amounts of appropriate survival factors are present. In fact, Stromberg and coworkers (1985) showed that the survival of adrenal medulla grafts in the striatum could be markedly improved by infusing NGF along with the grafts. In addition, effects of these grafts on apomorphine-induced rotations were markedly increased, although it has been suggested that the increased behavioral effect seen in this study (Stromberg et al. 1985) might not be directly related to the increased chromaffin cell survival (Pezzoli et al. 1988).

Clinical Studies

Adrenal medulla transplantation was the first procedure to be tried in human patients in the "modern era" of neural transplantation. In 1982, two patients with Parkinson's disease received adrenal medulla grafts into the brain. The operation involved removal of each patient's own adrenal gland, dissction of the adrenal medulla, and transplantation of fragments of adrenal medulla into the striatum. The tissue was placed inside a steel springlike carrier for implantation. Initially, both patients responded positively to the procedure. The improvement was of very short duration, however, lasting no more than two weeks. Presumably, the transplanted chromaffin cells survived only transiently, and the improvements disappeared as the transplanted cells died. Results of this study first appeared in the literature in 1985 (Backlund et al. 1985), although news of the procedure was first reported in 1981 (e.g., Sullivan 1981).

The tissue was transplanted into the caudate nucleus rather than into the lateral ventricle, even though animal studies up to that time suggested better survival of adrenal medulla grafts in the ventricle compared with the striatum. There were two reasons for this choice. First, there was the logical reason that if the beneficial effects involved secretion of chemical substances, it would be much better if the tissue was transplanted directly into the striatum rather than into the ventricular system, where much of the secreted chemical substances could be "washed away" into the CSF. Second, there was the very practical problem that tissue transplanted into the ventricle could easily become dislodged and block the flow of CSF, causing hydrocephalus.

On the positive side, there were apparently no serious detrimental effects of the procedure. Thus, two additional patients (a total of four) received adrenal medulla grafts using similar procedures, but with improvements including omission of the steel spring as a tissue carrier. The outcome was measured more systematically for these two patients, and indeed there was also some improvement, which lasted for about two months (Lindvall et al. 1987). Again, however, there was no long-term, sustained improvement.

The next development was by far the most dramatic, and eventually the most controversial. In 1987 Madrazo and coworkers transplanted adrenal medulla into two Parkinson's disease patients using an improved procedure. Or, at least logically, it seemed to me to be an improvement at the time. In this case, an opening was made through the skull and cortex in order to visualize the wall of the lateral ventricle. A small cavity was then made in the wall of the ventricle. Tissue from the adrenal medulla was placed into this cavity and anchored with steel clips to prevent it from being dislodged. Thus, the graft was in contact with the ventricular CSF as well as the striatum. From the animal literature available at the time, this procedure would seem to be more akin to transplantation of adrenal medulla to the ventricles, which leads to improved chromaffin cell survival. In contrast, direct stereotaxic injection of adrenal medulla into the striatum, which results in little or no tissue survival, had been used in the prior human trials.

Results of the Madrazo et al. study were quite dramatic. Over the course of several months, there was a substantial improvement in the patients' clinical state. For two to eight months, the patients, who had been severely disabled, became able to live relatively independently. Several relatively objective tests were also performed. For example, the patients were asked to draw circles, and the ability of patient 1 to perform this task improved markedly over the course of nine months. In comparing this result with the earlier trials by Backlund et al. (1985) and Lindvall et al. (1987), in which the patients improved rapidly but the improvement was not sustained, the improvements seen in the study by Madrazo and coworkers developed much more slowly. This kind of time course is inherently less likely to be a simple placebo effect, in that it is hard to imagine a placebo effect that would take months to develop. That is, if the patients expected a benefit, and improved based on their expectations, one would expect that benefit to occur relatively soon after the surgery, especially since the earlier patients had shown a pattern of rapid improvement. The gradual development of improvements over several months was quite unexpected.

In 1989, a more systematic study was published that included a total of 18 patients tested at three different medical centers: the Rush-Presbyterian-St. Luke's Medical Center in Chicago, the University of South Florida, and the University of Kansas, Kansas City (Goetz et al. 1989). Results of this trial have been described in great detail in a series of publications

(Goetz et al. 1989, 1990, 1991; Olanow et al. 1990). This trial duplicated the Madrazo et al. surgical procedure quite exactly. In it, the patients were evaluated very thoroughly and systematically, using standardized clinical rating scales. A major difference in the evaluation was that the patients were tested during both the "on" and the "off" states, whereas Madrazo evaluated his patients without regard to whether they were "on " or "off." (Patients with Parkinson's disease who are being treated with L-DOPA generally experience "on" states, in which they are able to function relatively normally, alternating with fairly sudden transitions to "off" states, in which the L-DOPA medication does not seem to work.) A second difference is that the patients received the same dosages of L-DOPA before and after transplantation.

Clinical Evaluations—A Digression

Before proceeding to discuss the results, we should consider the merits of the two procedures for clinical evaluation: (1) measurement of clinical state without regard to whether the patients are "on" or "off" and (2) separate measurements of clinical condition during "on" and "off." On the one hand, it seems better and more thorough to consider the patients' disease severity in the "on" and "off" states, as was done by Goetz et al. Ignoring whether the patients were "on" or "off" would not seem to be an ideal method for evaluating the outcome of the procedure. There is, however, a valid counterview. Suppose that the procedure alters the *nature* of the "on" and "off" cycling. In fact, the "on" and "off" transition is not always sharply defined; suppose that this becomes even more so following transplantation.

In support of this latter possibility, it has been observed in almost all of the various types of clinical transplantation trials that the duration of "on" and "off" periods is altered as the patients improve. Suppose that what is really happening is that the patients are still in "off" after transplantation, but are somewhat better *during* the "off" state (this does in fact occur), so that they *believe* they are in the "on" state. Determination of whether the patients are in "on" or "off" is made by the patients themselves. Therefore, all measurements of "on" and "off" durations could be contaminated by changes in clinical status during each of the periods.

In fact, the transition between "on" and "off" is not always sharp and abrupt, but is often somewhat gradual. Thus, an improvement during "off" could easily appear to be an increase in the duration of "on." Therefore, in fact, an increase in "on" durations is essentially the same as an improvement in clinical state during "off" periods.

In conclusion, the ideal way to evaluate the patients would be to measure their performance (motor function) at one-hour intervals throughout an entire day, and either average these measures or study the scores as a whole. None of the clinical studies, as far as I know, for either adrenal medulla or fetal brain tissue transplantation, have used this kind of procedure. Therefore, this issue is relevant for all of the clinical studies of transplantation in Parkinson's disease, because changes in "on" and "off" durations have been one of the most consistent clinical findings.

Now Back to the Clinical Studies

The results of the Goetz et al. study (1989) can be interpreted in different ways. On one hand, improvements did occur. The amount of improvement was not to the degree that had been expected by the medical community from the reports by Madrazo and coworkers, who had claimed that the procedure produced an "excellent amelioration of most of the clinical signs of Parkinson's disease." Parkinson's disease was still present in the patients who had received grafts, even though in the Goetz et al. study their dosages of L-DOPA were not reduced. Since that study was the most systematic and complete study of adrenal medulla transplantation using the Madrazo et al. technique, the results can be considered definitive.

The results from the Hoehn and Yahr (1967) rating scale (see table 11.1 for a description) are an interesting and simple means of examining the results. For the original 18 patients, at 18 months after transplantation (Olanow et al. 1990), the Hoehn and Yahr scale had improved from an average of 4.1 before transplantation to 3.5 at 18 months, during the "off" stage. During the "on" stage, the improvement was from 3.1 to 2.7 at 18 months. These improvements are rather small, and neither difference is statistically significant. Thus, the patients still had severe

Table 11.1
The Hoehn and Yahr scale

Stage 0.0: No signs of Parkinson's disease

Stage 1.0: Unilateral involvement only

Stage 1.5: Unilateral and axial involvement

Stage 2.0: Bilateral involvement without impairment of balance

Stage 2.5: Mild bilateral involvement with recovery on retropulsion (pull) test

Stage 3.0: Mild to moderate bilateral involvement; some postural instability but physically independent

Stage 4.0: Severe disability; still able to walk or stand unassisted

Stage 5.0: Confined to wheelchair, bedridden unless aided

Parkinson's disease after the surgery and a major change in their clinical status did not occur.

On the other hand, the data can be viewed in a manner that emphasizes the improvements. With another simple rating scale, the Schwab and England (1969) scale (see table 11.2), the patients did not improve much during the "on" stage. During the "off" stage, however, the improvement was considerable: from a mean of 30 before transplantation to 55 six months after transplantation (figure 11.3). These scores remained improved, at a mean of 42, even after 18 months. Moreover, the patients were in the "on" state *more of the time*, so that the mean total improvement in their overall functioning during the course of an average day, based on the Schwab and England scale, was about 50 percent (W.J. Freed, Poltorak, and Becker 1990). A 50 percent improvement is indeed significant: certainly a change of that magnitude could make a substantial difference in the lives of the patients. Note, however, that these scales are not linear or quantitative, so that the 50 percent figure should not be considered to indicate that the patients are necessarily 50 percent better.

If one rereads the above two paragraphs, it is obvious that even apparently objective data can be interpreted differently: Did the patients improve significantly, or didn't they? It all depends on how you look at it. I would say that the improvement seen after adrenal medulla grafts was probably enough to be detected statistically, but was not enough to change the disease substantially.

Table 11.2
The Schwab and England scale for rating the severity of Parkinson's disease

90–100%	Completely independent. Able to do all chores without slowness, difficulty, or impairment. Essentially normal. Unaware of any difficulty.
80–90%	Completely independent. Able to do all chores with some degree of slowness, difficulty, and impairment. Might take twice as long. Beginning to be aware of some difficulty.
70–80%	Completely independent in most chores. Takes twice as long. Conscious of difficulty and slowness.
60–70%	Completely independent. More difficulty with some chores. Three to four times as long in some. Must spend a large part of day with chores.
50–60%	Some dependency. Can do most chores but exceedingly slowly and with much effort. Errors; some impossible.
40–50%	More dependent. Help with half, slower, etc. Difficulty with everything.
30–40%	Very dependent. Can assist with all chores but few alone.
20–30%	With effort now and then does a few alone or begins alone. Much help needed. Part invalid.
10–20%	Nothing alone. Can be a slight help with some chores. Severe invalid.
0–10%	Totally dependent, helpless. Complete invalid.

Reproduced from Schwab and England (1969, 153).

It has frequently been implied that Madrazo was grossly incorrect, or even intentionally misleading, in his presentation of his clinical results. In fact, there were inconsistencies in the data reporting. Results of rating scales from the same patients were given differently in different reports by Madrazo and coworkers at different times, so that his group cannot have been strictly objective in their data reporting. Even so, it seems that Madrazo was not entirely incorrect in his assessment of the patients. Optimistically, he overstated things slightly. Nevertheless, more extensive trials, involving very systematic assessments of clinical outcome, reported reasonably similar improvements. Thus the results reported by Madrazo were not entirely fallacious. Due to the nature of the assessment technique, there were some apparent differences in the outcome and some differences in degree of improvement.

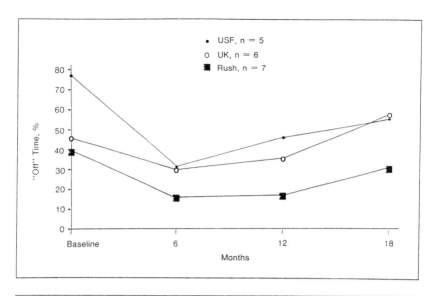

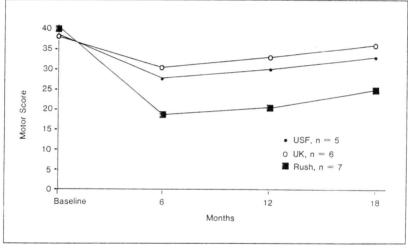

Figure 11.3

The time course of improvement seen in patients who received adrenal medulla grafts for Parkinson's disease. A total of 19 patients (18 of whom are represented) were included in the study, conducted in three medical centers. The upper graph shows percentage of time in "off," and the lower graph shows ratings on the motor subscale of the UPDRS. Results from each of the medical centers are shown separately (USF = University of South Florida; UK = University of Kansas; Rush = Rush-Presbyterian-St. Luke's Medical Center, Chicago). The largest improvements, and the only improvements that were statistically significant, were from the Rush subgroup. The improvements were maximal at three to six months after transplantation, and declined gradually thereafter. (From Olanow et al. 1990, with permission.)

Although the degree of improvement is, of course, important for clinical application, to me the argument about this seems rather like quibbling over semantics in view of the fundamentally surprising result that the patients actually did improve to a degree that was detectable from clinical ratings. The Parkinson's disease did not go away, of course. There is no question about that. Moreover, the clinical improvements diminished rapidly, starting about eight or nine months after surgery, and there were so many serious side effects (including deaths; see, e.g., Fazzini et al. 1991; Lewin 1988; Macias et al. 1989) that adrenal medulla transplantation is not a viable treatment for Parkinson's disease.

The actual clinical application of adrenal medulla transplantation, ultimately, is mostly limited by (1) the short duration of improvement, one year or so; (2) the questionable mechanisms of graft effects; and (3), most important, the high frequency of psychological, psychiatric, and medical side effects (e.g., Lewin 1988), as well as frequent deaths. The psychological and psychiatric side effects are especially disturbing. The question of *how much* the patients improved is (of course) important, but presumably the amount of improvement could be increased by subsequent research if there were no other problems associated with the procedure; for example, a method for obtaining excellent graft survival was described in Dubach and German in 1990 (see chapter 4, figure 4.4). In other words, if there were no side effects, sustained improvement were seen, and we knew how the grafts worked, a useful clinical procedure could probably be developed eventually, even if the improvements seen in the initial studies were fairly small. These are big "ifs," however, and further clinical use of adrenal medulla transplantation for Parkinson's disease is thus improbable.

In addition to the clinical studies discussed above, there were numerous others, mostly involving small numbers of patients (e.g., Allen et al. 1989; Kelly et al. 1989). Several trials, such as those conducted in Monterrey, Mexico, Madrid, and Havana, involved relatively large numbers of patients. Most of these studies will not be discussed in detail here (see "Further Reading"). The results of these studies were generally consistent with those discussed above. Further clinical studies of adrenal medulla grafts in combination with NGF infusions, or combined with grafts of peripheral nerve, generally have not produced dramatic improvements (e.g., Olson et al. 1991), perhaps with the exception of a single patient reported by Date and coworkers (1995). The consensus is that (1) some improvement did take place in many patients, although in some studies there was little overall change; (2) the improvements were transient, and mostly began to disappear within one year; and (3) the incidence of side effects, including deaths, medical complications, and psychological and psychiatric side effects, was unacceptably high. A considerable number of patients died.

Postmortem Findings

A number of patients with adrenal medulla grafts have died under circumstances that permitted their brains to be examined carefully. Examination of the brains of patients with adrenal grafts postmortem is perhaps—or at least it would seem to be—the ultimate means of finding out what is going on. Even here, unfortunately, the results are not entirely conclusive. For one thing, the improvement seen after adrenal medulla grafts disappears after a period of time, but generally the patients do not die until after the improvements have dissipated. Thus, the question of what was going on in the brain when the clinical improvement was present remains unanswered. There is often also some question about the degree of improvement, with some differences of opinion being present. Also, the preponderance of autopsy cases has been from patients who did not improve at all after the surgery. Finally, the number of autopsy cases is small, and each one has involved a different set of circumstances. Nonetheless, in the human autopsy cases that were examined, the consensus has been that the adrenal chromaffin cells did not survive, or survived poorly at best.

One case, described by Jankovic and colleagues in 1989, is unique and quite important. This patient showed persistent and marked, albeit very limited, improvement in motor function that persisted until he died, eight months after transplantation, apparently of cardiac arrhythmia. In addition to motor improvement, this patient showed some cognitive impairment after the surgery, which improved gradually even though some confusion remained until the time of death. The rating scales used did not detect major changes; improvements were seen only for certain rating scales, and they were somewhat unremarkable. The patient's wife, however, noted that he was able to arise and ambulate without assistance, even at night and during "off" periods. For example, he could get up and go to the bathroom at night without assistance, whereas he was unable to do so before the surgery. Postmortem examination of the graft revealed necrotic tissue, with no surviving chromaffin cells and no evidence of sprouting of fibers around the graft. Remember that both slight motor improvement and cognitive confusion were still present when the patient died. Since the graft, or at least the chromaffin cells in the graft, did not survive, the motor improvement as well as some of the psychological side effects may have been due to brain injury and to the tissue reaction to the presence of a graft.

This case remains the only one in which an autopsy was performed while the patient was still showing improvement. Even though neither chromaffin cell survival nor sprouting of dopaminergic fibers was present, it appears that neither is essential for the grafts to produce improvement in human patients. Therefore, despite some subsequent cases in which chromaffin cell survival and/or sprouting of fibers was seen, the most conservative conclusion is that neither contributes substantially to the clinical improvement. In fact, even when chromaffin cells were found to have survived, they were very few in number. Likewise, the TH+ fiber sprouting that has been seen involves only a small part of the striatum.

In addition to the Jankovic et al. case, there have been three reported autopsy cases in which the graft was necrotic (Dohan et al. 1988; Forno and Langston 1989; Peterson et al. 1989). In two of these, the patients showed no improvement, and in the other, the improvement had disappeared some time prior to the patient's death. Two postmortem cases revealed adrenal medulla grafts that contained surviving chromaffin cells, as indicated by immunostaining for chromogranin, a structural component of chromaffin granules (Hurtig et al. 1989; Waters et al. 1990). In the Waters et al. case, the tissue had been embedded in a steel spring. In these cases, the cells did not contain tyrosine hydroxylase, the catecholamine biosynthetic enzyme; thus the chromaffin cells were not biologically functional in that they could not produce catecholamines.

In two postmortem cases, tyrosine hydroxylase immunoreactive fibers were found adjacent to the chromaffin cell grafts (Hirsch et al. 1990;

Kordower et al. 1991). These fibers apparently had been stimulated to grow into the area by the presence of the graft, or conceivably by the tissue injury caused by graft implantation. This fiber ingrowth, although substantial, did not cover a large part of the striatum, and it is not clear whether it could account for the clinical improvements. In any case, these patients remained improved at the time of death.

In one of these cases (Kordower et al. 1991), a few surviving tyrosine-positive chromaffin cells were found. This patient showed the longest duration of clinical improvement (18 months) and the longest survival interval (30 months) of any patient who has been autopsied. Nevertheless, the clinical improvement seen after transplantation had entirely disappeared about a year prior to the patient's death. The number of surviving chromaffin cells was very few, probably not enough to explain the clinical improvement (although there could have been more cells surviving when the improvement was still present). Interestingly, despite motor improvement, this patient was plagued with severe psychiatric problems, including depression, auditory hallucinations, paranoia, and social withdrawal.

Thus, the consensus of the postmortem studies has been that only occasional chromaffin cell survival was found, with some evidence of sprouting of dopaminergic neurites adjacent to the grafts. Evidence for involvement of either in the clinical effects is weak. One must suspect that the clinical improvement which was seen is likely to have been due to brain injury or a local tissue reaction to the presence of a graft. If chromaffin cells are present, they may be more likely to produce psychiatric problems than clinical improvement in Parkinson's disease.

Conclusions

From animal data, it certainly seems that it should be possible to obtain adrenal chromaffin cell graft survival in human patients, but there is a serious question about whether this would be advisable. The array of peculiar side effects seen in human patients after adrenal medulla transplantation raises the issue of whether substances produced by adrenal chromaffin cells perturb normal brain functioning. If this is the case, one might well expect that even more severe and frequent psychiatric and psychological changes might result, along with increased motor improvement, from increasing grafted adrenal chromaffin cell survival.

On an even more general level, one might suspect that if the trophic (i.e., cell-nourishing) environment of the striatum has to be radically changed in order to support the survival of foreign cells that do not "belong" in the striatum, then such measures also might be likely to precipitate abnormal striatal functions. Although this is certainly speculative, it seems likely that inappropriate biochemicals could cause inappropriate behaviors. Thus, the introduction of cells that produce a random configuration of biochemically active substances into crucially important brain structures might generally be expected to cause undesired behavioral and functional aberrations. Ultimately, therefore, various heroic techniques to improve the survival of chromaffin cells (or other cell types that might be considered in the future) after intrastriatal transplantation may not be useful for the treatment of Parkinson's disease. Pain treatment, on the other hand, remains a potentially useful application for transplantation of adrenal medulla (see chapter 14). Odd side effects have not yet been encountered.

Further Reading

Calne, D. B., and McGeer, P. L. (1988). Tissue transplantation for Parkinson's disease. *Canadian J. Neurol. Sci.* 15: 364–365.

Date, I. (1996). Parkinson's disease, trophic factors, and adrenal medulla chromaffin cell grafting: Basic and clinical studies. *Brain Res. Bull.* 40: 1–19.

Freed, W. J., Poltorak, M., and Becker, J. B. (1990). Intracerebral adrenal medulla, grafts: A review. *Exp. Neurol.* 110: 139–166.

Gash, D. M., and Sladek, J. R., Jr. (1989). Neural transplantation: Problems and prospects—where do we go from here? *Mayo Clin. Proc.* 64: 363–367.

12

Studies in Subhuman Primates

There are several specific reasons for performing preliminary experiments in subhuman primates rather than using only rodents; all of these reasons are related to the much greater similarity between the primate and human brains. In general, there are practical reasons for primate experiments, for example, development of surgical methods, and there are theoretical reasons, such as controlled studies to determine whether the procedure is efficacious. Controlled studies, in which tissue other than fetal mesencephalon is employed for transplantation in the control group, are not feasible in human patients. Without such controls, it is very difficult to be certain about the efficacy of the procedure. In general, primate experiments have achieved the first purpose fairly efficiently, but so far have been less successful for the second.

The general principles of neural transplantation developed in rodents have been quite applicable to primates; there do not seem to be large biological differences that influence the nature of the methods used. Factors such as the types of needles used for tissue injection, age of the tissue, preparation of tissue for transplantation, and media used for tissue preparation and transplantation seem to apply similarly to all species. Therefore, rodent studies have been very useful even for working out fairly specific details about neural transplantation methodology.

Up to 1995, there had been several published studies of fetal substantia nigra grafts in monkeys using Parkinson's disease models, but no individual study was complete or conclusive. Limitations of these studies were that there were few controls, usually one or two, or none, and that in most cases the controls did not receive surgery or tissue implantation of any kind, which allowed for the possibility that the observed improvements could have been related to tissue damage associated with surgery. There were also experimental design issues: in most of the experiments, the animals were not tested "blind," nor were they randomly assigned to treatments. Although behavioral improvements were seen, there was a great deal of doubt about the results, based largely on the possibility that the animals were simply recovering spontaneously from treatment with MPTP (the toxin used to induce the Parkinson's disease-like syndrome; see chapter 8). Since human clinical trials have been in progress for some time, and the studies in monkeys have been part of the basis for human trials, these experiments have engendered considerable controversy (Landau 1990, 1993; W.J. Freed 1994). Although there have been quite a few published studies on monkey models (e.g., Annett et al. 1990, 1993; Bakay et al. 1985; C.R. Freed, Richards, et al. 1988; Redmond et al. 1986; Sladek et al. 1986; Fine et al. 1988), only two will be considered in detail here.

Bankiewicz, Plunkett, and Coworkers

Most of the subhuman primate experiments, including early studies with small numbers of animals, have been more or less in agreement about the following: (1) that grafts sent new dopaminergic fibers into the host brain, and (2) that this reafferentation is associated with clinical improvement in the animals. There is, however, a dissenting series of experiments by K. Bankiewicz, R. Plunkett, and coworkers (Bankiewicz et al. 1990, 1991; Plunkett et al. 1990). Bankiewicz and coworkers (1990) reported on experiments in monkeys in which grafts contained dopaminergic neurons, but the neurons did not send fibers into the host brain, at least not to a noticeable extent. Instead, the fiber growth from transplanted dopaminergic neurons was *within* the transplant. The reason that the typical projection of fibers from graft into host brain did not occur is uncertain, but it seems likely that it is because cavities were produced in the brain two to five weeks prior to transplantation. This procedure probably caused a glial scar to develop around the transplants. Such a barrier could have prevented dopaminergic fibers from penetrating into the host brain.

Even under these conditions, some behavioral improvement was seen. Controls, which received no surgery, did not improve. A later study, using animals that received other kinds of grafts (cerebellum or spinal cord), also observed improvements similar to those produced by the dopaminergic neurons. The implication of this observation is that the improvement seen was due either to host brain injury or to the induction of sprouting of host fibers around the site of the transplants.

Although this cannot be properly considered a controlled study, since the animals that received spinal cord and cerebellar (control) grafts were tested at a later time, the two procedures produced similar results. Thus, it appears that the improvements seen in this series of experiments were due not to reafferentation of the brain but rather to some nonspecific effect, such as tissue injury.

It should also be mentioned that the behavioral measure of improvement used in these experiments was decreases in apomorphine-induced rotation. It may very well be the case that nonspecific effects (e.g., tissue injury) are capable of alleviating simple behavioral measures of this type, while more complex tests of motor function (such as observational measures or tests of motor dexterity) may require grafts to form specific connections with the host brain in order for improvement to be detected. It should also be mentioned that studies by Marshall and Ungerstedt (1977) showed that apomorphine-induced rotation can be decreased simply by destroying part of the striatum.

Although it is tempting to conclude that the effects seen in this study are merely related to brain injury, there was some evidence that the effects of grafts were somewhat more complex. The major reason for this conclusion is the observation—which is interesting for other reasons as well—that one animal showed evidence of graft rejection (Bankiewicz et al. 1990). This animal had received grafts from two fetuses; perhaps one of these was immunologically incompatible with the host. Curiously, for this animal, behavioral improvement was seen initially but disappeared by six months, perhaps corresponding to rejection of the graft. Thus, the effects seen in this study may require the graft to be present, and thus may involve more than simply damage of the host brain. Parenthetically, there has been a second report of rejection of a fetal brain tissue graft in a monkey (C.R. Freed, Richards, et al. 1988).

Overall, the experiments of Bankiewicz and coworkers tend to suggest that at least some effects of transplants in primates can be nonspecific, probably related either to the release of trophic factors from transplanted brain tissue into the host brain, or to brain injury in some form. There has subsequently been some controversy related to these experiments—for instance, it has been claimed that all effects of transplants in primates are merely due to brain injury (Landau 1993). The available evidence, however, mainly suggests that the effects of transplants in *this* study are due to brain injury. Since the grafts did not reafferent the brain in the Bankiewicz experiments, little can be concluded from them about other experiments in which reafferentation of the host brain was seen. Therefore, these results are also consistent with the hypothesis that specific beneficial effects of SN grafts are based on the development of new connections with the host brain.

These studies, therefore, do not necessarily support the conclusion—which has sometimes been made—that grafts produce improvements in primates only through nonspecific mechanisms. The grafts did not produce reafferentation of the brain in this study, and reafferentation of the brain is probably required for specific graft-mediated improvement to occur.

Experiments of J. Taylor and Associates

This group, located at Yale University and the Chicago Medical School, which includes Jane R. Taylor, John R. Sladek, D. Eugene Redmond, and others, has performed transplantation experiments in large numbers of animals, starting in 1986. The results show that under appropriate conditions, transplanted dopamine neurons survive and send neurites into the host brain fairly extensively. Although several primate studies have included small numbers—usually one or two—of controls, only one experiment that has so far been published can actually be described as a controlled study (Taylor et al. 1995). An earlier report, by this same group, showed positive behavioral effects in animals that received fetal substantia nigra grafts, while control animals that received other types of tissue grafts did not show improvement (Taylor et al. 1990, 1991). Although this earlier study was the most extensive study at the time, it was a collection of results from animals tested at different times over a number of years, and thus cannot properly be considered a controlled experiment.

More recently, a very thorough and quite definitive report on transplants in subhuman primates has been published (Taylor et al. 1995). This particular experiment warrants consideration in some detail. The study included a total of 29 primates; testing of this number under identical conditions is in itself a remarkable accomplishment. The animals received grafts by stereotaxic injection of small blocks of tissue (about 1 mm^3) into the brain using a 19 gauge needle. Large numbers (thousands) of dopaminergic neurons consistently survived in the transplants, and the study showed unequivocal histological evidence for crossing of fine dopaminergic fibers from the graft into adjacent parts of the host brain.

Animals were tested behaviorally by standardized observational techniques. This involved daily observation of the animals, during which their spontaneous behaviors were recorded and scored for the presence of Parkinson's disease-like abnormalities. Examples of the abnormalities detected by this method included tremor, difficulty eating, delayed movements, impaired grooming, and general poverty of movement. Various tests were employed to ensure that the observational measurements were reliable.

The animals' evaluation by observational techniques is advantageous, since the outcome measures therefore did not rely on the induction of behavior by a drug or on simple stereotyped motor functions. The most prominent abnormal feature of the animals, consistent with Parkinson's disease, was prominent motionlessness and immobility, and lying facedown on the floor of the cage. Behaviors were scored in terms of frequency: severely parkinsonian animals had scores in the range of 50, about 60 percent of which consisted of facedown/immobility, and 75 percent of which was comprised of an aggregate of "facedown/immobility," "poverty of movement," and "freezing/motionlessness." Animals were studied for approximately six months after MPTP treatment before receiving transplants, to ensure that the behavioral deficits were stable, and were followed for eight to nine months after transplantation.

The results were dramatic: there was clear evidence that improvement was induced selectively by the fetal transplants of substantia nigra from

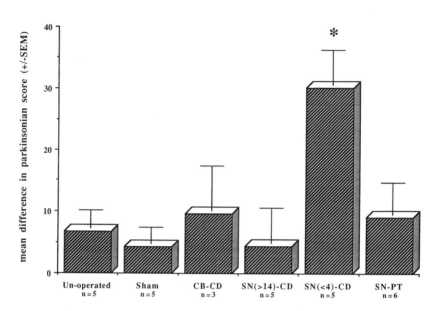

Figure 12.1
Effects of fetal substantia nigra grafts in a subhuman primate model of Parkinson's disease. Numbers on the vertical axis indicate decreases in total parkinsonian scores, so that higher numbers represent greater improvements. Substantial improvements were seen only in the animals that received SN grafts from fetuses in an early developmental stage, approximately 38–44 days (less than 4 cm crown-rump length). The asterisk indicates that the improvement in this group, (SN (<4)-CD), was statistically significant. The other groups are (1) unoperated, animals that received no surgery; (2) sham, animals that received injections of fluid only; (3) CB-CD, animals that received control grafts of cerebellum into the caudate nucleus; (4) SN(>14)-CD, animals that received grafts of more mature substantia nigra; (5) SN-PT, animals that received grafts of substantia nigra into the putamen. (From Taylor et al. 1995, with permission.)

the younger fetal donors. Tissue from fetal donors of approximately 44 days or younger was effective, while tissue from older donors, 80 to 165 days, was no more effective than control tissue (see figure 12.1). The overall improvement seen in the animals that received the immature SN grafts was more than 50 percent, and developed mainly over the course of two to three months after transplantation, with some additional improvement thereafter (figure 12.2). No noteworthy improvements were seen in the groups that received grafts of cerebellum or injections of fluid

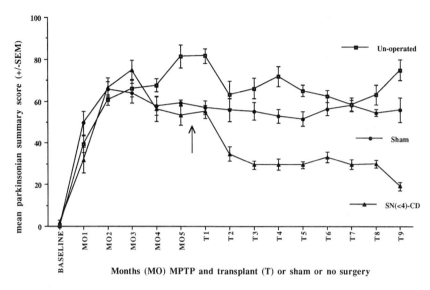

Figure 12.2
The time course of improvement in parkinsonian scores in monkeys that received substantia nigra grafts, compared with unoperated animals or sham-operated controls that received injections of fluid only. The numbers on the vertical axis indicate total parkinsonian scores, so that decreases indicate improvements. The animals that received early stage substantia nigra grafts (SN(<4)-CD) initially became worse from one to two months after MPTP lesioning (MO1 and MO2), and stabilized from three to five months after MPTP (MO3, MO4, and MO5). Improvement was fairly stable for the nine months of observation (T1–T9). (From Taylor et al. 1995, with permission.)

only (figure 12.1). The dopamine neurons in the grafts from younger fetal donors survived and produced fibers that extended into the host brain (figure 12.3).

The study by Taylor and coworkers (1995) is the first clear demonstration in a higher animal that transplants of fetal dopaminergic neurons can alleviate Parkinson's disease-like symptoms. Control grafts were not effective, showing that the effects were not due to tissue damage, nonspecific secretion of chemical substances by grafted fetal tissue, or the host brain's reaction to tissue implantation. Moreover, the improvement that occurred was evaluated by observation of the animals' spontaneous behavior, which probably indicates a generalized functional improvement rather than a restricted change in a single aspect of motor function, for

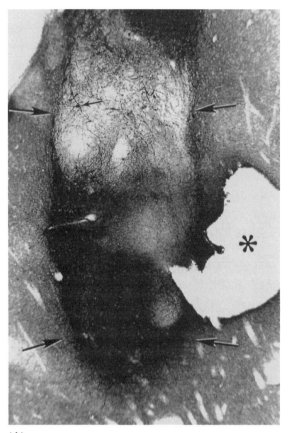

(A)

Figure 12.3
Transplanted dopaminergic neurons in a subhuman primate, with neurites extending into the host brain. The section is stained to show the catecholamine-synthetic enzyme tyrosine hydroxylase. This graft (outlined by large arrows in A) of dopaminergic neurons in a parkinsonian, MPTP-treated monkey, is characterized by the presence of thousands of tyrosine hydroxylase-stained neurons that are so densely packed they are difficult to discern in the low-power view (A). Some are seen individually (small arrow), and can be distinguished more clearly at higher magnification in (B). Extensive fiber outgrowth extends from the graft and is responsible for an elevation of dopamine in the surrounding tissue of the host brain, as measured biochemically in a microdissected sample, seen as a blank area indicated by an asterisk (*). (From studies by a consortium of investors including John Sladek, Gene Redmund, Robert Roth, Tim Collier, Jane Taylor, John Elsworth, and others. Photographs courtesy of John Sladek, Chicago Medical School.)

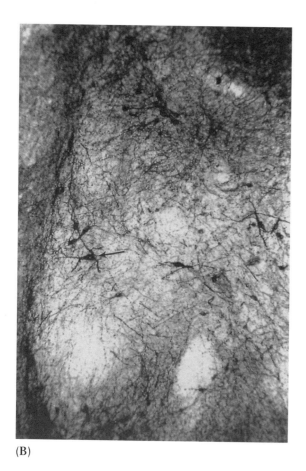

(B)

example. These data are very encouraging for the application of fetal transplantation to human patients with Parkinson's disease.

Further Reading

Dunnett, S. B., and Annett, L. E. (1991). Nigral transplants in primate models of parkinsonism. In: *Intracerebral Transplantation in Movement Disorders,* O. Lindvall, A. Bjorklund, and H. Widner (eds.), pp. 27–51. Elsevier, Amsterdam.

Freed, W. J. (1991). Substantia nigra grafts and Parkinson's disease: From animal experiments to human therapeutic trials. *Rest. Neurol. Neurosci.* 3: 109–134.

Freed, W. J. (1994). Special correspondence. *Neurology* 44: 573–574.

Ridley, R. M., Baker, H. F. (1991). Can fetal neural transplants restore function in monkeys with lesion-induced behavioural deficits? *Trends Neurosci.* 14: 366–370.

Ridley, R. M., Baker, H. F., Dunnett, S. B., and Annett, L. E. (1994). Special correspondence. *Neurology* 44: 573.

Taylor, J. R., Elsworth, J. D., Roth, R. H., Collier, T. J., Sladek, J. R., Jr., and Redmond, D. E., Jr. (1990). Improvements in MPTP-induced object retrieval deficits and behavioral deficits after fetal nigral grafting in monkeys. In *Neural Transplantation,* S. B. Dunnett and S.-J. Richards (eds.), pp. 543–559. Elsevier, Amsterdam.

13

Fetal Brain Tissue Transplantation in Parkinson's Disease: Clinical Studies

The idea of transplanting fetal dopaminergic neurons into the brains of patients with Parkinson's disease is the idea that got this field off the ground, and development of a successful clinical procedure would be the culmination of research in this field. Although there has been a great deal of work on transplantation in other disorders, Parkinson's disease is still the prototype. Parkinson's disease in general, and clinical studies of dopaminergic neuron transplantation, are discussed in greater detail because currently this is the most realistic application of brain tissue transplantation to a human disorder, and also because of the possibility that some readers may consider receiving this procedure.

Well in excess of 200 human patients with Parkinson's disease have received fetal tissue transplants in trials conducted in (among other places) Mexico, Sweden, the United States, Cuba, England, Poland, China, France, Canada, and Spain. In most patients, at least some improvement has been seen—although that fact alone doesn't mean much, since "improvement" has been reported or claimed to have been produced by almost every procedure, applied to almost every disease, for which transplantation has been tried. In Parkinson's disease, for example, adrenal medulla grafts appear to produce at least some improvement (chapter 11) even though there is little evidence that the grafts survive. Also, in some cases, grafts were reported to produce improvement in Parkinson's disease trials, but later studies showed that the grafts were from donors too mature for the dopaminergic neurons to have survived.

In the present chapter, some of the human trials of human fetal mesencephalic tissue transplantation in Parkinson's disease will be described in some detail. In addition to discussing the most thorough and modern clinical studies, I have included some of the earlier and more flawed trials. At the present time, although definitive conclusions are not possible, some postmortem studies have been highly encouraging. A final answer will probably, and unfortunately, have to wait for a sufficient number of deaths to allow for correlations between transplant viability measured postmortem and clinical improvement. Nevertheless, there are least strong indications, and tentative conclusions can be made. The status of this endeavor has been markedly clarified by two autopsy cases from the University of South Florida study showing conclusive evidence of transplant survival in human patients. This study will therefore be discussed first.

University of South Florida Study

It now appears that this study will be the standard, at least for the time being, by which other studies are judged, mainly because of fortuitous circumstances that led to the availability of two brains under nearly optimal conditions for autopsy. One patient, who had shown considerable improvement, died 18 months after transplantation, while in the hospital, due to a pulmonary embolism related to surgery for sequelae of an unrelated ankle fracture (Kordower et al. 1995, 1996). The brain was obtained within four hours and processed for histochemical staining under nearly optimal conditions. Large numbers of transplanted dopaminergic neurons were found to have survived and extended processes into the patient's brain (figure 9.5). There was little, if any, indication of damage, cell degeneration, or tissue necrosis of any kind. Details of this clinical trial are discussed below. A second patient died more recently, also of unrelated causes and also approximately 18 months after transplantation, and the graft in this patient also showed good survival of dopaminergic neurons (Kordower et al. 1998). The implications of these cases are profound: at the very least, they demonstrate that the surgical approach being employed is viable, and that transplants in humans behave quite analogously to transplants performed similarly in primates and even in rodents. Moreover, even though it has not been proven statistically, it seems likely that at least some of the improvement seen in these patients was related to survival, growth, and physiological functioning of the transplanted tissue.

Complete clinical results from this study have not yet been published; however, as of 1995, results from four patients had been reported in detail (Freeman, Olanow, et al. 1995). Several aspects of the procedure that was employed are noteworthy. One was the use of young fetal donors, 6.5 to 9 weeks postconception. A number of fetal donors (three or four for each side of the brain) were used for each patient, in order to ensure that substantial numbers of cells survived transplantation. Tissue was implanted in several sites about 5 mm apart in the putamen, in an attempt to "saturate" its posterior part with transplants. This distribution of tissue, and the fact that up to eight donor fetuses were used for each patient, meant that a considerable number of cells were transplanted into each subject. Fetuses were stored for up to 48 hours under refrigeration, in a special "hibernation" medium, so that enough tissue could be accumulated for transplantation. The patients were immunosuppressed with cyclosporine for six months.

At six months after transplantation, there were indications of substantial clinical improvement by several measures. Generally, there were improvements in rating scale measures of levels of function during "off" periods, and not during "on" periods. There were also substantial increases in "on" time and marked decreases in "on" time with dyskinesia. No improvements during the "on" phases were seen. These changes developed over the six months following transplantion. Although substantial, they were not obviously larger than the those seen after adrenal medulla grafts. Also, the pattern of clinical changes and time course did not differ from that seen after adrenal medulla grafts in any obvious manner. One possible exception, however, is that there were improvements in dyskinesia in two of the four patients that developed very rapidly, within one month. This is a possible difference from the effects of adrenal medulla grafts. Of course, the fact that the changes were not obviously different from those after adrenal medulla transplantation does not necessarily mean that the improvements were meaningless or should be dismissed out of hand. However, it is a sign that they should be interpreted with caution. Thus, even though we know that at least some of the grafts survived, a healthy degree of skepticism should be maintained.

When the transplants were examined postmortem, there was a remarkable degree of tissue survival and a near absence of an adverse reaction of the host brain. In the first patient, approximately 210,000 dopamine neurons were found, with numerous surviving neurons in each transplant site. Although this probably represents only about 5 percent of the number initially transplanted, it represents about 50 percent of the number normally present in the healthy human brain (remember that several fetuses were used for transplantation in each patient). Also, despite the survival of neurons in many locations, considerable parts of the putamen remained deafferented. The dopaminergic neurons were in excellent and normal-appearing condition, with numerous processes extending into the host brain. However, the lack of varicosities (beadlike areas of enlargement) along the cell processes was evidence that the transplanted neurons were still somewhat immature at the time of death. It was suggested that this apparent slowing of maturation might be related to the Parkinson's disease process in some manner. Although there was some evidence of gliosis in the host brain, there was no glial barrier surrounding the graft, so that, in the words of the authors, there was a "seamless," continuous integration between the graft and the host brain. Results from both patients were similar (figure 9.5).

The results of the postmortem examination of this graft showed that the methods used for tissue preparation and transplantation in the University of South Florida study are consistent with good graft survival. It is tempting to assume that the clinical improvements seen in this study were related to physiological effects of these surviving grafts. Although this is perhaps likely, it is not proven, and we should be somewhat cautious about concluding that the effects seen at six months after transplantation were definitely due to surviving transplanted neurons. Thus, although the University of South Florida study is not the most extensive study, and the patients have not yet been followed clinically for a particularly long period, it is very significant because we know that the grafts survived in at least the two patients examined postmortem, and probably in other patients as well.

One additional aspect of this study merits some discussion. A topic that we have not yet considered to any great extent is the possibility that the grafts would be rejected. In general, there is some protection of fetal brain grafts from rejection, but the necessity for using immunosuppression in human patients to avoid graft rejection is still controversial. Although in rats and even in monkeys, grafts made under similar circumstances survive quite well, there is the possibility that, compared with animals, the human immune system would be somewhat more effective in rejecting brain grafts. An approach used by several groups has been to employ an immunosuppressive drug (cyclosporine) for a limited period of time (e.g., six months) following transplantation, based on the supposition that this would prevent immune system sensitization during the period of wound healing associated with graft surgery. The patients in the University of South Florida study received low dosages of cyclosporine for six months after transplantation. Thus, for both of the patients who died, the grafts had survived for approximately one year after cyclosporine had been discontinued. In neither case was there any evidence of graft deterioration or of an obvious rejection response.

The second patient was examined for the presence of several markers that specifically indicate immunologically functional cells (Kordower et al. 1997). Here there was evidence of a minor ongoing immunological response to the grafts: activated microglia and some T cells. Therefore, it is possible that there is a very low-level, ongoing immune response to the presence of brain allografts in at least some human patients. Possibly this low level response could expand and eventually result in graft damage, or even destruction, although this seems improbable, given the fact that the patients died a year after cyclosporine had been discontinued. Such an event, if it occurred, could have adverse consequences that extend beyond loss of the graft per se, perhaps to damage of adjacent tissues as well. It does not appear that this observation requires any major readjustment of the approach to human transplantation at the present time; however, it does serve as a reminder that we need to be wary, and that immunological issues regarding human transplantation have not been entirely resolved. To be conservative, I would think that the use of cyclosporine in human brain tissue grafts should probably be continued for at least the six-month interval that currently is employed most frequently.

The implications of the University of South Florida autopsy cases are profound. First, these findings indicate that the general approach is working, so that the clinical results provide a good test of the principle. It also appears that the predictions and extrapolations made from animal studies are not overly optimistic; in fact, experiments in rodents and sub-human primates seem to be good indicators of the effects that can be expected clinically. Thus, the techniques now being used, at least at the University of South Florida, probably are sufficiently effective to provide a very good test of the general approach of fetal tissue transplantation in Parkinson's disease.

Yale University Study

This group has performed some of the most extensive and systematic clinical trials, especially in that the procedures used have been tested fairly extensively in subhuman primates. A major feature of the clinical trials performed by this group has been the use of a type of control/comparison group that receives no surgery, but instead the best available medical treatment and the same testing protocol as the surgery group. After one year, the control/comparison group also received transplantation surgery. This permits comparisons between the patients who received transplants and the control/comparison group, who did not receive surgery. When the patients were being evaluated, their heads were covered with a surgical cap, so that they could be observed without revealing whether or not they had received surgery. They were videotaped during a structured examination, so that all of the patients could be independently rated "blind."

Although it does not rule out nonspecific effects of surgery, the strategy of using a control group that does not receive transplants for the first year at least allows for comparison of transplantation with alternative treatment, as opposed to simple comparisons with the patients' state before transplantation. This is a major improvement. The use of a nontransplanted comparison/control group also avoids the potential problems that might be associated with the use of control surgery. However, the crossover design, in which the comparison patients receive transplants after one year, limits the period of observation to one year. Since the controls also received transplantation, after a one-year delay, comparisons to the control group could not be made subsequent to one year.

The initial published study by this group (Spencer et al. 1992) included results from four patients who received transplants (case patients) and three nonoperated controls. The donor tissue was obtained from fetuses of 7, 10, 10, and 11 weeks' gestation. Although most data suggest that donor tissue should be younger than 11 weeks, the time of 10 weeks of gestation is on the borderline of being viable for transplantation. The tissue was stored, frozen in liquid nitrogen, prior to transplantation.

The second transplanted patient, who received tissue from an 11-week gestational fetus, died four months after surgery. It turned out that this patient had striatonigral degeneration rather than Parkinson's disease, even though he had responded to L-DOPA early in the illness. He had not improved markedly following transplantation. The graft had surviving neurons that contained neuromelanin (which is characteristic of human dopaminergic neurons), but the grafted neurons did not express tyrosine hydroxylase, the characteristic enzyme indicative of dopamine production. Only a single tyrosine hydroxylase-containing neuron was found (Redmond et al. 1990). It is also likely that the lack of tyrosine hydroxylase-expressing neurons was at least partly due to the relatively late gestational stage of the fetus that was used.

The remaining three patients survived up to the 18-month evaluation point, and showed signs of improvement by certain measures. Evaluations were of two types, rating scales and measures of motor function. There were improvements in the transplanted patients according to two of the rating scales that assess "activities of daily living" (ADL): these were the Schwab and England scale and the Unified Parkinson's Disease Rating Scale for ADL and motor function. Several additional scales did not demonstrate improvement. There were also, however, some improvements in the controls. In most cases, the improvements seen in the transplanted patients, according to the rating scales, were not dramatically larger than those seen in the controls. There was a 25 percent improvement in the UPDRS ratings for the controls after one year, and a 30 percent improvement in the three transplanted patients after 18 months.

The measures of motor function also showed similar trends; however, for these measurements the difference between transplanted patients and controls was more distinct. Distinct signs of improvement were seen on the tests of pronation-supination, foot tapping on both sides, and thumb-index finger tapping. Tests of walking, however, were the exception; walking tended to become worse in the transplanted patients compared with the controls. For the pronation-supination test (see glossary), for example, the transplanted patients improved by about twofold; there was essentially no change in the nontransplanted patients.

Subsequent to this initial report, this group has studied 12 additional patients, and has made several improvements. Notably, in the more recent patients, tissue from younger donors (six–nine weeks' fetal age) has been used, and for the most recent five patients, tissue was transplanted bilaterally into both the caudate and the putamen (Redmond et al. 1998). In general, there were improvements in many of the patients. Surprisingly, however, the later patients, who were less severely ill and who received transplants from younger donors, tended to show less improvement than the earlier group. In addition to the patient who died after four months, discussed above, three more patients died. None of these had improved. In one case, autopsy was refused. One patient died 27 months after transplantation, and in this patient there were signs of possible graft rejection. The fourth died after 37 months, and no surviving dopaminergic neurons were found.

This series of studies has been perhaps the most systematic, in that procedures had been tested in primates prior to human application, and that the clinical study was carefully and systematically executed. There are, however, some drawbacks. One is that for the first few patients, the donor tissue was more mature than what is probably optimal for use in human transplantation, an issue that became clarified from animal data only after the trial had been initiated. A second is that tissue was transplanted into the caudate nucleus only, rather than into both the caudate and the putamen, for all but the last five cases. Another potentially problematic technical issue is the use of tissue that had been stored in a frozen state prior to transplantation. Although the freezing technique was studied prior to use in humans, and there are certainly advantages to being able to use stored tissue, some loss of tissue viability probably resulted from this manipulation.

An interesting aspect of this study is that the psychiatric status of the patients following transplantation surgery was systematically investigated (Price et al. 1995). Unlike adrenal medulla transplantation, which often was found to cause psychiatric disturbances (psychosis, delirium) shortly after transplantation, fetal mesencephalic tissue grafts produced few psychiatric abnormalities during the postoperative period. There were, however, some psychiatric disturbances that occurred longer after the surgery. In general, however, these later developing symptoms appeared to be somewhat related to the patient's expectations regarding the surgery; for example, disappointment that the parkinsonian symptoms had not improved more. Improvements in rating scales and motor function tests do not necessarily translate into changes that make a real difference in the lives of the patients. It is probably worth noting that patients' expectations regarding the outcome of surgery may tend to be unrealistic, even if researchers are careful to explain that the procedure is experimental. Transplantation as a therapy is invasive and dramatic, and the patients will quite naturally hope that the improvement seen will be correspondingly notable.

Three of the nine patients developed major psychiatric problems. In one case, a patient who had previously experienced occasional panic attacks developed a more serious panic disorder with agoraphobia, about one month after transplantation, that appeared to be related to the development of seizures. This improved with drug treatment, but nine months after transplantation, this patient developed a major depressive episode, which also responded to drug treatment. A second patient developed a major depressive episode about six months after surgery, and a third patient developed a major depressive episode after a little more than a year. Major depressive problems in three of nine patients represents a very high incidence. Whether these were caused by direct effects of the transplants, or were interactions between transplant effects or the ongoing disease and patients' disappointment about the outcome, or some combination of the above, is unclear.

Overall, there were improvements in both the transplanted and control groups, although for some measures greater improvements were seen in the group that received transplants. Several of the differences between the improvements seen in the control and transplanted groups were fairly substantial. The use of a comparison group that does not receive transplantation is an excellent method to objectively test the effects of transplantation, without the requirement of subjecting patients to the control surgery. The fact that improvements were seen in the controls, who did not undergo surgery, should be borne in mind in relation to evaluating effects of various transplantation procedures in other studies.

Studies from Lund, Sweden

The studies by Lindvall and coworkers, at Lund University in Sweden, include some of the earliest, and some of the most technically sophisticated, clinical trials. This group has now performed transplantation procedures in at least 10 patients, including 2 with parkinsonism induced by the toxic drug MPTP. In all cases, tissue from several fetuses was transplanted by stereotaxic injection as a crude suspension; that is, the tissue was partly dissociated, so that some cells remained as clumps. Tissue was also injected into several sites, usually three in the caudate and three in the putamen, or in the putamen only, and in most cases on both sides of the brain. The patients were temporarily immunosuppressed with both cyclosporine and prednisolone. All of the patients received grafts from relatively immature donors, eight weeks' gestation or earlier.

In the first two patients, only minor improvements were seen (Lindvall et al. 1989). Subsequently a number of procedural improvements were made, which seemed to result in a better outcome. For example, in the first two patients a simple saline solution was used as a vehicle for injecting the tissue into the brain, whereas for later patients a tissue culture medium was used. Animal experiments suggested that the results might be better if smaller needles were used to implant the tissue. Although this sounds rather trivial, it is actually not so obvious: smaller needles may bend when inserted, which can cause obvious problems in human neurosurgery. Also, although it is a simple change, the requirement for using small needles is not really obvious a priori. In fact, one might imagine that smaller needles would produce greater damage to the cells, by forcing them through a smaller opening. Another important change is that more tissue was used in the later trials. Calculations based on the limited numbers of surviving cells in animal experiments suggested that better results might be obtained by using multiple fetuses for transplantation. Another improvement consisted of targeting the transplants entirely to the putamen, which is the area most severely affected by degeneration in Parkinson's disease.

In the third patient, the results of which were published in a paper by Lindvall and coworkers in 1990, more substantial improvements were seen; however, the results were inconclusive, as the clinical effects over the first several months were not remarkable different from those seen after adrenal medulla transplantation (W. J. Freed 1990; see also comments below). The improvements seen in this third patient, and a fourth patient who received similar surgery, were thought to be related to the procedural changes mentioned above. Thus, it was presumed that the improvements were related to better survival of the tissue and integration with the host brain.

The most remarkable change, perhaps, is that in the fourth patient, progressive, long-term improvement was seen. This patient showed improvement from 4 to 10 months after surgery, then additional improvement after a year. The percentage of time in "off" was about 70 percent before transplantation, and afterward decreased to about 40 percent and stayed at that level up to about 12–14 months. Then a second phase of improvement began, with additional improvements in "on"-"off" times and rigidity developing from 12 to 30 months after transplantation. In this patient, by 30 months after transplantation the percentage of time in "off" was zero, and rigidity of the left side (contralateral to the graft) almost entirely disappeared (figure 13.1). This patient remained remarkably improved, with only mild symptoms, for the fourth and fifth year after surgery. During the sixth postoperative year there was a slight worsening, but the patient was still markedly better than before transplantation. Normally, Parkinson's disease is inexorably progressive. Such a long-term, progressive improvement strongly suggests long-term maturation of the graft and/or development of connections with the host brain.

Additional evidence of functional integrity of the graft in Patient 4 is that fluorodopa uptake, evaluated by PET scanning, was increased in the striatum in an area corresponding to the area receiving a transplant (figure 13.2). In areas of the brain that did not receive transplants (e.g., the

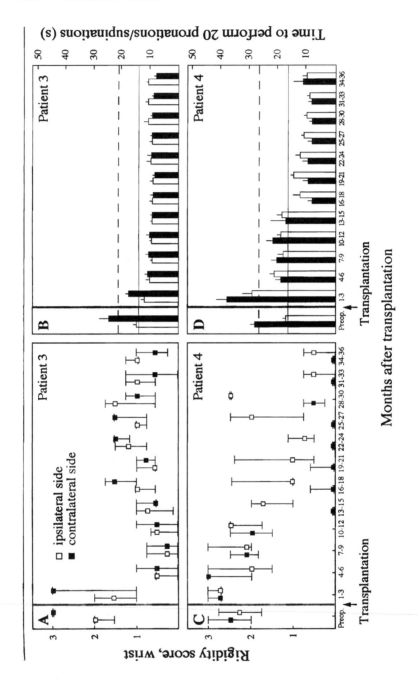

caudate and the opposite side of the brain), there was a continued decline in fluorodopa uptake, corresponding to ongoing degeneration. In the putamen that received grafts, the decline in fluorodopa uptake was prevented, and fluorodopa uptake was nearly normal both three and six years after transplantation. Although not in themselves entirely conclusive, these PET scan findings provide strong support for the idea that the functional improvements were related to physiological effects of the transplants.

A total of six patients with idiopathic Parkinson's disease received grafts using these improved procedures: patients 3 and 4, and four additional patients (numbered 7, 8, 9, and 10 in their series) who received

---

Figure 13.1

Effects of transplantation of fetal tissue in two patients with Parkinson's disease, from experiments by Lindvall and coworkers (1994). The graphs show results from patient 3 and patient 4. The graphs on the left show scores for wrist rigidity, and the graphs on the right show scores for time to perform 20 pronations/supinations (turning the hand palm up-palm down-palm up, etc.). For both measures, decreased scores represent improvements. Data are shown for three years after transplantation.

For patient 3, most of the improvement occurred within the first four months, with scores generally stable thereafter. There was somewhat more improvement on the contralateral side, where most of the improvement would be expected; note that the scores were worse on the contralateral side before transplantation, but after transplantation scores for both sides were similar. There was no indication of progressive deterioration in this patient, which might be expected over the course of three years in untreated Parkinson's disease.

Patient 4 showed a very interesting pattern of improvement that is quite distinct from most other patients with Parkinson's disease who have shown improvement after various kinds of transplants. There was no improvement in pronation/supination scores for the first three months, and little improvement for the first year (D). For rigidity scores, there also was no improvement for the first year (C). However, this patient did show decreases in "off" times of at least 50–60 percent beginning after four months; this is not shown. Starting one year after transplantation, this patient showed progressive improvements in both pronation/supination scores and rigidity. Particularly notable is that rigidity on the contralateral side improved markedly, to normal levels, starting one year after transplantation, and remained at normal levels through three years after transplantation. Of the six patients tested using similar methods, this patient showed the most striking overall pattern of long-term improvements (Wenning et al. 1997). (Reproduced from Lindvall et al. 1994 with permission.)

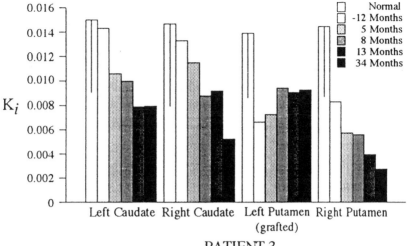

PATIENT 3

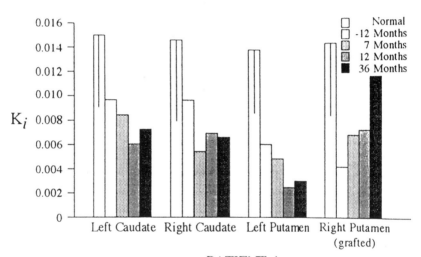

PATIENT 4

Figure 13.2
PET scanning results, showing measurements of [^{18}F]-fluorodopa uptake for patients 3 (top) and 4 (bottom) from Lindvall et al. (1994). Each group of five or
six bars indicates data from one brain region. The first bar in each group indicates
normal values (from other, normal subjects), and the remaining four or five bars
show fluorodopa uptake over the course of time (12 months before transplantation, and 5–36 months after transplantation). In most brain regions, a progressive
decline in fluorodopa uptake was seen. In patient 3, where the left putamen was
grafted, the fluorodopa uptake does not decline after 8 months, and actually
shows a small increase. In the right putamen of patient 4, where fetal cells were
grafted, there is no progressive decline, and fluorodopa uptake actually recovers
to nearly normal values between 12 and 36 months after transplantation. (Courtesy of Lindvall et al. 1994, reproduced with permission.)

transplants between 1993 and 1994 (Wenning et al. 1997). Two of these patients experienced clinically significant improvement, while in two others only minor improvements were seen. All patients received grafts on one side of the brain only. Overall, there were dramatic improvements in the response to L-DOPA, and moderate improvements in measures of motor function. The improvements in clinical state were generally stable and did not disappear from the first to the second year after transplantation. Perhaps the most consistent and remarkable indication that the grafts were physiologically functional is that PET scanning revealed increases in fluorodopa uptake in the grafted putamen, in contrast with a continued decline in the nongrafted putamen on the other side of the brain.

These data are very encouraging for clinical use of neural transplantation, in that the effects seen are consistent with the changes that might be expected from grafts that become physiologically integrated with host brain function. The clinical improvements were only partial, but only one side of the brain was grafted. The time course was extended, and improvements seen during the first year did not dissipate during the second. Thus, at least in this respect, the clinical changes were qualitatively different from those seen after adrenal medulla grafts and were probably not just reflections of brain injury or disruption. Further procedural refinements are thus likely to lead to clinically useful transplantation procedures.

MPTP-Induced Parkinsonism
Using similar methods, transplantation was performed in two additional patients who were unique and quite interesting. These patients, rather than having Parkinson's disease per se (idiopathic Parkinson's disease, which means that the disease is of unknown cause), were severely affected with MPTP-induced parkinsonism, having taken MPTP that had been synthesized by amateur chemists in illicit attempts to produce a synthetic form of heroin (see chapter 8). Transplantation was performed on both sides of the brain.

In these patients, there was evidence for substantial improvement, some of which took place over a very long time. Overall, the improvement was rather dramatic, although mixed. One test of motor function was the pronation/supination test. This test indicated that improvement took place in one patient, whereas the second patient became worse (table 13.1). The most telling result, perhaps, was the test of walking ability, which would seem, logically, to be a good general indicator of Parkinson's disease motor disability. Both patients showed a rather marked improvement in walking from before to after transplantation. The walking test indicated that the improvement developed mainly subsequent to three months after surgery, with continued improvement for at least one year. The time required for each patient to walk 14 meters before and at various times after surgery is shown in table 13.2. Results from Parkinson's disease rating scales were roughly parallel to the results from the walking test: both patients showed marked improvement, with most of the improvement developing between six months and two years after the transplantation surgery.

Table 13.1
Pronation/supination test (number of wrist turns in 30 sec; average of right and left hands during "off" state)

	Before Transplantation	1–3 Months	4–6 Months	7–9 Months	10–12 Months	22–24 Months
Patient #1 (#5 in series)	6	2	5	6	14	25
Patient #2 (#6 in series)	23	42	25	19	15	14

From Widner et al. 1992.

Table 13.2
Time required to walk 14 meters (during "off" state), with one turn

	Before Transplantation	1–3 Months	4–6 Months	7–9 Months	10–12 Months	22–24 Months
Patient #1 (#5 in series)	44 sec	38 sec	32 sec	31 sec	33 sec	18 sec
Patient #2 (#6 in series)	30 sec	23 sec	18 sec	19 sec	13 sec	13 sec

From Widner et al. 1992.

In patients with MPTP-induced parkinsonism, there are several ways in which interpretation of the results is simpler than with idiopathic Parkinson's disease. Especially, the onset and cause of the disease are defined, and they took place at a known time point. Thus, there was no question about whether the disease might be progressing—that is, becoming more severe—while the grafts were developing. Also, there is no concern about the presence of some unknown agent that killed the patient's own dopaminergic neurons in the first place, and that might kill the transplanted dopaminergic neurons as well.

Denver, Colorado

The clinical studies by C. R. Freed and coworkers were among the first, and are quite extensive. New methods have been developed for these experiments as well. A "blind" controlled study, which has some controversial aspects, has been funded by the National Institutes of Health. The last patient in this controlled study received surgery in January 1998; the study was completed in February 1999 and initial results were presented in April of 1999 (C. R. Freed et al. 1999). Although the patients will continue to be followed after that point for as long as possible, the blind part of the study was finished in January 1999 (C. R. Freed, personal communication, October 1998). This research program is likely to form a significant part of the basis for future decisions about clinical use of neural transplantation, and these studies will, therefore, be described in some detail.

For most of the patients, the technique employed involves extrusion of long, thin "noodles" of tissue by pressing the tissue out of a syringe (figure 13.3). The initial patient studied by C. R. Freed and associates (1990), however, received transplants of dissociated cells.

Fetuses of seven to eight weeks' gestational age, which is within the range for probable good survival of dopaminergic neurons, were used for all cases. Compared with the studies by Lindvall and coworkers, C. R. Freed and coworkers have relied upon distribution of a limited amount of tissue to a larger number of sites within the striatum, instead of increasing the number of fetuses and amount of tissue used. Thus, relative to

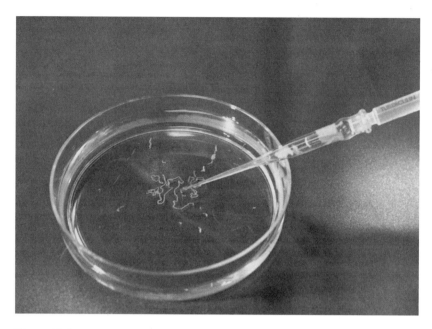

Figure 13.3
Illustration of the preparation of "noodles" of fetal brain tissue employed for human transplantation in the studies by Curt Freed and coworkers. (From C. R. Freed et al. 1991, with permission.)

the approach of Lindvall and coworkers, Freed has used fewer fetuses (recently, as many as four) but focused on delivery and distribution.

As in the studies of Lindvall et al., C. R. Freed has attempted to employ smaller needles for injection of tissue into the brain. Larger needles were employed initially to prevent deflection of the needle when it was inserted into the brain. Later experiments employed smaller or tapered needles, with larger-diameter sections above the transplantation area and the part entering the brain smaller in diameter. The needle used in Freed's initial study in 1988 was 1.5 mm in diameter, whereas the needle used in his later experiments was only 0.6 mm diameter, with a larger sleeve used for stiffening.

In 1992, C. R. Freed and coworkers reported detailed results of transplantation in seven patients with Parkinson's disease. These studies are particularly noteworthy for the comprehensive nature of the assessment.

Improvements were seen in six of the seven patients according to a number of different measurements. Each patient was assessed repeatedly, using videotapings made in their homes. Improvements in facial expression, postural control, gait, and bradykinesia occurred in each of the five patients who received bilateral implants into the putamen. The first subject to receive a transplant developed considerable improvements at long time periods after transplantation, including a particularly notable improvement in walking speed starting one year after transplantation (figure 13.4); see discussion below.

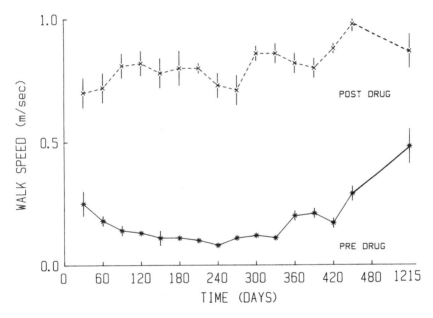

Figure 13.4
Long-term improvement in a patient with Parkinson's disease who received a transplant of dopaminergic neurons. The patient was equipped with a photocell-based apparatus that allowed him to test his walking speed at home. The graph shows walking speed both before and after drug treatment; larger numbers represent improvement. Walking speed continued to become slower for one year after transplantation, perhaps representing continued progression of the disease. Beginning at one year, however, progressive and dramatic improvements in walking speed began to emerge. It is not likely that these improvements were related to practice, since people normally walk, and any practice effect would probably develop before one year. (From C. R. Freed et al. 1992, with permission.)

This first patient received the dissociated cells rather than "noodles," implanted in the right caudate nucleus and putamen only. This surgery, the first performed in the United States, was done in November 1988. This patient showed some improvements during the first 9–15 months after the operation, including improvements in functions of the hands, with more improvement in the left side, opposite the transplant.

Walking speed was measured, during both "on" and "off" phases, using an automated apparatus in the patient's home. During the first year after the operation, walking speed did not improve. But when studied over a longer period, it started to show improvements, beginning about one year after transplantation and continuing up to 40 months (figure 13.4). By several measures, continued improvement developed in this patient from one to three years after transplantation. This first patient continued to improve for about four years after transplantation, with some of the improvement slowly disappearing from four to six years following transplantation. Fluorodopa PET scanning, which was done at 9 and again at 33 months, indicated that the graft continued to develop. This observation is consistent with the possibility that the transplant continued to become integrated with the host brain over an extended period of time, and to produce corresponding improvements in behavior.

The first seven patients were evaluated by the Activities of Daily Living Scale, which rates general functional capacity on a 0 to 52 scale, where 52 represents a complete absence of the ability to carry out daily activities (e.g., getting dressed and eating), and 0 represents completely normal function. Six of the seven patients were evaluated according to this scale. They showed an overall improvement in these scores during both "on" and "off" phases, with most of the improvement taking place during the three months after surgery and some additional improvement occurring between three and six months. These patients were studied for an extended period of time, and in general the maximal improvements were seen two to four years after transplantation (C. R. Freed et al. 1998).

A unique aspect of the clinical studies by C. R. Freed is that immunosuppression, consisting of cyclosporine A treatment, was used in alternating patients. Freed has felt that that immunosuppression should not be used automatically, because immunosuppressive treatment itself causes risks, and that there is no direct evidence that immunosuppression would be required for a single operation. At present, 8 of his patients have been immunosuppressed and 15 have not. No apparent benefit of immunosuppression has been seen, and five of the eight immunosuppressed patients did not improve.

Several problems have occurred. One patient died following a stroke that occurred during surgery; this patient turned out to have striatonigral degeneration rather than Parkinson's disease. Distributing tissue by implanting grafts into a large number of sites increases the risk of damaging a blood vessel with the implantation needle. To minimize this risk, Freed and coworkers now transplant by inserting the needles through the forehead rather than the top of the head. This permits tissue to be transplanted into the same number of sites with only 4 needle passes rather than the 16 previously used. Another patient died of hemorrhage 30 days after transplantation. Two patients with cognitive difficulties became much worse after transplantation: one of them had impaired memory, and the second had dementia and delusions, after transplantation. Thus, any patient with a cognitive abnormality is now excluded from consideration for receiving a brain graft in this study.

C. R. Freed has undoubtedly been one of the most controversial figures in brain tissue transplantation research. He has had a tendency to proceed in a manner that engenders controversy; for example, he performed the first clinical trial of neural transplantation in the United States in 1988, initiating his study during the fetal tissue research ban by using private funding while the Panel on Fetal Tissue Guidelines was still deliberating. There were some who felt that he should have awaited the recommendations of this panel before beginning. Subsequently, others (such as myself) were concerned about the absence of immunosuppression use with his first patients (C. R. Freed et al. 1991), although this does not seem to have led to any problems. Also, the use of sham surgery has aroused a great deal of controversy. Of course, there are two sides to each of these issues.

There are many positive aspects to Freed's studies, including the very thorough clinical assessments, the use of very frequent in-home clinical testing, the use of early gestational donors (which is almost certainly important for success), and the development of novel techniques for transplantation.

Denver/New York Collaborative Study

The improvements seen in the studies by C. R. Freed and his associates led to the initiation of a larger, controlled trial funded by the National Institutes of Health. Certainly, the improvements that were reported are significant enough that additional study is justified. Several aspects of this new proposed study, however, are quite controversial.

When complete, the study will include 40 patients, 20 of whom will receive fetal ventral mesencephalic tissue, and 20 who will receive control surgery. The control surgery will consist of skull drilling only, without implantation of tissue. Half of the patients in each group will be under 50 years of age, and the other half will be older than 50. Once selected for the study, patients will undergo evaluation, then be assigned to receive either a transplant or sham surgery strictly at random. The experiment and all of the details about assignment of patients to treatment groups have been planned very carefully, so that neither the patients nor those doing the ratings know whether any particular patient is to receive a transplant or is a control. Even the surgeons will not know which treatment the patient is to receive until after the patient is anesthetized and prepared for surgery, the actual time for the start of the transplantation procedure. The surgery, of whichever type, will then be completed, using methods essentially like those used in the previous studies by C. R. Freed and coworkers. The patients will be extensively evaluated following surgery, but no one involved in the evaluation, including the patients, will know whether or not they received a transplant. The evaluation will be carried out for one year, after which the patients will be informed whether they received sham or active transplants. At that time, the sham patients will be given the option of receiving active transplants. Of course, this unique and quite remarkable procedure has aroused a great deal of controversy.

A number of objections to this study have been raised by several individuals. Some of them were discussed in a letter published in *Science* (Widner 1994) and an article published in *Science* the preceding week (Cohen 1994). Foremost among these objections is the complaint that the particular approach used by C. R. Freed and his colleagues may not be the best one, and if the trial does not work, the entire field will be tainted or, at least, will receive less attention. As quoted by J. Cohen (1994, 600), John Sladek said, "We legitimize fetal tissue transplants by getting a new president in the White House, and then we put all our eggs in one basket. We're worried about what will happen if that basket falls apart." Widner (1994) also expressed concerns about excessive concentration on a single approach.

This, although it is a—sort of—strategic (rather than an ethical) issue, is a legitimate concern. It is especially so if phrased with a slightly different emphasis, related to the topic discussed in the section "Studies from Lund, Sweden" in this chapter. Has this particular approach been sufficiently developed to warrant spending the amount of money and resources that it will cost? As discussed earlier, postmortem data have become available that suggest the methods being used for the study at the University of South Florida are highly effective. Also, there are potential approaches involving coadministration of growth factors or cotransplantation with peripheral nerve cells, for example. Will one of these come along in the next year or two, and render the study obsolete shortly after it is finished? I don't know the answer; at some point, one must start. A collective decision has been made, by C. R. Freed and the National Institutes of Health, to start now.

An additional objection is the opinion that sham surgery is unethical in any circumstance. To perform sham surgery, including opening the skull, exposes the patients to some of the risk of surgery without the potential benefits that may be imparted by transplants. Furthermore, if—for example—the control patients elect to not receive transplants, they would then have been subjected to the surgery and would not receive any possible associated benefits. On the other side of this issue, however, is the point that if we do not perform sham surgery, how will we *ever* know whether or not the procedure is working? If we continue on indefinitely without initiating controlled studies, in the long run a great many more patients may be subjected to transplantation even if it does not work. Is it better to subject an aggregate 200 or even 2,000 patients to a possibly ineffective procedure, not knowing it to be ineffective, or to perform sham surgery in 20? Further, if positive benefits are not found using this relatively "lenient" experimental design (i.e., effects related to nonspecific tissue injury could produce positive results), then transplantion is almost certainly not producing a meaningful clinical improvement. Thus, there are good arguments in favor of conducting a controlled study. Certainly it would be valuable if, indeed, it would answer the question of whether transplants "really" work. Unfortunately, this study might not provide definitive answers.

Personally, I do have a number of concerns about this study, but mostly not for the reasons that have so far been expressed. First of all, no study of comparable sophistication has been performed in subhuman primates. It does not seem to me that it makes sense to perform a large-scale, double-blind controlled study in humans when no comparable study has been performed in primates. Ideally, I would have opted instead for spending the money to perform a large-scale controlled study in subhuman primates, using exactly the methods proposed for use in humans. The feasibility of such a study has been demonstrated (Taylor et al. 1995).

A second (and very serious) problem is that skull drilling is not an ideal control procedure. Skull drilling will turn out to be a good control procedure if the results of the study are negative. Of course, it allows for improved blinding of the observer. However, the limitation of studies of neural transplantation is mainly, in my opinion, that nonspecific effects may occur. There is a consensus that some improvement is seen, with a specific time course. I do not believe that these observations are entirely spurious, or related to the expectations of patients and staff or to the testing itself. It is also improbable that these nonspecific effects are related to skull drilling. Thus, if the results of this study are positive, we won't know much more than we do now—except that the clinical improvements seen after neural transplantation are not due to skull drilling. However, as far as control groups are concerned, it's probably the best that can be done.

The danger is that the study will be over-interpreted: If the results of the study are positive, which is more than likely, the improvements seen could still be related to implantation of tissue into the brain and associated cellular reactions, disruption of the blood-brain barrier, or nonspecific cellular damage. Such effects could not be discriminated by this clinical trial, and of course a controlled study in humans in which cellular damage in the brain was intentionally produced in the control group would certainly be unethical.

Another problem is that the period of active study is too short. I think it is quite likely that the "real" effects of neural transplantation (i.e., effects that are not just by brain injury, etc.) begin to appear only after one year. It seems that transplantation of tissues, including adrenal medulla and fetal brain tissue, into the brain by means of several methods all produce fairly similar improvements for a few months. The time course of this improvement is generally from three to six months after surgery. Perhaps the effects of adrenal medulla transplants are related to nonspecific injury, and those of fetal dopaminergic neurons are more physiological, but we can't be sure of this. Since the control group will be maintained for only one year, specific changes that take place after longer intervals will not be detected. In other words, improvements in the transplanted patients that occur after one year cannot be evaluated by comparison with the control group. The patients will continue to be followed for as long as possible, but the controlled part of the study lasts for only one year.

Finally, a controversy related to financing has arisen. The *New York Times* reported that patients have paid up to $40,000 for transplantation surgery. The motivation for personally paying the costs for receiving fetal tissue is, presumably, to avoid the 50 percent probability of receiving sham surgery. In an article in the *New York Times* on February 8, 1994, it was stated that patients could avoid the 50 percent possibility of receiving sham surgery by paying the $40,000 cost of the operation, and being part of C. R. Freed's "private" study. However, this is not strictly accurate, in that the sham-operated patients will get the option of receiving transplant surgery at the end of the one-year period, or waiting until the end of the entire trial to receive surgery, and will receive the transplantation surgery at no personal cost at that time. Moreover, the sham subjects have priority in receiving transplants at the completion of the study. This aspect of the trial would definitely *not* seem to present any potential conflict of interest. Especially since the controls can choose to wait until they find out whether the surgery worked before receiving transplatation, they perhaps have the best option of all!

At the time of the writing of this book, all of the patients in the study have received surgery, and preliminary results have been presented (C. R. Freed et al. 1999). The results were generally positive. The patients who received active transplants showed greater improvements than the controls by some measures; the groups were significantly different by more objective measures of outcome (e.g., clinical ratings and objective tests). The subjective outcome measures gave less clear results; that is, the placebo patients also believed that they were doing much better. Patients older than 60 years as a group did not show significant improvement. Improvement continued after 12 months, when the "blind" was broken. Thus, the results are quite encouraging, although it is still possible that some of the clinical changes are related to nonspecific effects of tissue implantation. This study is therefore useful, but it does not provide a definitive answer as to whether the effects of the grafts are specific, and physiological, or related to tissue injury. Thus, again, this study should not be over-interpreted.

Mexico City (Madrazo and Coworkers)

This study is unique in that tissue was transplanted into the wall of the ventricle, using methods similar to those that had been used by this group for transplantation of adrenal medulla. Like several other studies, this one has the deficiency of having used grafts from relatively mature donors, 12 to 14 weeks' gestation. Although there has not yet been postmortem verification, it is within the realm of possibility that the mode of transplantation, to the wall of the lateral ventricle, promoted survival of relatively mature dopaminergic neurons. Almost certainly, even with this possible advantage, 12 to 14 weeks of gestation is too mature for survival of dopaminergic neurons. There were four patients in the study, aged 45 to 52. Rating of the patients by the Unified Parkinson's Disease Rating Scale in the "off" state suggested that there was an improvement of about 50 percent during the first eight months after transplantation, and that this improvement remained stable as long as the patients were followed, for 19 to 32 months (Madrazo, Franco-Bourland, Aquilera, Ostrosky-Solis, Madrazo, et al. 1991). Assuming that dopaminergic neurons mainly did not survive in this study, we should be cautious about interpreting improvements seen in other studies.

Havana, Cuba

A large number of patients have been studied by this group. The 30 patients included in a report published by Molina and coworkers in 1991 received transplants between January 1988 and April 1990.

Tissue donors were aged 6 to 12 weeks of gestation. Methods of transplantation involved an open microsurgical approach to the lateral ventricle with implantation of solid tissue fragments, similar to the methods used by Madrazo and coworkers. The procedure was performed quite rapidly, so that the average time from abortion to tissue implantation was between 25 and 70 minutes (average = 45 min), which would be a favorable factor for graft survival. The use of solid tissue fragments allows for the use of slightly more mature donor tissue, so that it is possible, or even likely, that dopaminergic neurons survived transplantation in some cases.

There was a substantial overall improvement in these patients, which was generally similar whether evaluated by rating scales or by tests for motor function, activities of daily living, hypokinesia, rigidity, posture, and tremor. Generally slight, and in some cases significant, improvement was seen after two weeks, with continued improvement up to six months. From six months up to two years after transplantation, no further improvement was observed. Improvements during both "on" and "off" phases were seen, although somewhat larger improvements were seen during the "off" phases, so that after six months the differences between the "on" and "off" phases were markedly diminished.

The studies from Cuba have received somewhat less attention in the United States than have the American and Swedish studies, to a large extent because details of procedures and results have not been communicated as extensively or in sources that are readily accessible to American scientists or the general public. From the information available, the studies seem to have been fairly systematic. There are several pieces of information that could add to the value of these studies, including procedural details and information on the exact age of fetal tissue used for each case. Results of quantitative tests, such as the pronation/supination test, which have not yet been published, could assist in comparing results of these experiments with those of other studies.

Birmingham, England

This group was one of the first to report on effects of fetal transplants in humans (Hitchcock et al. 1988), in a letter published in the *Lancet*. Details of the study were later published by Henderson et al. in 1991. Ventral mesencephalon from fetuses of 11 to 19 weeks' gestational age was used. The tissue was partially dispersed mechanically; that is, it was not dissociated into individual cells, but agitated to form clumps of cells that could be injected through a syringe. This dispersed tissue, in a volume of between 0.5 and 2.0 ml, was stereotaxically injected into the right caudate nucleus using a plastic syringe and needle. Because of the relatively crude technique used for tissue preparation and transplantation, the large volumes of material injected, and the relatively mature state of the donor tissue, it is thought that few transplanted neurons are likely to have survived. Transplants were made into the right side only. The procedure was performed under local anesthesia. This program has not been continued since Dr. Hitchcock died in 1992.

Histochemical examination of postmortem brain samples from some of the patients who have died, by K. Bankiewicz (published as Hitchcock et al. 1994), suggested that a few cells containing the tyrosine hydroxylase enzyme (TH) characteristic of dopaminergic neurons, as well as a number of cells that were positive for neuromelanin (a marker of substantia nigra pars compacta neurons), were in fact present in the area of the transplants. Nevertheless, these cells stained weakly for TH, and were not well differentiated, having formed few or no processes that reafferented the host brain (figure 13.5). Thus, notwithstanding the presence of a few TH-containing cells, it does not appear likely that the improvements seen in these patients were related to the development of a new dopaminergic afferentation of the brain. The presence of melanin at relatively short intervals after transplantation is perhaps also an indicator that the cells were aging at an accelerated rate, since melanin is normally present in human dopaminergic neurons, but not until at least several years of age. It was also noted in the histochemical studies that there were fairly substantial cavities in the striatum, apparently produced by the mechanical stress of injection of large volumes of tissue.

In view of the probable brain injury produced by transplantation and the probable lack of graft survival, this study makes an interesting comparison with others. What were the effects of these grafts on the patients? Although the rating scales and measurement methods used by this group unfortunately were not the same as those used by other groups, there were enough similarities to allow for several comparisons. First, most of the improvements were seen over the course of three to six months following transplantation. The magnitude of the improvement, on the Northwestern University Disability Scale and the Webster Rating Scale, were about 25 percent to 35 percent in the "off" state, and 22 percent to 28 percent in the "on" state, although comparisons between different scales are not very useful.

Most telling was the time required to perform 20 pronation/supinations with the hands, which improved over three to six months (figure 13.6). The percentage improvement in the pronation/supination test was about 36 percent for the left side and 18 percent for the right side after six months (mean of six patients). Since the transplants were made only on the right side, the improvement on the left side is the more relevant. The maximum improvement on this test was seen at 6 months, with a slightly poorer performance after 12 months. This is quite similar to the improvements observed by Lindvall and coworkers (1992), for example, during the first year. For the Lindvall et al. study, the first patient (patient 3 in their overall series) improved on this test by 54 percent for the right side and 29 percent for the left side at six months. Patient 4 became worse by 35 percent for the right side and improved by 15 percent for the left side. In the second of the two MPTP patients studied by Widner and coworkers (1992), there was also a similar improvement in pronation/supination during the first year, whereas the first patient did not improve until after one year.

Few transplanted dopaminergic neurons are likely to have survived in the Hitchcock et al. study. This again leads one to the almost inescapable conclusions that (1) a similar improvement occurs up to the first

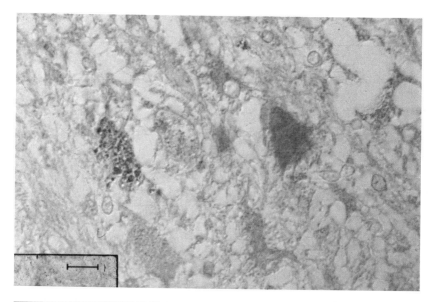

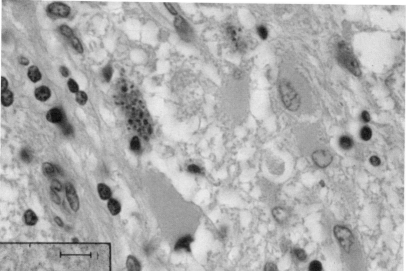

Figure 13.5
A histochemical examination of brain from patients who received grafts in the study by Henderson and coworkers (1991), clinical results of which are shown in figure 13.6. These brains showed evidence for survival of only a few poorly developed dopaminergic neurons, and most of these neurons contained neuromelanin. The upper panel shows a cell weakly positive for tyrosine hydroxylase. The dark particles in the lower panel are neuromelanin from the same patient. Neuromelanin would not normally be expected to accumulate in dopamine neurons of this age, indicating probable accelerated aging and deterioration of the transplanted cells. (Photographs courtesy of K. Bankiewicz, National Institutes of Health.)

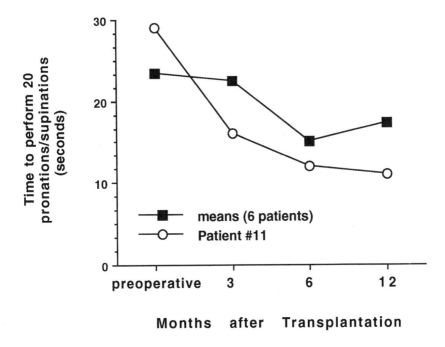

Figure 13.6
Effects of transplantation of fetal tissue on tests of pronation/supination, from studies by Henderson, Hitchcock, and coworkers (data from Henderson et al. 1991). Improvements were observed even though the grafts in these patients were performed under conditions that do not lead to substantial survival of transplanted dopamine neurons. The most probable explanation for these improvements is that slight brain injury, and effects related to the glial reaction of the brain to the implantation of cells, can lead to some functional improvement. The data shown are times to perform 20 pronations/supinations with the left hand (transplants were made on the right side), so that decreases indicate improvement. The black squares indicate the means for the last six patients tested, and the white circles indicate the results for patient 11, who showed the best response.

year, at least by some measures, regardless of the tissue or transplantation technique that is used, and (2) this early improvement is unlikely to be related to physiological function of the transplanted neurons; rather, it is probably related to host brain trauma. This is a very pessimistic view, I will admit, but again, we should be very cautious about overinterpreting improvements, especially those seen during the first year after transplantation.

In this study, fetal brain tissue was removed from relatively mature fetal donors, dispersed, and injected into the brain with relatively large volumes of culture media. As in the other clinical studies, the tissue used for transplantation contains many types of cells other than dopaminergic neurons, and the dopaminergic neurons in a dissected tissue such as was used would not comprise more than about 2 percent of the total cell population. Various experiments by this group showed that some viable cells, of undetermined nature (probably glia), are present in the preparations that were used. Living cells probably were implanted, but were likely to have been mostly glial cells and perhaps other kinds of neurons. The specific procedure used by this group was not tested in animals in any systematic manner.

Warsaw, Poland

Although this study included only a few patients, and they received tissue that was somewhat more mature than optimal, the study is of interest mainly because of the unique methods used (Zabek et al. 1994). Essentially, a device that permitted fragments of tissue to be inserted into the wall of the lateral ventricle stereotaxically, without a requirement for open surgery, was developed. The net result was the implantation of tissue into the caudate nucleus, penetrating through the ventricular ependyma and in contact with cerebrospinal fluid, similar to the procedure developed by Madrazo and coworkers in Mexico City. There is, however, no evidence from animal studies that such a procedure would be more effective than comparable methods—or, in fact, that it would work at all.

The tissue used for transplantation was obtained from 11–12 week gestational donors, which is too mature for survival of dopaminergic neurons. Consistent with this notion, the first patient to receive a transplant died after four months. The death was not related to the surgery (the patient died from choking). The graft was in generally good condition and contained surviving neurons, but no dopaminergic neurons were present.

Three patients received transplants, and results were reported for up to 12–30 months for them. Substantial improvements were seen in each patient. The time course of improvement was such that initial improvements were seen at three months and additional improvement was present after six months. In the first patient, no changes were seen from 6 to 30 months after transplantation. In the other two patients, some additional improvements were seen between 6 and 12 months. There was little evidence that additional improvements took place beyond one year.

This carefully conducted study would have been more interesting were it not for the fact that the donor fetuses were too mature to expect good tissue survival. If this identical study had been performed with eight-week-old fetal tissue, we would probably conclude that the improvements seen were related to integration of the grafts with the host brain. Since the improvements were quite substantial anyway, we should be suspicious of similar improvements in all studies, even when the conditions are optimal for the survival of dopaminergic neurons. Still, there is a possibility that a few surviving dopaminergic neurons were present in these grafts, since conditions were similar to or better than in the Birmingham studies. The human brain with Parkinson's disease might favor neuronal survival more than animal or tissue culture conditions, although this seems improbable at present.

Burlington, Massachusetts, Studies with Pig Donor Tissue

One study that is currently in progress, in the form of an open (nonblind) safety trial approved by the Food and Drug Administration, involves transplantation of fetal pig neurons into human patients. If it were possible to employ fetal pig neurons in place of human tissue, the development of a human clinical procedure might, perhaps, be greatly facilitated. This possibility was originally suggested by Freeman and coworkers in 1988. In addition to avoiding the requirement for obtaining primary human tissue obtained through abortions, the use of pig donors would allow for thorough screening of the animals, maintenance of the animals under controlled conditions, and breeding timed to obtain tissue exactly when desired.

The principal problem, of course, is that donor tissue from pigs might be rejected by the human immune system. Grafts from different species (xenografts) are more vigorously rejected than grafts within the same species (allografts), and grafts from pig to human are between widely disparate species, a situation that might be expected to result in a vigorous immune response. Even in the brain, grafts between widely separated species (e.g., from rabbit to rat) are more rapidly and completely rejected than grafts between related species (mouse to rat) (Dymecki et al. 1990).

As we have discussed previously, grafts within the brain are somewhat less likely to be rejected than grafts elsewhere, and brain tissue grafts are probably somewhat less immunogenic than other tissues. Since a drug that is quite effective in preventing graft rejection (cyclosporine) is available, transplantation of pig neurons into the human brain has been considered acceptable, using cyclosporine immunosuppression. This is not entirely unreasonable—recall that there is some debate concerning whether cyclosporine is needed at all for allografts, and continuous use of immunosuppression by cyclosporine for human allografts is probably somewhat overkill. It is likely, therefore, that pig transplants would survive in human patients immunosuppressed by cyclosporine. Discontinuation of cyclosporine treatment after six months, as has been done for human donor tissue, probably could not be done with pig-to-human grafts.

So far, twelve patients have received the procedure (Deacon et al. 1997), without untoward problems. A single patient died 12 months after transplantation, and the brain was examined. Pig neurons and glial cells were found, fibers had extended from the graft into the human host brain, and the graft was in generally good condition.

A second controversy has arisen regarding the possible transmission of pig retroviruses to humans through this procedure (Schumacher et al. 1997). The genomes of all mammalian species contain occult viral genomes, which usually remain dormant and do not become activated, but conceivably could give rise to complete and infectious viruses under unusual conditions (i.e., after being transplanted to a different species). There is no evidence that this has occurred, but it is certainly a theoretical possibility that should be considered and monitored.

Despite the somewhat daunting problems of immune reactions and the potential for viral transmission, in the long-term the use of fetal pig neurons for transplantation is a very attractive possibility. The logistics of the procedure—being able to obtain tissue from thoroughly characterized animals precisely when needed—is very attractive. Eventually, it should be possible to produce pigs with decreased immunogenicity for human transplantation, either through genetic engineering or simply by selective breeding. Proviral genomes can be detected, and ultimately any problematic viral sequences could perhaps be eliminated, disabled, or simply monitored to assure that they are not reactivated. It may be many years before these improvements are accomplished, but certainly a therapeutic procedure that depends upon elective abortions—as neural transplantation for Parkinson's disease would otherwise do—is not likely to be used for large numbers of subjects. The use of pig tissue is a very attractive means of overcoming this limitation.

Conclusions

Before talking about anything else, I should emphasize that there is still a lingering doubt about the nature of the clinical improvements seen in human patients. Remember that grafts are quite effective in decreasing rotational behavior in rats, but much less effective when more complex tests, which measure functions such as skilled motor coordination, are used. In fact, it often seems that the more the behavioral test truly measures deficits in coordinated motor function, the less likely it is to show that improvements are produced by transplants. Often, no effects of transplants of dopaminergic neurons are found with these tests. This may reflect the limited degree to which transplanted dopaminergic neurons reconstruct host brain circuits. Also, although there has been one quite thorough controlled primate study, it is the only such study, and the number of animals in that study was fairly small. Another one or two double-blind, controlled experiments in primates could help a great deal. In light of this, when the clinical changes seen in humans are examined carefully, they are suspiciously similar to effects of adrenal medulla grafts in humans, which are probably doing little more than stimulating a reaction of the host brain to injury—or some such change far less interesting than restoring dopaminergic input to striatal neurons.

Long-term improvement, after one year, has been seen in some human patients, and this effect is likely to represent bona fide function of the transplanted cells. But, as of the writing of this book, the evidence is still very thin. The demonstrated survival of grafts in some of the human patients is encouraging, but we should not be misled into thinking that the clinical improvement must be real because the grafts survived; these are two quite different things. In fact, some improvement has been observed in one patient who received a fetal tissue graft that was found on autopsy to contain no neural tissue (Folkerth and Durso 1996). "Controlled" clinical studies that have recently been completed (C. R. Freed et al. 1999) are not likely to resolve the issue, because they employ only low-level control procedures (see table 5.1)—of course, the more sophisticated control procedures cannot be used in human subjects.

Therefore, in considering transplants for Parkinson's disease in humans, we have to realize that some or all of the clinical work has probably been premature. It is, perhaps, surprising that primates have played a relatively minor role in the development of the procedures that have been used in humans. Although some clinical programs have used primates to develop viable surgical procedures, this has been far from universal. Although the principles of neural transplantation were developed mainly in rat models, there are many details regarding surgery and methodology that could have been perfected in subhuman primates to a much greater extent than has been done. There is no case in which a controlled study in primates has preceded a comparable study in humans. There has, in fact, been only one extensive controlled study in subhuman primates (Taylor et al. 1995), and most of the procedures currently being used in humans differ from those used in that study to varying degrees. One must wonder whether—or, from my own experience, I would say that certainly—the increasing expense and regulatory restrictions regarding animal research in general, and primate research in particular, have made it easier and less expensive to proceed directly to human subjects. This is certainly unfortunate.

Let's forget about all the above concerns for a moment; perhaps we should hope for the best. Whenever a clinical trial is initiated using a new procedure, there will always be some degree of uncertainty. If we were to wait until we were as certain as humanly possible, clinical trials of fetal tissue transplantation in Parkinson's disease would probably not have been started yet. A conservative research program to prepare for human transplantation trials might involve a controlled, blind trial in perhaps 40 monkeys (similar to the study by Taylor et al. 1995), using procedures matched to those planned for human use to as great a degree as possible. Additional issues that might be worked out more thoroughly in animals would be the requirement for immunosuppression and the number of fetuses and distribution of tissue that are needed. Although these issues were explored in rats to some extent, they were not entirely worked out in animals (which would have required subhuman primate studies) before human trials were initiated. To some extent, they are not entirely worked out even now. We can reasonably ask two questions, therefore, about the clinical studies to date: (1) Are we farther along in the development of a clinical procedure by virtue of the patients who have already been transplanted? (2) Have the patients themselves benefited from the surgery, in aggregate?

To address the first issue, we certainly are farther along in the development of an effective human procedure than would be the case if no transplants had yet been done. The experience that has been gained from now hundreds of human procedures has helped to improve the methodology. Interest in the topic has also been engendered by human studies. Moreover, autopsies have provided a great deal of information that could not have been obtained by any other means. Unfortunately, in at least two cases, autopsies have revealed apparent errors in tissue preparation, resulting in inclusion of nonneural tissues in the grafts (Folkerth and Durso 1996; Mamelak et al. 1998). The positive experience has, however, been obtained from the more carefully planned trials only. Studies that have—for example—used tissue that is too mature for dopaminergic neurons to have survived have provided us with little useful information. The human studies conducted under conditions where the grafts do not survive can be used for comparison with the better studies, but this certainly is not worthwhile for the patients, and the studies are usually too dissimilar to make meaningful comparisons (except that there always seems to be improvement, so we ought to be cautious).

It seems likely that at least some of the patients are better off. This is, of course, difficult to evaluate. Patients have died as a consequence of transplantation surgery. Other patients who have died, including those for whom the most important autopsy data were obtained (Kordower et al. 1995), died of causes unrelated to the transplantation surgery. Many patients have shown improvement, sometimes substantial and lasting for years. The negative side effects of fetal substantia nigra transplantation have been minimal. There also are many patients subjected to transplantation procedures that could not have produced viable grafts, and for these patients we would have to assume that the improvements experienced were probably not worthwhile.

If we (meaning the overall scientific community) could have done a little bit better in terms of planning and choosing the most carefully thought-out transplantation programs, the results would probably be considerably better. In contrast, the results of adrenal medulla transplantation in human patients were much less positive. Although improvements were seen, there were more deaths and serious side effects (including psychological and psychiatric disturbances), and the improvements were short-lived, mostly disappearing by one year. The clinical consensus seems to have been that the adrenal medulla transplantation procedure was not worthwhile.

The situation seems to be quite different for transplantation of fetal substantia nigra. For the first patients, as individuals, and for those subjected to less-than-ideal procedures, transplantation was probably not worthwhile. Thus, the inescapable conclusion is that a significant number of human patients have been subjected to experimental procedures that have had little chance of success because of poor planning or insufficient animal experimentation. With some reservations, I would say that for patients who now are receiving transplants using state-of-the-art procedures, the benefits probably outweigh the risk. At this point, however, the procedure is still experimental, and more definitive conclusions will probably be possible within a few years.

Further Reading

Freed, W. J. (1991). Substantia nigra grafts and Parkinson's disease: From animal experiments to human therapeutic trials. *Rest. Neurol. Neurosci.* 3: 109–134.

Freed, W. J. (1993). Neural transplantation: Prospects for clinical use. *Cell Transplant.* 2: 13–31.

Garry, D. J., Caplan, A. L., Vawter, D. E., and Kearney, W. (1992). Are there really alternatives to the use of fetal tissue from elective abortions in transplantation research? *N. Eng. J. Med.* 327: 1592–1595.

Kassirer, J. P., Angell, M. (1992). The use of fetal tissue in research on Parkinson's disease. *N. Eng. J. Med.* 327: 1591–1592.

Kolata, G. (1994). Parkinson patients set for first rigorous test of fetal cell implants. *New York Times,* February 8, p. C-3.

Lindvall, O. (1994). Neural Transplantation in Parkinson's disease. In *Functional Neural Transplantation,* S. B. Dunnett and A. Bjorklund (eds.), pp. 103–137. Raven Press, New York.

Olanow, C. W., Kordower J. H., and Freeman, T. B. (1996). Fetal nigral transplantation as a therapy for Parkinson's disease. *Trends Neurosci.* 19: 102–109.

Tivol, M. (1993). Experiment in hope. *Washington Post Magazine,* October 17, pp. 16–43. This is an interesting relation of the experience of receiving a fetal transplant at Yale University by a woman with Parkinson's disease.

IV

Using Transplants to Influence Localized Brain Functions

14

Pain

The adrenal medulla was initially employed as an alternative tissue source for transplantation in Parkinson's disease models, simply because adrenal chromaffin cells secrete catecholamines and have some neuronlike properties. As discussed in chapter 11, it was thought that adrenal chromaffin cells might thus be capable of substituting for fetal neurons from the substantia nigra as a transplantation source.

In addition to catecholamines, however, adrenal chromaffin cells also produce and release a number of peptide molecules, including the endogenous opiate peptides met-enkephalin and leu-enkephalin. Many neurons, and chromaffin cells as well, that release a classical neurotransmitter (e.g., catecholamines) also release a peptide as a cotransmitter. This observation led to the development of adrenal medulla transplantation as a possible treatment for chronic pain by Sagen, Pappas, and coworkers.

What are "endogenous opioids"? It was discovered that opiate drugs, so called because they are derived from opium, exert their effects on the brain by binding to proteins on the surface of cells called opiate receptors. Then an obvious paradox developed: it seemed peculiar that the brain would contain a receptor molecule designed to interact with an artificial compound. The vast majority of individuals live their entire lives without being exposed to opiate drugs. Why should the brain be designed to interact with such compounds? Thus, a search for compounds normally present in the brain that interact with these receptors was undertaken, and the endogenous opioids were found as a result (see "Further Reading" at the end of this chapter for additional details).

Endogenous opioids comprise a series of peptides, 5 to 30 amino acids in length, that are produced in the brain by the processing of larger

Table 14.1
Endogenous opioid peptides

Precursor	Number of Amino Acids in Precursor	Some Opioid Peptide Products	Number of Amino Acids in Opioid Peptide	First Five Amino Acids in Opioid Peptide
Proopiomelanocortin (POMC)	267	β-endorphin	31	y g g f l
		γ-endorphin	17	y g g f l
		α-endorphin	16	y g g f l
Proenkephalin A	269	met-enkephalin##	5	y g g f m
		leu-enkephalin ##	5	y g g f l
		peptide E	25	y g g f m
Prodynorphin or Proenkephalin	256	β-neoendorphin	10	y g g f l
		Dynorphin A1-17	17	y g g f l
		Dynorphin B	13	y g g f l

y, tyrosine; g, glycine; f, phenylalanine; l, leucine; m, methionine.

precursor peptides (table 14.1). Although a large number of these opioid peptides exist, met-enkephalin and leu-enkephalin appear to be the most widespread and important in brain and spinal cord function. Opioid peptides are widespread in the brain, and are thought to subserve a wide variety of functions, some hypothetically. These functions include learning, memory, and mood. Most important, however, the endogenous opiates can inhibit pain perception.

The endogenous opioids are indeed potent analgesics, being active in very low concentrations. The discovery of these substances has not, however, been of any immediate or direct value for clinical treatment of pain. There are a dismayingly large number of obstacles to the pharmacological use of these substances. One is that the dependence and tolerance associated with chronic use of opiate drugs cannot, apparently, be avoided by the use of opioid peptides. A second problem is that endogenous opioid compounds are rapidly degraded, so that they would be effective only if they could be administered continuously. In contrast to opiate drugs (such as morphine), they are not easily delivered to the brain. When administered systemically, they do not cross the blood-brain barrier. Moreover, even if they could be administered systemically, they would influence all circuits in the brain that employ opioids, just as opiate drugs do. Opiate drugs produce sedation, euphoria, and other effects in addition to relief of pain, and the endogenous opioids appear to produce a similar range of effects. No means of overcoming these obstacles has appeared, and in fact, very little has been developed in terms of therapeutic use of either endogenous opioids or any other endogenous peptide compound (of which there are very many).

Indeed, there are already very good drugs that act on opiate receptors, for example, morphine and heroin. Although these drugs are excellent analgesics, clinical use is extremely limited because they produce tolerance and dependence, probably in large part due to their effect on widespread brain circuits, not only those that are modulating the pain. Therefore, despite the excitement and interest associated with the discovery of endogenous opioids in the early 1970s, the discovery of these substances did not lead directly to the development of a means for therapeutic use. In fact, the first real possibility for a direct therapeutic use of endogenous opioids therapeutically involves transplantation.

A key piece of information in using transplantation to administer opioid peptides is knowing where in the brain and/or spinal cord opiate drugs act to alleviate pain. Studies have been performed to determine where in those sites opiates act to alleviate pain. One type of study was based on administering small amounts of opioids—initially opiate drugs and later opioid peptides—directly into various regions of the brain and spinal cord. Additional studies involved an anatomical search for locations where opiate receptors were located in high concentrations (see Cooper et al. 1996; Iversen and Iversen 1981; or S. Snyder and Childers 1979 for additional details). Two regions were found to be of predominant importance. The first is the periaqueductal gray, adjacent to the cerebral aqueduct in the brain stem. The second is the dorsal horn of the spinal cord. The periaqueductal gray appears to be a major site for the central processing of pain-related information. The spinal cord, by contrast, is the site where primary fibers that transmit pain from the periphery terminate. In both areas, small amounts of either opiate drugs or peptides can inhibit pain. In the spinal cord, the inhibition is locality-specific; that is, there will be inhibition only of such pain as is transmitted via the appropriate regions of spinal cord. Injection of opiates into the periaqueductal gray, on the other hand, apparently inhibits all forms of pain, regardless of where the pain originates.

Jacqueline Sagen, George Pappas, and Mark Perlow at the University of Chicago, beginning in 1986, showed that adrenal medulla transplants were capable of alleviating pain in rat models (Sagen, Pappas, and Perlow 1986; Sagen, Pappas, and Pollard 1986; Sagen et al. 1990; Sagen et al. 1991; Sagen et al. 1993; Sagen and Wang 1990). The first experiments involved transplantation of adrenal medulla into the spinal cord. It was found that either rat adrenal medulla or isolated bovine adrenal chromaffin cells were capable of alleviating acute pain in rats, mainly when release was stimulated by nicotine. In some experiments, adrenal medulla was also transplanted into the periaqueductal gray, but most experiments have concentrated on transplants into the spinal cord.

Although the previous discussion has emphasized endorphins, we should note that catecholamines can also stimulate analgesia when injected into the spinal cord and periaqueductal gray. In fact, catecholamines (actually, norepinephrine agonists) and opiates, when injected together, act synergistically to produce analgesia, so that the two classes of compounds combined produce a much greater effect than either alone (Drasner and Fields 1988; Yaksh and Reddy 1981). This being the case, adrenal chromaffin cells may be nearly ideal for inducing analgesia, since they release large amounts of norpinephine in addition to endogenous opioids. Studies by Sagen and coworkers suggest that the analgesic effect of adrenal medulla grafts was, in fact, due to the combined effects of released catecholamines and enkephalins (Sagen et al. 1991).

Since the analgesic effect was blocked by the opiate antagonist naloxone, and inhibited by the catecholamine antagonist phentolamine, it appears that both opioids and catecholamines are involved in pain inhibition. Increases in met-enkephalin and catecholamines were found in the cerebrospinal fluid (CSF) of animals with these adrenal medulla grafts. Increases in met-enkephalin in the CSF of patients that received adrenal medulla grafts for Parkinson's disease (Drucker-Colin et al. 1988) and later for pain (Winnie et al. 1993) also have been reported. Thus, the pain-inhibiting effect is probably due to the combination of catecholamine and opioid peptide release.

Dr. Sagen and her coworkers have explored possibilities for employing adrenal medulla grafts from a different species to induce pain relief in rats. For these experiments, bovine (cow) chromaffin cells, which are very effective in producing and releasing met-enkephalin, were used. For consistent and long-term survival of these grafts, immunosuppression, using the drug cyclosporine to prevent graft rejection, is required. A relatively short-term course of immunosuppression, however, appears to be sufficient to allow for long-term xenograft survival. Thus, when chromaffin cells from bovine donors were transplanted into rats, and the host animals were immunosuppressed for only two weeks, the transplanted cells survived indefinitely. In general, it appears that grafts in the brain are most susceptible to rejection during the first two weeks after implantation. During this period, the blood-brain barrier is healing, tissue reactions to injury are subsiding, and antigenic material is being released from grafted cells that do not survive the implantation. As was seen with chromaffin cell grafts transplanted from rats to rats, bovine chromaffin cells were found to produce analgesia, especially when stimulated with nicotine.

In addition, Sagen and coworkers have examined the effects of adrenal medulla transplants in models of chronic pain. The serious nature of chronic pain, as an illness in itself, is often underestimated. The nature of chronic pain is such that it becomes amplified by long duration of occurrence. That is, pain of an intensity that is perceived as mild during short exposure gradually becomes more serious when exposure to the pain is prolonged. Chronic pain can become entirely debilitating, and may result in weight loss and appetite depression, irritability, hyperventilation, and sleep disruption. In most cases, when pain management is a clinical problem, it is chronic pain that is prolonged for weeks or months, whereas most forms of acute pain are easily managed with standard analgesics. Syndromes associated with long-term severe pain, to give a few examples, include cancer, neuralgia (nerve damage) and neuromas (abnormal growth of peripheral nerve fibers), phantom limb pain, and arthritis.

Sagen and coworkers have also investigated adrenal medulla transplantation in chronic pain models in animals, in one study using an arthritis model (Sagen et al. 1990), and in a second study using a peripheral neuropathy model (Hama and Sagen 1993). In the first model, arthritis was induced in rats by adjuvant administration. Adjuvants are materials that enhance immune responses; thus, in immunology, adjuvants are administered locally in order to produce inflammation and autoimmune reactions. In this case, adjuvant was employed to provoke an autoimmune response involving the joints. In this chronic pain model, animals show pain-elicited vocalizations and chronic loss of body weight. Adrenal medulla from rat donors transplanted into the spinal cord alleviated, by about half, the loss of weight seen in control animals (controls received transplants of muscle tissue). The pain-associated vocalization was not significantly decreased by the adrenal medulla grafts; however, nicotine (which stimulates release of both catecholamines and opiates from adrenal chromaffin cells) markedly decreased vocalization in the animals with adrenal medulla grafts but not in the controls (figure 14.1). Thus, in this experimental paradigm, adrenal medulla grafts in the spinal cord alleviated chronic pain somewhat, but with additional nicotine stimulation a pronounced effect was obtained. Both naloxone (an opiate antagonist) and phentolamine (a catecholamine antagonist) were able to block the analgesic effect of nicotine. Naloxone completely blocked the effect, while the effect of phentolamine was only partial, suggesting that opioids are required and that catecholamines contribute to the analgesic effect of released opioids in this chronic model.

In one sense, the requirement for nicotine stimulation to obtain pain inhibition from adrenal medulla grafts could be useful. If these grafts are used in humans, nicotine or other drugs could be used to stimulate graft efficacy only when needed. In some cases, pain might be intermittent, and the analgesic effect could be adjusted as needed. Nicotine could be administered during severe pain episodes or during waking hours, or the analgesic effect might be enhanced if a graft was not sufficiently effective in a particular patient. In case of overly effective grafts—for example, if side effects or sedation occurred—it might be possible to block some of these effects. There may be additional possibilities for pharmacological manipulation of the analgesic efficacy of adrenal medulla grafts. Pacheo-Cano and coworkers (1990) observed enhancement of the pain-suppressing effects of adrenal medulla grafts by dibutyryl cyclic AMP. In addition to stimulation by nicotine, Sagen and Wang (1990)

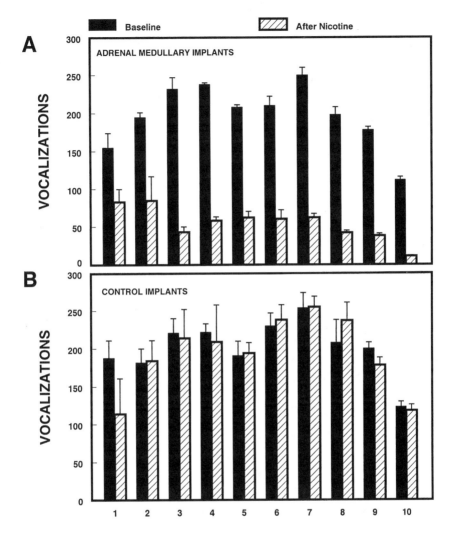

Figure 14.1
Effects of adrenal medulla grafts on arthritis pain induced in rats by adjuvant administration. In this chronic pain model, animals show pain-elicited vocalizations and chronic weight loss. Adrenal medulla from rat donors transplanted into the spinal cord alleviated, by about half, the loss of weight that was seen in control animals (not shown). The pain-associated vocalization was not significantly decreased by the adrenal medulla grafts alone (solid bars in A); however, nicotine (which stimulates release of both catecholamines and opiates from adrenal chromaffin cells) markedly decreased vocalization in the animals with adrenal medulla grafts but not in the controls. Each pair of bars represents data from a single rat, before and after nicotine administration. There were 10 animals that received adrenal medulla grafts (A) and 10 controls (13). From Sagen, Wang, and Pappas 1990, with permission.

found that the duration of action of the analgesia could be prolonged by administration of kelatorphan, which inhibits metabolic degradation of enkephalins by inhibiting the enzyme enkephalinase. Thus, there is a potential for modulation of the efficacy of the grafts by simple pharmacological manipulation. This is a particularly attractive feature of this transplantation model, especially regarding the possibilities for use in humans.

What about use in human subjects with chronic pain? At first glance, one might question this application on the grounds that potent analgesics already are available, so why resort to such an invasive and potentially risky procedure? Further examination, however, supports a much different view. Weak analgesics such as aspirin and ibuprophen are indeed effective, but are not sufficient to treat severe or prolonged pain. Pain is not only an abstract concept but also the major source of suffering in a number of diseases. The purpose of pain, as a biological phenomenon, is to alert an individual to the presence of a potentially damaging effect. When, however, pain is present as an accompaniment of chronic disease, it serves no useful purpose but demoralizes the patient, and may cause as much or more debilitating effect than does the disease itself.

Opiates such as morphine are, of course, effective, but are addictive, lead to tolerance when used chronically, and produce sedation and other undesirable side effects (e.g., respiratory depression) when administered systemically. In fact, administration of opiate drugs directly into the spinal cord via implanted mechanical pumps has been used, on a limited basis, as a means of circumventing some of these problems. There are considerable problems with the use of mechanical pumps, including risk of infection (often associated with refilling or recharging them), the necessity of refilling them, and the somewhat bulky and inconvenient nature of the device. Basically, this involves having a device at least the size of a hockey puck implanted under one's skin, and refilling it periodically. Thus, there are good reasons to consider development of more effective and specific treatments for chronic pain, even if they are invasive and there is some risk involved. Adrenal medulla transplantation has considerably greater potential than mechanical drug-delivery pumps for use in severe, chronic pain.

Early reports on adrenal medulla transplants for chronic pain did not show them to be successful, although these studies were not reported in detail (Vaquero et al. 1988). In the study by Vaquero et al., cancer patients with chronic pain received adrenal medulla grafts in the spinal cord, with little or no relief from pain. It is not clear that the techniques employed by this group were optimal; for example, purified cell populations were not used, and the methods may not have resulted in a high cell survival rate.

More recently, the possibility of using adrenal medulla transplants for chronic pain treatment in human cancer patients has been explored further by Sagen and coworkers (Sagen et al. 1993; Winnie et al. 1993). The subjects were cancer patients with severe pain and a life expectancy of less than one year. In this case, although no primate experiments were done previously, it seems to make good sense to proceed directly to humans. On one hand, there are considerable difficulties with testing procedures that involve the production of chronic pain symptoms in primates, and conditions of chronic pain are difficult to assess accurately in animals. Another factor is the population in which this procedure has been tested. By attempting this procedure in cancer patients with a poor prognosis, there is little risk associated with the possible failure of the procedure, and successful transplants have the real possibility of improving the lives and condition of these patients.

For the patients who were selected, effective pain control could not be maintained even with escalating doses of narcotic drugs. Three subjects had colon cancer, a fourth had breast cancer, and the fifth subject had Gardner's syndrome, which involved multiple tumors and gastric obstruction. Human adrenal medulla tissue was obtained from a tissue bank. The adrenal medulla was dissected, cut into small pieces, and held in culture for three to seven days prior to transplantation. The tissue was transplanted into the cerebrospinal fluid space in the lumbar region of the spinal cord, by injection through a large needle. As in the animal experiments, the patients were immunosuppressed with cyclosporine for two weeks, starting the day prior to transplantation.

It is, of course, difficult to measure the severity of pain directly, since pain is experienced by the individual patient. In the studies by Sagen and her coworkers, pain was measured in two ways. First, the patients were

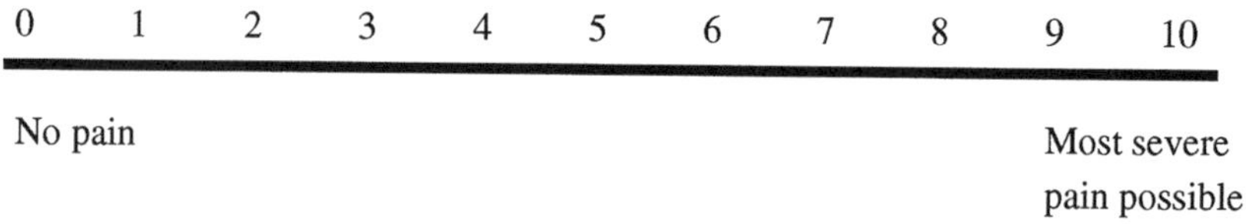

0	1	2	3	4	5	6	7	8	9	10

No pain   Most severe
                                                               pain possible

Figure 14.2
The visual analog scale employed to assess pain on a 0–10 scale in the studies
by Sagen et al. (1993). Patients are asked to describe the severity of their pain
by marking a point on this scale.

asked to rate the severity of their pain, using what is called a "visual
analog scale." This method involves showing patients a scale, and asking
them to mark an indication of the severity of their pain on the scale (figure
14.2). This is inherently subjective, as is any direct measurement of pain.
A second measure was amount of analgesic drugs used. Each of the patients was using substantial amounts of narcotic drugs prior to surgery,
mainly morphine. The patients were able to control their intake of narcotics, using them as needed to alleviate their pain. Thus, the amount of
narcotics used provided a second measure of effectiveness of the transplants in alleviating pain.

Remarkably, whenever pain scores increased or decreased, narcotic intake changed almost exactly in parallel. This tends to validate the two
measures; certainly, if narcotic intake was decreased for some spurious
reason (e.g., difficulty in obtaining the drug), one would expect pain to
increase rather than decrease. Conversely, it did not appear that decreases
in pain scores were caused by increased narcotic use. Interestingly, these
patients apparently were not self-administering narcotics for their eu-
phirogenic effects, nor were they using these drugs in excess.

In two of the patients, the procedure was essentially a failure. The patient with breast cancer showed gradual alleviation of pain over the
course of about five weeks after the transplant, but the pain returned
shortly afterward. By 10 to 12 weeks after transplantation, her pain and
narcotic intake were about the same as before the transplant. The patient
with Gardner's syndrome reported no improvement one month after the
procedure, and then became uncooperative and hostile, so that no further
data were available.

In the remaining three patients, however, the results were extremely
encouraging. Each of them had colon cancer. Each was using morphine

or a morphine derivative prior to the transplantion surgery, and was nonetheless experiencing severe pain, rated 6–9 on the visual analog scale. Remarkable improvement was obtained in all three. Gradually, over the course of 5 to 10 weeks, their pain scores decreased. From 10 weeks after surgery until their deaths, these patients remained essentially pain-free even while using little or no narcotic drugs (figure 14.3). Increases in met-enkephalin and norepinephrine in the spinal CSF were found, although the same changes were not seen in all of the patients. These changes in CSF are, nonetheless, generally consistent with the clinical findings. Although this study is preliminary and there are some caveats, the improvement in quality of life that this represents is indeed remarkable. Additional patients have now been tested, also with positive results (Pappas et al. 1997), and there is evidence that the grafts survived for one year (Bes et al. 1998).

It has been pointed out that these studies have several limitations (Foley and Yaksh 1993). One is that the baseline pain experienced by the patients, prior to transplantation surgery, was measured only once or over a very short time span. If the patients were referred for surgery during episodes of acute and severe pain, the pain might have responded spontaneously, not because of the transplants. Thus, Foley and Yaksh suggested that pain scores should have been measured for at least a few days prior to surgery. Otherwise, it is not clear that the improvement was due to the transplantation rather than spontaneous remission. Another issue is the relationship between CSF and clinical findings. Since animal studies had been done in rats only, and no data on larger animals were available (even though primates present difficulties, experiments could have been done in other animals, such as dogs or sheep), there were no animal data that could be used to evaluate the changes in CSF met-enkephalin and catecholamines as representative of the presence of surviving cells. Ultimately, a double-blind controlled trial will probably be required, and this study thus should be regarded as preliminary in nature. Nevertheless, it is certainly encouraging!

There have been several follow-up studies of human subjects. In one study, performed in Switzerland by E. Buchser and coworkers (1996), cancer patients received adrenal chromaffin cells transplanted into the spinal cord. In this case, the cells for transplantation were obtained from calves. In order to prevent graft rejection, the cells were transplanted

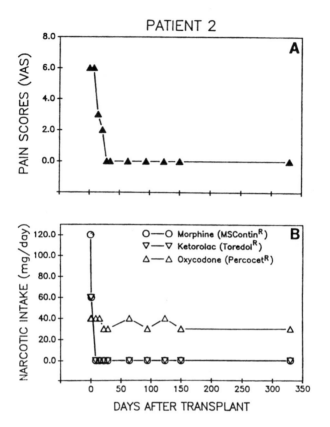

Figure 14.3
Progressive decreases in pain scores (figure 14.2), shown as dots with solid lines, and narcotic intake (triangles with broken lines) in two of four cancer patients after receiving adrenal medulla grafts into the spinal cord. In patient 2 there was a sustained improvement, whereas pain scores and narcotic intake returned to baseline levels after 60 days in patient 3. (From Sagen et al. 1993.)

in a semipermeable capsule that allows small molecules (such as met-enkephalin and catecholamines) to escape and thereby influence the host spinal cord. The nature of the membrane surrounding the grafts is such that passage of cells and large molecules that mediate immunological re-sponses to grafts is prevented. This general encapsulation approach is under development by a private corporation based in Rhode Island, CytoTherapeutics, Inc., for possible use in a number of disorders. Thus, in theory, molecules produced by the graft that could sensitize the

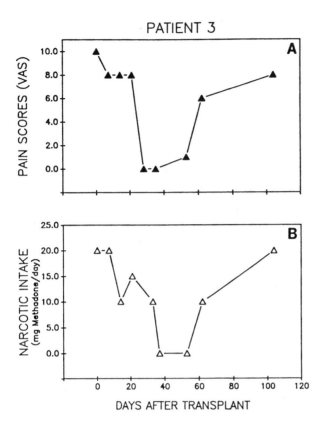

immune system do not escape, and immune "effector" cells (such as macrophages and T lymphocytes) that could destroy the graft, as well as antibodies, cannot enter in any appreciable quantity. The encapsulated cells were transplanted into the spinal cord under local anesthesia, using a simple, minimally invasive procedure.

The effects of the implants in this study were examined over a relatively short duration, mostly between 41 and 85 days. Three of the seven patients had the implants removed electively, and four were removed postmortem. There were substantial, although variable, reductions in pain scores and morphine dosages. Three of the seven patients had reductions in self-rated pain scores of at least 80 percent, on at least one of the two rating systems. Two patients had no reductions in pain scores. The three patients showing very large decreases (>80 percent) in pain scores were not receiving morphine and were studied for between 43 and 85 days. One patient survived for an extended period after the device was removed, and did not show a significant worsening of pain during that interval. Overall, the beneficial effects of the transplants were somewhat variable and the study was quite short in duration; nevertheless, the results were quite promising.

In some model systems, such as for repair of visual system deficits, it is clear that transplants must produce new connections with the host brain in detail in order to be effective. In Huntington's disease and spinal cord injury, this is probably true as well. In Parkinson's disease, it is not entirely clear. In pain, however, it seems clear that simple release of biochemicals from the graft can be effective, without any requirement whatever for the formation of new synapses with host cells.

There are also interesting possibilities for genetic engineering of cells for use in pain treatment (chapters 22 and 23). One possibility is that instead of using normal chromaffin cells for transplantation, other cells could be engineered to produce norepinephrine and enkephalins. Transplants of immortal serotonin-producing cells have been found to alleviate pain in an animal model (Eaton et al. 1997). Another possibility is that chromaffin cells could be genetically altered so that they can be grown in tissue culture, and all that would be required would be for them to produce norepinephrine and enkephalins. Any deficits in these cells' functions could be corrected by genetic engineering. Possibly even the production of opioids by normal chromaffin cells could be enhanced, or engineered so that production is under the control of hormones or other drug modulators. Since these functions of chromaffin cells are relatively simple (production and release of norepinephrine and met-enkephalin), perhaps treatment of pain will be the first case to which new technological advances are applied in neural transplantation.

A second reason that pain is an attractive application of neural transplantation technology is the potential usefulness of the method. For pain treatment, what is required of neural transplants is quite simple, yet what can potentially be accomplished may be quite useful. Few would argue that alleviation of the suffering of cancer patients is not a worthwhile or compelling goal. In the long run, there are additional pain syndromes that present treatment difficulties and might be amenable to treatment through this or similar techniques. Phantom limb pain, neuromas, and pain due to nerve injury are examples. Many such syndromes cannot be treated effectively by conventional techniques, and might ultimately be amenable to treatment using cell transplants. Thus, it would not be surprising to see the use of neural transplants in this area to become explored very extensively, and perhaps become a very significant clinical application over the next ten years.

Further Reading

Cooper, J. R., Bloom, F. E., and Roth, R. H. (1996). *The Biochemical Basis of Neuropharmacology*. Seventh edition. Oxford University Press, New York.

Czech, K., and Sagen, J. (1995). Update on cellular transplantation into the CNS as a novel therapy for chronic pain. *Prog. Neurobiol.* 46: 507–529.

Iversen, S. D., and Iversen, L. L. (1981). *Behavioral Pharmacology*. Second edition. Oxford University Press, New York.

Snyder, S. H., and Childers, S. (1979). Opiate receptors and opioid peptides. *Ann. Rev. Neurosci.* 2: 35–64.

15

Hypothalamus and Pituitary

The hypothalamus is a small region located at the base of the brain, above the pituitary. In general, it participates in the control of homeostatic functions: regulation of blood pressure, metabolic processes, hunger, thirst, motivational processes, aggression/predatory functions, fluid and electrolyte balance, sexual differentiation and sexual function, body temperature, daily activity cycles (circadian rhythms), and immune function. Physiologically, the hypothalamus interacts with the endocrine system and the autonomic nervous system, and may be thought of as mediating functions that are connected to basic physiological maintenance systems. There are also homeostatic functions (for example, circadian rhythms) that are controlled by the hypothalamus but not primarily through endocrine systems.

The various hypothalamic nuclei accomplish these regulatory processes in two ways: (1) through influencing pituitary hormone secretion and (2) through neural connections with other brain regions. The hypothalamus is relatively small, considering the large number of functions it performs, but these functions are relatively simple, and are very similar in both lower animals and man. Indeed, the endocrine system of a rat is similar to that of humans in complexity, whereas the cerebral cortex of humans is vastly more complex than that of rodents.

The entire endocrine system is under control of the hypothalamus through the pituitary gland, which secretes hormones that regulate various bodily functions. There are two major divisions of the pituitary, the neurohypophysis (more or less corresponding to the posterior pituitary) and the adenohypophysis (anterior pituitary). For the adenohypophysis, hormone secretion is controlled by a second set of substances, releasing hormones, which are produced by the hypothalamus and carried to the pituitary via small, specialized blood vessels. The neurohypophysis is an extension of the hypothalamus itself, and secretion of hormones from it by the direct release from axonal terminals. Large cells, called *magnocellular* neurons, located in the supraoptic and paraventricular nuclei of the hypothalamus, release the hormones vasopressin and oxytocin directly into capillaries.

There have been a considerable number of studies of neural transplantation involving hypothalamic and pituitary functions; not all of these will be covered in this book (see table 15.1). What will be described is a selection of interesting experiments, in order to provide an overview of the types of studies and manipulations of hypothalamic function that may be possible via transplantation. Since a number of hypothalamic functions involve localized secretion of biochemicals, the alteration of hypothalamic function by neural transplantation is a goal that can be readily achieved. In fact, the earliest studies to show a functional interaction between neural systems and a graft involved transplantation of pituitary tissue into the hypothalamus. In these experiments, the pituitary was removed and transplanted into the hypothalamus. Some of the endocrine deficits produced by pituitary removal (called hypophysectomy) in these experiments were found to be alleviated by pituitary grafts in the hypothalamus (Halasz et al. 1965).

In the modern era of neural transplantation, experiments by D. Gash, J. Sladek, and C. Sladek were the first to examine functional properties of grafts in the hypothalamus (Gash et al. 1980). Their studies employed Brattleboro rats, which have a deficiency in secretion of the antidiuretic hormone (ADH, or vasopressin). This hormone acts primarily on the kidney to promote fluid retention, and plays an important role in fluid and electrolyte balance. In addition, vasopressin is important in blood pressure regulation. Because of the lack of vasopressin, the kidneys of Brattleboro rats cannot concentrate their urine. This results in a high rate of fluid loss, so these animals must drink large amounts of water in order to maintain fluid balance.

In the study by Gash and coworkers (1980), the anterior region of the hypothalamus, containing the vasopressin-producing magnocellular

Table 15.1
Some applications of neural transplantation involving pituitary and hypothalamic functions

Function	Model	Manifestation	Tissue Transplanted	First Study
Abnormal ADH secretion (vasopressin deficiency)	Mutant rat strain	Polydipsia, polyuria (diabetes insipidus)	Anterior hypothalamus, containing vasopressin magnocellular neurons	Gash et al. (1980)
Gonadotropin-releasing hormone deficiency	Mutant mouse strain	Underdeveloped reproductive organs	Improved reproductive behavior and organ development	Krieger, Gibson, et al. (1982)
Blood pressure	Spontaneously hypertensive vs. normal rats	Hypertension	Fetal hypothalamus	Eilam et al. (1991)
Autoimmunity	Strain susceptibility	Arthritis, inflammation	Hypothalamus	Misciewicz et al. (1997)
Circadian rhythms	Lesions of the suprachiasmatic nucleus	Loss of circadian rhythms	Restoration of cycling	Drucker-Colin et al. (1984)

neurons, was dissected from normal rat fetuses (i.e., animals that did not possess the genetic deficiency in vasopressin production) and transplanted into the hypothalamus. In a few (about 20–25 percent in different experiments) of the recipient animals, transplants of hypothalamic tissue from normal animals into the Brattleboro animals were able to restore the animals' ability to regulate urine osmolality, a measure of fluid retention capacity. As a result, there were decreases in the excessive water consumption. Later experiments showed that in order to be effective, it was necessary for the graft to contain vasopressin neurons near the portal blood vessels at the base of the hypothalamus, perhaps thereby facilitating vasopressin release into the bloodstream.

The grafts were, however, effective in only a minority of the animals, and in some subsequent experiments none of the transplanted animals recovered. Later, these investigators used another model, in which the neurohypophysis was removed. This causes about 75 percent of the magnocellular neurons to degenerate. Using this lesion model, recovery was obtained in about half of the transplanted animals. As a general summary of these findings, it might be concluded that it is possible to obtain recovery of vasopressin deficiency with hypothalamic transplants; however, this probably requires a very specific combination of circumstances, involving the degree of deficiency in the host and survival of adequate numbers of transplanted vasopressin neurons in a precise anatomical position. Thus, it may be difficult to obtain these circumstances consistently and predictably.

Although vasopressin deficiency is present in small numbers of human subjects, it can be treated by administration of antidiuretic hormone and is not a life-threatening disorder. In addition, there are several reasons that vasopressin deficiency is not a good candidate for application of transplantation to human disease. As discussed above, the effects of transplants are inconsistent, even in animal models. From a surgical standpoint, hypothalamic transplants would be difficult to perform safely and predictably, because of the many crucial regulatory centers that are nearby in the hypothalamus and could be disturbed by surgery. Pure populations of vasopressin neurons cannot be obtained, so tissue dissected from the hypothalamus would contain other types of neurons that might in themselves cause regulatory dysfunction. Finally, it would be very dif-

ficult, perhaps impossible, to remove a hypothalamic transplant if undesirable effects were obtained. Thus, there has not yet been a compelling
reason to employ transplants in humans for this disorder. Nonetheless,
the value of these experiments is that the feasibility of the approach, both
as a research tool and perhaps as a therapeutic procedure, has been
shown. Since that time, many interesting possibilities related to hypothalamic tissue transplantation have been developed. Although none have
yet been conceived of as being therapeutic possibilities, this is not out of
the question at some future date.

Sexual Function and Differentiation

A considerable number of experiments have examined effects of hypothalamic tissue grafts on the development of reproductive function and
on differentiation of male versus female sexual behavior patterns. Not
all of these experiments will be described here; the references at the end
of this chapter can be consulted for further details.

One very extensive series of experiments involved the use of animals
with a deficiency in the production of hormones that influence the development of the reproductive system. These animals have a deficiency in
the production of gonadotropin-releasing hormone, or GnRH, which is
produced in the hypothalamus and exerts its effects in the pituitary. The
effect of GnRH is to cause the release of two additional hormones,
follicle-stimulating hormone (FSH) and luteinizing hormone (LH). These
hormones are necessary for development of the reproductive organs, so
in animals with deficiencies in these hormones, the reproductive system
fails to develop normally. Particular manifestations of this deficiency include underdeveloped testes and spermatogenesis in males, and unde-
veloped ovaries and ovulation in females. The animals with GnRH
deficiency also do not exhibit normal mating behavior.

In a series of experiments, Dorothy Krieger, Marie Gibson, and their
coworkers showed that with transplantation of hypothalamic tissue containing the GnRH-producing neurons, they were able to reverse the hypo-
development of the reproductive system. Krieger and coworkers (1982)
found that following transplants, more normal development of the reproductive organs ensued. Gibson, Krieger, and coworkers (1984) showed

that animals with GnRH deficiency were able to mate and become pregnant after receiving transplants. Interestingly, there are other GnRH-producing neurons in the accessory olfactory bulb that are not normally involved in regulation of FSH and LH release. These neurons were able to reverse hypogonadism in animals with GnRH deficiency when transplanted to an appropriate location in the hypothalamus (Perlow et al. 1987).

There have also been experiments on regulation of sexual behavior, rather than reproductive function, by neural transplants. Of particular interest are experiments by Luine and her colleagues, on sexual behavior in female rats. For these experiments, hypersexuality was induced in female rats following damage to serotonin neurons in the hypothalamus produced by the serotonergic toxin 5,7-DHT. Such animals show increased sexual behavior that spontaneously returns to normal after 9–10 weeks. This hypersexuality could be greatly decreased, during the eight weeks prior to spontaneous recovery, by transplanting serotonin neurons into the hypothalamus (Luine et al. 1985).

These studies do not necessarily suggest any particular therapeutic application, although there are possibilities. For hormone-deficiency diseases, especially those related to pituitary deficiency, most of the effects produced by transplants can be more simply achieved hormonally.

Is it possible that transplants could be used for alleviating disorders that are manifested as sexual dysfunction of a very serious nature? Well, probably this won't happen, but we will discuss it anyway. There certainly are disorders of sexual function in humans. The hypothalamus is a difficult place for surgery, being located deep within the brain, close to many crucial centers. Are there any disorders serious enough to warrant an experimental surgical procedure in the hypothalamus? It is interesting to think about the possibilities. There are centers in the hypothalamus that influence both sexual behavior and aggression. We can at least think about the possibility of using tissue transplants to diminish sexual drive or aggression in rapists or other violent offenders. Such things might be possible. For example, say that it was found possible to block the sexual-aggressive urges that lead to rape or violent tendencies by transplanting some sort of tissue or cells into the hypothalamus. It might even be possible to block other sorts of criminal aggression hormonally, in a similar way. This is perhaps within the realm of technical possibility.

The availability of such a procedure would raise many societal issues (to say the least). First, we would have to consider whether transplants could be used in violent sex offenders when there is no direct evidence of an underlying neural disorder. Using transplants to alter the behavior per se would probably be objectionable, even if some evidence of brain dysfunction was found. This kind of issue has come up in the past, in the context of using neurosurgery to remove parts of the brain in violent individuals (chapter 7). Brain transplants would be slightly better, since parts of the brain would not be removed, but would nonetheless raise similar issues. Such a procedure might be perceived of by society as constituting cruel and unusual punishment, and certainly other objections might be raised. It would also have to be assumed that prisoners would not be able to freely make a decision to receive such a procedure. So this is not going to happen now.

Nonetheless, the rules of society can change. First, it certainly seems that rape and certain other kinds of violence could be considered disorders per se, rather than crimes, under only slightly modified conditions of our legal and medical systems. Thus, one potentially reasonable viewpoint would be that there is nothing wrong with treating these individuals by whatever means are possible, including tissue transplantation. Even if acts of violence are disorders, individuals prone to committing such acts would have to be confined, for the good of society. An efficacious treatment could decrease the need for confinement, and under only slightly different moral standards or societal conventions, treating violent sex offenders by means of neural transplantation could come to seem very humane and reasonable.

Suppose we continue to believe that these acts are crimes which should be punished rather than treated. Or perhaps they are crimes as well as diseases, which require both punishment and treatment. This is also possible. Then we accept the need for confining such individuals for a defined period of time. The possibility of employing hormonal treatments to prevent the urges (or whatever they are) leading to the crime affords no help, since there is no guarantee that the individuals will continue the treatment once they are released from confinement. However, a hypothalamic transplant would be quite a different situation. Such a transplant would not easily be removed. In fact, of all areas of the brain into which a transplant might be made, removal from the hypothalamus would be probably the most difficult. It might well be impossible to remove a hypothalamic transplant by surgical means.

Under only slightly different societal conditions, we might imagine transplants being used for violent sex offenders even if their acts continue to be thought of as criminal offenses. It might not be acceptable for society to sentence a convicted rapist or child molester to receive a transplant. Perhaps once sentenced to jail, however, the offender could be offered a transplant as an alternative. For example, you are sentenced to twenty years in prison. If you elect to receive a transplant, your sentence will be reduced to one year. Or the offender could be offered this treatment as a means of decreasing the chances for further problems. The prisoner has everything to gain (namely, freedom) and nothing to lose: if he prefers the punishment, it could be carried out as specified. The possibility of coercion could be mitigated by having the process monitored by an independent review board. The form that such a system would take is certainly unclear. Nonetheless, it it likely that there are at least possibilities for controversy about, if not actual use of, hypothalamic tissue transplantation in human patients.

Blood Pressure Regulation

This topic was first studied by Eilam and coworkers (1991). Additional studies by C. Murphy, R. Canbeyli, and B. Yongue (1992), published only in abstract form, will be discussed here for illustrative purposes. The latter group of investigators used for their experiments two strains of rats, the spontaneously hypertensive rat (SHR) and animals of the Wistar-Kyoto strain, from which the SHR rats were bred. The SHR rats have high blood pressure, whereas the WKY strain animals have normal blood pressure. Their experiments showed that transplanting tissue from SHR rats into the third ventricle, adjacent to the hypothalamus, caused elevations in blood pressure in the normal WKY rats. Transplants of hypothalamus from 19–20-day gestational SHR fetuses increased blood pressure transiently for 30–60 days, whereas transplants of cortical tissue from

19–20-day gestational SHR fetuses did not increase blood pressure. Curiously, when 15–16-day gestational tissue was used, transplants of both cortical and hypothalamic tissue were found to cause increases in blood pressure, and in both cases the increased blood pressure lasted indefinitely. In a subsequent experiment, Yongue and Canbeyli (1994) found that transplants from normal WKY rats tended to reduce blood pressure in animals that were susceptible to high blood pressure. The factors responsible for these effects are unknown, but it may be that the properties of SHR hypothalamus responsible for blood pressure regulation are a general property of the CNS, or that cortical tissue differentiates differently when transplanted into the hypothalamus, so that factors which influence blood pressure are produced. Although this topic has been explored only minimally, this is an excellent example of the use of grafts to study physiological regulatory mechanisms.

Immune Mechanisms

A recent observation suggests that alterations in systemic immune regulation can be influenced by transplants of tissue into the hypothalamus. Misiewicz and coworkers (1997) employed Lewis rats, which are highly susceptible to autoimmune inflammatory diseases, such as experimental autoimmune encephalomyelitis (EAE) and arthritis. In these animals, corticosteroid-releasing hormone production, which is regulated by the hypothalamus, is impaired. Corticosteroids are hormones produced by the adrenal cortex. Since corticosteroids tend to modulate immune function, animals deficient in corticosteroid production can be excessively reactive to immune stimuli, and thus are susceptible to autoimmune disease.

Lewis rats received hypothalamic tissue transplants from a different strain of rats, Fisher 344, which are resistant to autoimmune disease; these grafts produced a decrease in susceptibility to inflammatory responses. Other kinds of grafts, including spinal cord tissue from Fisher 344 rats, and grafts of hypothalamic tissue from other Lewis rats, also decreased inflammatory responses, although not to the same extent as the Fisher 344 hypothalamus grafts. Thus, in summary, excessive susceptibility to autoimmune reactions in particular rat strains can be reduced to some extent by grafts of hypothalamic tissue from autoimmune-resistant rats.

Circadian Rhythms

One of the most unusual and perhaps unexpected uses of neural transplantation is the alteration or restoration of circadian rhythms by transplants of the suprachiasmatic nucleus, first described by Drucker-Colin and coworkers in 1984. Before proceeding, however, I will explain what circadian rhythms are. Most animals, being either diurnal (active in daylight, like most birds and humans) or nocturnal (active in the dark, like rodents and many common small mammals, such as opossums, raccoons, and foxes) show daily rhythms in activity, being active for about half of each day. The periods of light "entrain," or directly influence, the animals' activity cycles. Underlying these cycles, however, animals also have an intrinsic activity cycle, which continues to run even if the entraining effects of light are removed. Thus, if animals are kept in continuous darkness, there will still be an activity cycle. This underlying cycle will not be exactly one day, but is usually more or less than a day by an hour or two—hence the name "circadian" (from the Latin *circa* for "about" or "in the vicinity of," and *dies* for "day"). When daily cycles of light and dark are present, the circadian rhythms are not evident because of the entraining effects of light. In humans, these circadian rhythms are evident, for example, during jet lag. When one moves across several time zones quickly, via air travel, one's circadian rhythms continue to run at the usual pace. Yet one is in a different time zone, where everyone else is working and living according to their own schedule (different from that of the traveler). It takes a few days for the jet traveler to become "entrained" to the schedule of the new time zone.

It was found, during the late 1970s and early 1980s, that a small nucleus in the hypothalamus, called the suprachiasmatic nucleus (SCN), is essential for maintaining circadian rhythms. When the SCN is destroyed, circadian rhythms are abolished. It was also found that the rhythmicity of neurons in the SCN is a self-contained function: even in tissue culture, SCN neurons continue to display rhythmic cycles of activity.

In 1984, Drucker-Colin employed animals with lesions of the SCN, which thus did not have circadian rhythms, to show that circadian rhythms could be restored by SCN transplants. Lehman, Ralph and co-workers expanded on this finding, examining the properties of the transplants in detail (Lehman et al. 1987; Lehman and Ralph 1994; Ralph et al. 1990; Ralph and Lehman 1991; Silver et al. 1996). These experiments showed that circadian rhythms in activity, eating, and drinking behavior could be restored by such transplants. As in other models of transplantation, immature tissue is required for transplant efficacy, and other tissues (e.g., fetal cerebellum or superior colliculus) are not effective. These experiments have shown that the circadian rhythm function of the SCN is entirely self-contained, not dependent on the influence of other nuclei or of a complex neuronal network.

A most interesting aspect of this area of research is several experiments in which two animals have circadian rhythms of different lengths and transplants have been made from one animal to the other. In all cases, the transplants restore circadian rhythms to the lesioned host animal, but they restore the rhythms of the *donor*. This phenomenon has been documented (Ralph et al. 1990; Vogelbaum and Menaker 1992). In one case (Ralph et al. 1990), hamsters with a mutation called *tau* were used. These *tau* mutant hamsters have a circadian rhythm of about 20 hours (compared with 24 hours for normal hamsters). Actually, homozygotes have a 20-hour circadian rhythm, while heterozygotes have a circadian rhythm of about 22 hours. Homozygotes have the mutation on both copies of their DNA, while heterozygotes have only one copy of the mutation.

As shown in table 15.2, the transplants restored circadian rhythms to the animals with SCN lesions, but they restored to these animals the circadian rhythm characteristic of the source of the donor tissue—not the rhythm to which the host animal was accustomed. Thus, normal hamsters could be converted to hamsters that behaved as the *tau* mutants did, simply by removing their suprachiasmatic nucleus and transplanting into them the suprachiasmatic nucleus obtained from a *tau* mutant animal. *Tau* mutants could likewise be converted to animals that behave as normals do (Ralph et al. 1990).

This unique experiment creates grounds for some interesting speculation. Most other forms of neural transplantation have been used to

Table 15.2
Altering circadian rhythms with SCN transplants

Type of Animal	Circadian Rhythm
Normal hamster	24 hours
Tau mutant	20 hours
Hamster with SCN lesion	none
Tau hamster with normal SCN transplant	24 hours
Normal hamster with *tau* SCN transplant	20 hours

From Ralph et al. 1990.

correct a specific deficit rather than to alter an individual brain functional property in some way. Suprachiasmatic nucleus transplants can, in effect, be used to transfer particular parameters of brain function from one individual to another. This kind of experiment tends to border on alteration of personality, as opposed to correction of a specific deficiency.

In order to illustrate this, let's translate this experiment to a human situation. First, it is necessary to translate the experimental phenomenon of circadian rhythms to situations that are evident in everyday life. Of course there is jet lag; however, jet lag is infrequent. Circadian rhythms probably play a role in other parts of our everyday lives as well. During a workweek or schoolweek schedule, circadian rhythms are not really evident, because our schedules are determined by our jobs or other activities (although for people with circadian rhythms longer than 24 hours, it may be harder to get up on time in the mornings). During vacation times, and to some extent on weekends, circadian rhythms become more evident. To illustrate: some individuals tend to be early risers; they get up at 4:30 A.M. without an alarm clock. These individuals probably have a circadian rhythm of less than 24 hours, say 20 hours. Others like to sleep late. Over the course of a week's vacation, they gradually adjust their schedules and eventually arise at 10 or 11 o'clock, even if they have had enough sleep, unless there is something that they have to do. These late-sleeping individuals probably have circadian rhythms of 26 or so hours. When not constrained by schedules, society, friends and family, or daylight, these people tend to sleep progressively later, and stay up later at night. It would be—or at least animal studies suggest that it would be—possible to change the circadian rhythms of a human subject by destroying the suprachiasmatic nucleus and replacing it with the suprachiasmatic nucleus from a donor with a circadian rhythm of a different length.

To make a specific speculation that is quite bizarre, even a little silly, one might imagine a married couple who do not get along because one is an early riser and the other likes to get up late. The couple, being wealthy and perhaps having had cosmetic surgery on their faces and bodies, decide to take decisive action to solve the problem. They generate a pregnancy, and use the fetus to solve the "problem." The fetal suprachiasmatic nucleus is divided in two parts, and half is transplanted into the hypothalamus of each parent (who, of course, had received suprachiasmatic nucleus lesions to eliminate their own circadian rhythms). Through (the miracle of modern) surgery, the couple then has been matched for circadian rhythms! Is incompatibility of circadian rhythm duration a disorder? Or is getting up late for work a disorder? Of course not today, but the rules of society can change. Emphatically, this is not recommended: it is certainly preposterous, and it would certainly be unethical by almost anyone's standards. Nevertheless, it could be *possible*.

The interesting aspect of this idea is that this kind of procedure begins to border on an alteration of personality by a "brain transplant." Even though circadian rhythm length is a very specific and circumscribed aspect of brain function, it is a component of brain function that certainly makes a contribution to personality. An individual who was otherwise identical, but suddenly changed from an early riser to a "night person," would be, to some degree, different from the person he or she had been before.

Conclusion

At first glance, the hypothalamus seems as though it might be the least interesting brain area as a site for brain tissue transplants. After all, the hypothalamus mostly influences regulatory functions, such as blood pressure or sexual activity. Why would it be interesting or worthwhile to influence these regulatory systems by brain transplants, rather than administering drugs or hormones systemically?

In fact, however, a wide range of quite disparate and interesting functions is regulated by the hypothalamus. Many of these functions interact with other parts of the brain, either directly, through connections between the hypothalamus and other brain regions, or indirectly, through peripheral systems. The hypothalamus has, in fact, long been a brain region of great interest to neuroscientists because of its important role in body weight regulation, fluid balance, sexual function, temperature regulation, and hormonal homeostasis.

Since many hypothalamic functions are mediated biochemically, and require less complex interconnections with other neurons, it may be relatively easy to influence hypothalamic function by using brain tissue transplants. Useful applications of hypothalamic tissue transplantation for disease may eventually become evident. Possibilities for producing controversial, and perhaps ethically questionable, alterations in brain function through transplantation in the hypothalamus are likely to appear as well.

Further Reading

Dunnett, S. B., and Bjorklund, A. (1994). *Functional Neural Transplantation.* Raven Press, New York.

Koutouzis, T. K., Emerich, D. F., Borlongan, C. V., Freeman, T. B., Cahill, D. W., and Sanberg, P. R. (1994). Cell transplantation for central nervous system disorders. *Crit. Rev. Neurobiol.* 8: 125–162.

Ralph, M. R., and Lehman, M. N. (1991). Transplantation: A new tool in the analysis of the mammalian hypothalamic circadian pacemaker. *Trends Neurosci.* 14: 362–366.

Sladek, J. R., Jr., and Gash, D. M. (1984). *Neural Transplants: Development and Function.* Plenum Press, New York.

16

The Cerebral Cortex and Stroke

The cerebral cortex, often called the neocortex or cortex, is the outer layer of the brain; it contains layers of neurons that interconnect with each other and with neurons in other brain regions. There are large tracts (such as the corpus callosum) that connect cortical neurons with other cortical neurons. In lower mammals (such as the rat), the neocortex is relatively small, though still a significant structure. In higher mammals (e.g., monkeys) and especially in human beings, the cerebral cortex is much larger, mainly in total surface area and complexity of interconnection rather than thickness. This is accomplished by the cortex becoming folded or convoluted; that is, it contains gyri (e.g., the posterior central gyrus), which are convolutions, separated by sulci (e.g., the superior temporal sulcus), which are folds or fissures. The cortex is relatively (although by no means entirely) homogeneous in structure from one region to another, containing a series of layers of cells that is similar in structure throughout.

On the one hand, one might assume that the connectivity of the cerebral cortex is so extensive that it is nearly inconceivable that even a small part of it could be restored to any useful degree by cortical tissue grafts. This tends to argue against the cortex as a site where neural transplantation would be useful. On the other hand, the cerebral cortex has a remarkable ability to recover from injury, and to some extent can repair itself. Thus, if even a little could be done to "help it along," a great deal of improvement might be possible.

One fact that makes the cerebral cortex an attractive site for neural transplantation is the nature of cortical injury. Many forms of cortical injury, such as that resulting from trauma or stroke (cerebrovascular accident), can be localized quite precisely. In many cases, the consequences of such injuries become less severe with passing time, representing a process of recovery. The changes that underlie this recovery are not entirely clear, but to some extent reorganization of cortical connections may be involved. Thus, if something could be done to improve the process of recovery from cortical injury, it might be possible to apply this procedure on a case-by-case basis. Since the structure of the cortex is relatively homogeneous (but only relatively—there are many differences between one region and another), it might be possible to apply more or less the same procedure for cortical injury in a number of locations.

Is it conceivable that neural tissue transplantation could ever be applied to cortical injury caused by trauma or stroke? Consideration of this issue raises a number of interesting and complex questions. For Parkinson's disease or Huntington's disease, all cases have similar manifestations and causes; thus a standardized and uniform procedure might be developed and applied wherever appropriate. This is quite unlike cortical injury. The cerebral cortex is much larger than any subcortical structure, so injury can appear anywhere and can have a wide range of manifestations, and each case is unique.

There is a large body of literature on transplantation of cerebral cortex in animals, as well as of relevant literature on the ability of the cerebral cortex to recover from injury on its own, without transplantation. Only a fraction of this literature will be described.

Transplantation of the Cerebral Cortex in Lower Animals

After it was found that fetal cell transplants were capable of producing functional improvement in an animal model of Parkinson's disease, it was generally believed that transplants were effective in this model because application of the neurotransmitter dopamine was all that was required. The complex circuitry of the cerebral cortex was not thought to be amenable to modification by brain transplants. Donald Stein and coworkers, then at Clark University in Worcester, Massachusetts, began to look at cortical transplants in the early 1980s, and observed that some functional effects could be produced by transplantation of neural tissue into the

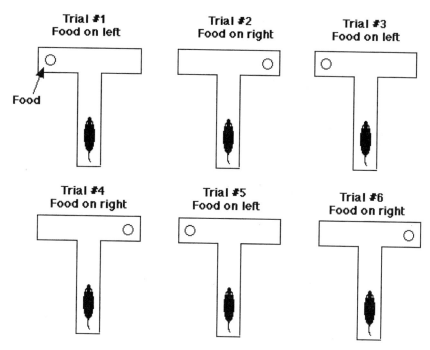

Figure 16.1
The T-maze side-alternation test used in rats. Animals are required to turn left or right in the maze. They are rewarded for turning in the direction opposite to the direction turned in the previous trial.

cerebral cortex. As it eventually turned out, these effects were more related to effects of glial cells than to transplanted neurons.

And, although it may not be possible to reconstruct major cortical circuitry via transplantation of new neurons, some modification of the outcome of cortical injury might be possible, and it even appears that some reintegration of new transplanted neurons into existing cortical circuitry following injury may occur under appropriate circumstances. In 1983, Labbe, Firl, and coworkers reported that grafts of cerebral cortex facilitated recovery from cortical injury in rats, using a test of memory-learning ability as a measurement. The test employed a T-maze, which is basically an alleyway with two arms. Animals can obtain a food reward by running down the alleyway and making either a right- or a left-hand turn (figure 16.1). The particular test used requires animals to run to one side on one trial, and to the opposite side on the next trial. Thus, when performing the test correctly, the animals turn right-left-right-left-right-left-right, etc. Consecutive turns to the same side are errors. Thus, if the animal turns right-left-right-left-left-right-left-right-left-right, it would have made nine correct choices and one error (figure 16.1).

Cortical injury was produced in rats by removing part of the frontal cortex of both sides of the brain. After recovering for a week, the animals received grafts of frontal cortex from fetal donors. The transplants were obtained from very mature fetuses, at day 22 of gestation (just prior to birth). A few days after transplantation, testing for T-maze behavior was started. The animals with transplants of neocortex improved, learning the T-maze test more rapidly than controls. The controls received cerebellar tissue grafts, and did not show improvement.

Several facets of these experiments (Labbe et al. 1983) suggested that effects of glial cells, probably related to trophic factor production, were responsible for the improvement in behavior. First, the donor tissue was taken from fetuses that were quite mature, at a stage of development when few neurons would be expected to survive transplantation, but glial cells could survive quite well. Later experiments by Kesslak, Brown, et al. (1986) found that even adult tissue grafts could produce improvement. Second, testing was begun only four to six days after transplantation, and although it was not clear exactly when the effects of transplants began to appear, it seemed that effects appeared quite early, before new connections between the transplants and the host brain could have developed. Third, in subsequent experiments, it appeared that effects of transplant showed a peculiar specificity: in a model of visual learning deficits produced by lesions of the occipital cortex (as compared with the spatial deficits produced by frontal cortex lesions), transplants of occipital cortex did not produce improvement. Surprisingly, transplants of frontal cortex did produce improvement in this model (Stein et al. 1985). These findings strongly suggested that transplants of frontal cortex are capable of producing a chemical substance which promotes functional recovery after certain types of cortical injury.

Direct evidence for a trophic type of effect was later obtained, by Kesslak and coworkers in 1986. These investigators employed a side-alternation test like the one used by Labbe and coworkers (1983), and tested three kinds of implants. The first was embryonic frontal cortex and, like Labbe and associates, Kesslak et al. found that this tissue produced improvement.

The second type of implant used was Gelfoam (a type of gelatin sponge) that had been removed from the site of cortical lesions (in different rats) after having been left in the animals for ten days. While it remains in the injury site, proteins accumulate in the Gelfoam. The Gelfoam pieces were then removed and placed in tissue culture dishes containing neurons. The Gelfoam accumulated trophic activity (i.e., proteins accumulated in the Gelfoam), as defined by the pieces' ability to increase the survival of cultured neurons. Astrocytes also migrated into the Gelfoam from the surrounding brain. These conditioned Gelfoam implants produced behavioral improvement when transplanted to the cortex of animals with lesions. Finally, transplants of cultured astrocytes produced improvement similar to that produced by cortical transplants or by the conditioned Gelfoam implants. These findings strongly support the conclusion that glial cells, or chemical substances produced by glial cells, are responsible for the improvements in maze performance produced by cortical tissue transplants.

The above provides the reason, in fact, that the chapter on cortical injury is included in part IV "localized effects." There is little—or probably no—evidence that cortical tissue transplants can produce behavioral improvement by restoring the complex connectivity that mediates the bulk of the functioning of the cerebral cortex. Instead, it seems likely that when cortical tissue transplants do produce behavioral improvement, they do so by secreting chemical substances that promote restructuring and recovery in circuits adjacent to the grafts.

Since the series of experiments by Labbe, Stein, Kesslak, Cotman, and their associates, a number of other studies have described effects of cortical tissue transplants in rat models. In some cases, transplants produce behavioral improvements after cortical injury, while in other cases, no improvements are seen. Whether or not cortical transplants "work" seems to depend upon a large number of factors, including the particular type of test and type of cortical injury that is used, and the type of tissue used for transplantation.

Especially important, apparently, is the time at which the transplants are made in relationship to the time at which the cortical injury occurs. When lesions and transplants are made at the same time (Kesslak, Brown, et al. 1986), or when there is a long delay between lesioning and transplantation, cortical transplants are generally not effective. Experiments by Kolb and coworkers (1988), and by Dunnett, Ryan, et al. (1987), found that transplants improved performance on a maze-learning test early after transplantation, but if the animals were tested at longer time intervals after transplantation, their performance was worse. This literature has been reviewed in detail by Kolb and Fantie (1994), and in general it appears that most of the effects of cortical grafts on recovery of function after injury are likely to be due to the secretion of chemical substances rather than to the development of new connections with the host brain.

One interesting series of experiments on cortical tissue transplantation that has obtained relatively consistent improvement employed a model of taste-aversion learning and lesions of the gustatory cortex. Taste-aversion learning, or conditioned taste aversion, is a specialized form of learning that occurs for the purpose of allowing animals to avoid ingesting substances which have made them ill. In its natural habitat, if an animal eats a new food and then becomes ill, it will learn to avoid that food. To test this type of learning in the laboratory, a specialized procedure has been employed (figure 16.2). Animals are allowed to drink a pleasant-tasting but novel beverage; often a saccharin solution, or water with chocolate, orange, almond, or other flavoring is used. Within a few hours, animals are injected with something that makes them mildly ill. Often lithium chloride is used, but drugs such as amphetamine may be used as well. Animals will then learn to avoid the novel fluid that they recently ingested, associating it with the illness they experienced. The animals do not, however, experience this as a conscious decision. (Even when humans experience this type of learning, it is probably not as a conscious decision.)

Bermudez-Rattoni and coworkers have studied effects of cortical tissue transplants on conditioned taste-aversion learning in rats (Fernandez-Ruiz et al. 1991; Escobar et al. 1989; Bermudez-Rattoni et al. 1987). For these studies, the gustatory neocortex was removed, which impairs the

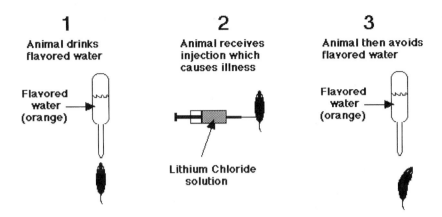

1
Animal drinks
flavored water

Flavored
water ──→
(orange)

2
Animal receives
injection which
causes illness

Lithium Chloride
solution

3
Animal then avoids
flavored water

Flavored
water ──→
(orange)

Figure 16.2
Conditioned taste-aversion learning. Animals are allowed to drink a novel but pleasant-tasting fluid, such as saccharin- or orange-flavored water. The animals are then injected with a drug that causes a mild illness, often lithium chloride. When the animals are then allowed access to the flavored water a second time, they avoid it. This avoidance is due to an association of the drug-induced illness with the flavored water; if the animal in the wild encountered a novel food or fluid that caused illness, this would permit the animal to avoid ingestion of this substance and thus avoid poisoning itself. This kind of learning has unique features that distinguish it from more common forms of conditioning, such as maze learning.

ability of rats to acquire a conditioned taste aversion. Then the corresponding area of cortex from fetal animals was transplanted into the area from which cortex had been removed. This procedure produced a significant recovery of taste-aversion learning two months after transplantation. Transplantation of tissue from other parts of the cortex produced no improvement, or possibly a slight improvement only (figure 16.3).

In this series of experiments, several factors suggest that the effects are due to specific properties of the transplants rather than to general tissue disruption or other nonspecific factors. First, significant improvement was not seen when tissue from other parts of the neocortex was transplanted into the lesioned area. Second, there was evidence that the transplants established connections with the host brain. The time course of the development of these new connections between the graft and the host brain roughly paralleled the development of behavioral improvement.

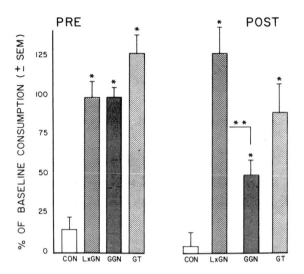

Figure 16.3
Effects of cortical grafts on conditioned taste aversion (figure 16.2). Rats were tested for conditioned taste aversion prior to transplantation ("pre") and eight weeks after transplantation ("post"). Numbers indicate percentage of baseline fluid consumption, so that decreases (lower numbers) indicate aversion to the fluid, and thus an ability to perform the test. Before transplantation, controls avoided the fluid while the other three groups all had lesions of the gustatory neocortex and thus performed poorly. The LxGN group did not receive a graft, and thus performed poorly after transplantation as well. The GGN group received grafts of gustatory neocortex. Conditioned taste aversion in these animals recovered, although not completely, as seen by the decrease in saccharin consumption compared with the LxGN group. The GT animals received grafts of fetal tectum as a control, and they did not recover. The two asterisks indicate that the decrease in fluid consumption in the GGN group is statistically significant, compared with the LxGN group. (From Escobar et al. 1989, with permission.)

Acetylcholine production by transplanted tissue appeared to be the major factor in the improvement of conditioned taste-aversion learning (Miranda et al. 1997; Lopez-Garcia et al. 1990). Interestingly, the grafts of gustatory neocortex, which produced behavioral improvement, released acetylcholine in response to stimulation, but control grafts (of occipital cortex) did not. Since NGF promotes development and growth of CNS acetylcholinergic systems, effects of NGF in this system were examined. NGF was found to accelerate the time course of improvement, but it did not change the ultimate degree of recovery (Diaz-Cintra et al. 1995).

NGF had no effect in animals without grafts, nor did it alter recovery in animals with grafts from other cortical regions (occipital cortex). This suggests that the production of acetylcholine by gustatory neocortex grafts is a key factor in the production of behavioral recovery in this model.

A few additional experiments should be mentioned in this connection. Experiments by Arendt and coworkers (1988) showed that memory deficits in animals produced by chronic alcohol treatment could be alleviated by grafts into the neocortex that contain acetylcholine. Later experiments by this group (Bruckner and Arendt 1992) showed that purified astrocytes also were effective, using the same model of alcohol-induced memory deficits. Another experiment, by Welner and coworkers (1990), found that adrenal chromaffin cells grafts in the cerebral cortex (which certainly could not have become integrated into the host neural circuitry) produced improvement in the T-maze alternation performance. These grafts also increased acetylcholine in adjacent parts of the cortex. In summary, these various experiments seem to point to an important role of acetylcholine in neocortical grafts that produce behavioral improvement.

One might suspect, therefore, that the cases in which cortical grafts can produce behavioral improvement are those in which increases in acetylcholine production are sufficient to cause behavioral improvement. In such cases, when grafts are successful in increasing acetylcholinergic activity, either by supplying acetylcholine or by augmenting the acetylcholine-producing ability of nearby host neurons, behavioral improvement may be seen. Or, more generally, when simple augmentation of some existing aspect of neuronal function (such as increased neurotransmitter release, or promotion of collateral sprouting) will suffice, behavioral improvement can be produced. Perhaps where other, more complex functions are needed—for example, replacement of entire circuits—cortical grafts are not as likely to be effective. Although consistent with available data, this conclusion is, at this point, merely speculative.

Selective Cortical Injury

Most of the studies that have been described thus far have approached the repair of cortical injury from the standpoint of attempting to obtain recovery of function—usually a learning or memory test—by some approach, and then of trying to determine how it worked. As it has turned out, for the most part, some of these experiments have partially succeeded in obtaining behavioral improvements, but these improvements do not seem to have been caused by complete integration of the grafts with the host cortical circuits. Perhaps this is for the best—the cortex certainly requires complex synaptic interconnectivity, and we may ultimately be much more successful in providing materials or chemical factors that assist the cortex in completing its own repairs (more or less) than in attempting to "rewire" the cortex (which may be more or less impossible).

A parallel approach to the repair of cortical injury might be to produce cortical transplants that become integrated into the host circuitry to as great a degree as possible, through gradual refinement of methods. Then, once the transplantation method has been optimized, the next step could be to determine whether these grafts can improve behavioral function. This approach is under way, although it has not yet obtained behavioral improvements.

Although there have been many experiments on integration of cortical tissue grafts with the host brain, certainly the most sophisticated so far have been the experiments by J. D. Macklis (1993). They involve a unique approach to the production of very locally restricted cortical injury. Rather than injuring the cortex by removing an area of tissue, specific populations of neurons are damaged with a unique toxic chemical. The way this works is as follows (see figure 16.4 for illustration). The chemical, clorin e_6, is injected in another part of the brain, near the terminals of some axons that originate from the neocortex (rather than injecting it near the cell bodies). Axons in the vicinity of the injection take up the toxin and transport it to their cell bodies. Other axons not coming from the neocortex also may take up the toxin.

Clorin e_6 is not normally toxic to neurons. It is toxic only when it is activated by laser light, which causes it to produce oxygen radicals. These oxygen radicals are toxic to neurons, but do not diffuse through tissue (they can diffuse less than one micrometer, which is less than the size of a neuron). Thus, clorin e_6 is toxic only when it is inside a

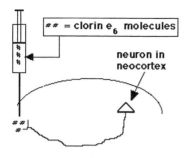

1. Clorin e$_6$ injected near axon
terminals

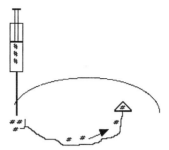

2. Clorin e$_6$ transported back to
cell bodies

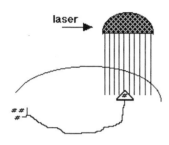

3. Clorin e$_6$ illuminated by
670 nm laser

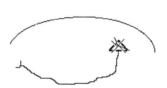

4. Clorin e$_6$ produces oxygen radicals
which kill target neurons

Figure 16.4
The method for destroying selected populations of neurons in the cerebral cortex used by Macklis (1993). The dye clorin e$_6$ is injected near the synaptic terminals of any target population of cortical neurons. This dye is transported by these neurons back to their cell bodies. When the dye is illuminated by a laser that can pass through tissue, oxygen radicals that kill the neuron are generated. These reactive oxygen radicals can diffuse only very short distances, and thus do not kill neighboring cells.

cell (in this case, a neuron) *and* only when the toxin is activated by laser illumination.

The next step is to illuminate a part of the neocortex with laser light of a particular wavelength has the ability to penetrate directly through brain tissue, for a distance of several millimeters, and activate the clorin e_6, which in turn damages the neurons in which the dye resides. The dye is present only in neurons that have axons projecting to the injection area, so only a fraction of cortical neurons in the appropriate area are injured. Glial cells, fibers, blood vessels, and most of the neurons in the vicinity are uninjured. This produces a very limited lesion, without extensive scarring and without stimulating repair processes such as gliosis, which can interfere with the normal brain structure.

Macklis (1993) reported on experiments that employed this model system to study the ability of transplanted neurons to become integrated with the host brain. These experiments used immature animals, 14–15 days old, as hosts for transplantation. Under conditions when cortical neurons from embryonic mice were transplanted adjacent to the areas of neuronal loss in the host cortex, some of the donor neurons migrated up to approximately 1 mm, to appropriate positions in the areas from which neurons had been lost. Moreover, the transplanted neurons that migrated developed shapes similar to normal pyramidal neurons, resembling the major population of neurons that had been destroyed. The transplanted neurons also began to send out processes. Thus, the transplanted neurons were able to become quite well integrated into the host brain structure, apparently occupying places that were vacated by neurons that had been destroyed.

Many control conditions were used, to demonstrate that this neuronal substitution could take place only under these selective lesion conditions. When larger lesions were made using kainic acid and when the host animals were not lesioned, or when other types of neurons (such as cells from the cerebellum) were transplanted, the transplanted neurons did not migrate into appropriate positions, nor did they assume a pyramidal shape. Thus, when a select population of neurons is removed, without injury to other brain components, transplanted neurons can to some degree substitute for the neurons that are removed—at least, in immature animals.

Can Cortical Transplants Be Used in Human Stroke Patients?

We now return to the issue posed at the beginning of this chapter. Again, there are two aspects to this problem. First, cortical transplants might be used to assist the cortex in completing its own repair and recovery processes. This seems to be a possibility, and in some animal experiments, improvements in behavior consistent with this kind of effect have been obtained. These effects are, however, capricious, in the sense that improvement is seen only for certain behavioral tests, and for certain conditions of testing. Recent experiments using modified tumor cells that have been treated to promote neuronal differentiation and inhibit growth, have observed behavioral improvements in animals (Borlongan et al. 1998), and a similar procedure has been tried in a human subject (cf. Fackelmann 1998). In some circumstances, such as when transplants are made at long time intervals after the injury, transplantation of cortical tissue into the site of injury can make matters worse, at least as judged by behavioral testing in rats. These results are, therefore, not especially encouraging for prospects of using cortical tissue transplantation in human subjects.

In addition, there is the possibility of attempting to reconstitute cortical circuitry, in such a way that the transplanted cortical tissue becomes part of the host cortical circuitry. In animals, this can be accomplished to some degree. The real question at this point, however, is whether functional recovery can be produced as a result of this reconstructed circuitry, as opposed to an incidental effect on adjacent circuits that are not part of the transplant. This approach also raises many ancillary issues: How can effects directly related to the cortical tissue grafts be sorted out, and separated from facilitatory effects on intact host circuits? If such behavioral recovery can be obtained, what would it mean for the integrity of the organism? We will return to these issues in the concluding chapter.

Further Reading

Chen, K. S., and Gage, F. H. (1994). Transplantation, aging, and memory. In *Functional Neural Transplantation,* S. B. Dunnett and A. Bjorklund (eds.), pp. 295–315. Raven Press, New York.

Freed, W. J. (1991b). Brain tissue grafting and human applications. *J. Neurosurg. Anesthesiol.* 3: 167–169.

Kolb, B., and Fantie, B. (1994). Cortical graft function in adult and neonatal rats. In *Functional Neural Transplantation,* S. B. Dunnett and A. Bjorklund (eds.), pp. 415–436. Raven Press, New York.

Sharp, F. R. (1993). Transplants for stroke patients? *Ann. Neurol.* 34: 322–323.

Sinden, J. D., Gray, J. A., and Hodges, H. (1994). Cholinergic grafts and cognitive function. In *Functional Neural Transplantation,* S. B. Dunnett and A. Bjorklund (eds.), pp. 253–291. Raven Press, New York.

Stein, D. G. (1991). Fetal brain tissue grafting as therapy for brain dysfunctions: Unanswered questions, unknown factors, and practical concerns. *J. Neurosurg. Anesthesiol.* 3: 170–189.

V

Circuit Reconstruction

17

Huntington's Disease

Background

Like Parkinson's disease, Huntington's disease, or Huntington's chorea, is a degenerative disorder that involves the loss of a restricted population of neurons. The neurons which are lost are largely those located in the neostriatum, although there are also losses of neurons in other brain regions. In a similar manner to Parkinson's disease, Huntington's disease develops in adults, although unlike Parkinson's disease, it develops in young adults and has a clear genetic basis. The abnormal gene responsible for Huntington's disease, IT15, is located at the end of chromosome 4 (Huntington's Disease Collaborative Research Group 1993; Goodfellow 1993). However, knowing the location of the gene responsible for Huntington's disease has not yet led to great advances in understanding or treating this disease, because no one knows exactly how the product of this abnormal gene causes Huntington's disease. We know this gene produces an abnormal protein, but we do not yet know how the abnormal protein leads to the death of neurons. This finding may ultimately yield information of therapeutic value.

Huntington's disease is a progressive neurodegenerative disorder with an onset often between ages 35 and 55. Symptoms may initially appear in considerably younger or older patients. It is a relatively rare disorder, appearing in approximately 50–100 per million individuals. The disease involves characteristic rapid, involuntary jerking or writhing choreiform movements, as well as rigidity, dystonia, and difficulty in speaking and swallowing. In addition to these abnormal movements, patients with Huntington's disease may develop personality changes and psychiatric symptoms, especially depression. The depression is probably secondary to the motor abnormalities, since it often develops prior to the appearance of any other symptom (Folstein 1989). The disease is inexorably progressive, eventually leading to death. There is no effective treatment, although neuroleptic drugs (dopamine receptor blockers) may produce slight, and temporary, reductions in symptom severity. Other potentially effective drug treatments, designed to slow progression of the disease, are being investigated.

A very detailed understanding of the genetic basis of Huntington's disease has been developed since the mid-1980s as the result of an extraordinary and concerted collaborative research effort. In 1993, it was found that the IT15 gene causes Huntington's disease when it terminates with an excessive number of trinucleotide repeats. This trinucleotide repeat consists mainly of a long string of CAGs, which code for the amino acid glutamine. This results in the addition of a long string of glutamines to the encoded protein, which has been called "huntingtin."

Normal individuals have the same protein, but with between 9 and 34 glutamines. If the number of glutamines is extended to 35 or more, the patient develops Huntington's disease. There may be some uncertainty when the number of CAG repeats is between 30 and 40. Generally, however, there is a rough correlation between the number of CAG repeats and severity of the disease. Patients with a large number of repeats, say more than 80, have an early age of onset and very severe disease.

There is strong evidence that the huntingtin protein causes disease by a gain of function rather than a loss of normal function. That is, it does something, in some way toxic, that the normal protein does not do. The main evidence for this conclusion is that homozygotes (patients with the abnormality in both copies of their DNA) do not have a more severe form of the disease than heterozygotes. If an absence of the normal functions of huntingtin caused the disorder, homozygotes (who would have none of the normal form of the protein) should have a very severe form of the disease. Thus, the presence of the abnormal protein is somehow damaging. Another interesting fact is that huntingtin is expressed in many tissues other than in the brain. Even within the brain, it is expressed not only in the striatum but in other places as well. Even expression in the striatum is not especially high. Therefore, it seems reasonable to guess that huntingtin containing more than 35 glutamine residues is somehow "toxic" for certain populations of neurons. In this context, "toxic" must be defined liberally: it could be something as indirect as an effect on transcription of an entirely separate factor.

It is a curious fact that the first signs of Huntington's disease usually develop in adulthood, well after the susceptible neuronal populations have been established, and well after most—probably nearly all—of the connections of these neurons with other cells have developed. Even the behavioral functions that are subserved by these neurons and their connections are well established prior to disease onset. Thus, even though the system is functioning normally, in midlife the abnormal form of huntingtin causes striatal neurons (and certain other neurons) to begin to degenerate. How this occurs is unknown, and on the face of it is quite mysterious. Currently, it seems most likely that the product of the abnormal gene interacts with other proteins in the striatum to form insoluble aggregates which eventually accumulate and become toxic (Li et al. 1995; Martindale et al. 1998).

In 1976, it was discovered by Coyle and Schwarcz, and by McGeer and McGeer, that the neurotoxic chemical kainic acid, when locally injected into the striatum, produces death of striatal neurons. Prior to that, it had been known for some time that kainic acid and several other compounds, which stimulate receptors for the neurotransmitter glutamic acid, were capable of destroying neurons. These "excitotoxic" chemicals excite (or activate) neurons by opening ion channels that are coupled to glutamate receptors. Opening of these ion channels causes a movement of electrically charged ions across the cell membrane into the cell, resulting in its activation. Normally, when neurons are activated by synaptic inputs, the ion channels coupled to glutamate open only briefly, and only a relative few open at any one moment. When these channels are activated by injection of glutamate or kainic acid, many channels are opened for long periods of time. This apparently disturbs the ionic composition of the cell, and may culminate in cell death through a mechanism that has been termed excitotoxicity. Kainic acid was noted to produce a pattern of cell death and biochemical changes in the striatum which resembles that seen in Huntington's disease (McGeer and McGeer 1976; Coyle and Schwarcz 1976).

Because of this similarity, animals with lesions of the striatum induced by kainic acid, or sometimes by the related compounds ibotenic acid and quinolinic acid (Beal et al. 1991; Sanberg, Calderon, et al. 1989), have been used to test experimental therapies. Rodents, and recently primates, with excitotoxic lesions of the striatum have been used as animal models for experiments on neural transplantation. Since 1976, there has been considerable speculation as to whether Huntington's disease is actually caused by excitotoxicity or a similar phenomenon. Although this continues to be a reasonable possibility—quinolinic acid in particular is a candidate for the damaging agent (Beal et al. 1991)—direct evidence that this is the case is incomplete. There are other possible mechanisms through which striatal neurons might be damaged.

There have been two kinds of transplantation studies related to Huntington's disease. One kind aims to prevent the degenerative changes in Huntington's disease models. For such studies, cells that produce a neurotrophic factor are transplanted to the striatum. The neurotrophic factors that have been used in this manner are, mainly, nerve growth factor (NGF) and ciliary neurotrophic factor (CNTF). Subsequent to transplantation of growth factor-producing cells, an excitotoxic substance is injected into the striatum and the extent of damage is measured. Both NGF and CNTF have been found to alleviate striatal lesions produced in this manner. (Some additional details on these experiments are presented in chapter 23.) Although these experiments are very promising, they depend on how accurately the excitotoxic lesion model reflects the actual cause of injury in Huntington's disease, which is unknown.

The second type of experiment on neuronal transplantation and Huntington's disease aims to reconstruct the striatum *after* it has been damaged. For this type of experiment, the route through which damage occurs is of less importance, since the end result (the neurons are lost) is the same. Thus, the model is sufficiently similar to the human condition—at least, the scope of degeneration is similar to that seen in humans—that excitotoxic lesions of the striatum provide a very useful model for studies of reconstruction of the striatum by neuronal tissue transplantation.

Nevertheless, it should be emphasized that animals with excitotoxic lesions of the striatum do not show motor abnormalities that are similar to those seen in humans with Huntington's disease. These animals do show motor changes and behavioral deficits: they may be hyperactive, or show impaired coordination or deficits in maze-learning ability. Most of the tests for the functional impairment associated with excitotoxic lesions that have been used do not have very good face validity; that is, the impairments do not appear to be very similar to the motor symptoms of Huntington's disease. Therefore, one of the main challenges in this area has been the development of tests for functional impairment in animals that provide reasonable means of measuring the ability of transplants to restore the behavior to normal, and that appear likely to be capable of predicting clinical effectiveness in humans.

Transplantation and Reconstruction of Circuits

Compared with Parkinson's disease, there are several significant obstacles to the use of transplantation as a treatment for Huntington's disease. Certain aspects of Parkinson's disease physiology seem to favor transplantation therapy. For instance, the dopaminergic neurons in the substantia nigra (SN) fire at a fairly constant rate; in fact, at least superficial examination suggests that these neurons seem to function with little change in response to the environment. Thus, repair of this system might conceivably be accomplished even if the transplanted neurons are deprived of most of their normal inputs. Second, the SN dopaminergic neurons project mainly to a relatively restricted region of the brain, the caudate putamen.

In contrast, the *medium spiny projection neurons* of the caudate putamen, the most important population of neurons that degenerates in Huntington's disease, form part of a complex circuit that presumably would have to be reconstructed, at least in part, to obtain therapeutic efficacy (figure 17.1). Significant components of the damaged circuitry include at least inputs from the cerebral cortex and substantia nigra to these neurons (which are certainly essential); other relatively minor, but probably still important, inputs (including inputs from neurons in the striatum); and important output pathways to both the globus pallidus and the substantia nigra. Thus, the medium spiny neurons form part of a relay circuit that integrates inputs from several places, at least two of which are quite far apart (cerebral cortex and substantia nigra pars compacta), and sends

Afferents from cortex

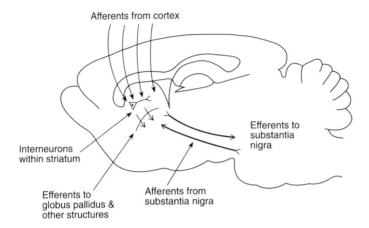

Efferents to
substantia
nigra

Interneurons
within striatum

Efferents to
globus pallidus &
other structures

Afferents from
substantia nigra

Figure 17.1
Schematic representation of the connections formed by striatal neurons. At least
some of these connections would have to be replaced to obtain functional restoration by transplantation of neurons into the striatum following striatal injury.

major outputs to two additional places, which also are quite far from
each other (globus pallidus and substantia nigra pars reticulata). In addition, the outputs from these neurons comprise links in a highly complex
circuit.

In Parkinson's disease, by contrast, it seems that (a) the inputs to dopaminergic neurons are not essential, at least for some aspects of behavior,
and (b) some of the inputs to these neurons arise from the place to which
the neurons project (the striatum). It may be that these unique features
of Parkinson's disease are a reason that grafts are at least partly effective,
and that the neurons can be placed into the striatum.

In Huntington's disease, the affected neurons almost certainly perform
a complex integrating function. At least some of these circuits would
probably have to be restored, at least partly, in order to obtain improvements. The particular circuit that is thought to be most important
in the abnormal movements of Huntington's disease involves the GABA-
mediated inputs to the globus pallidus, and in all probability at least some
of this circuit would have to be repaired. The important conclusion from
all of this is that although there is some evidence that fetal transplants
can produce some improvements in animal models of Huntington's dis-

ease, it is not certain that such transplants would result in therapeutic improvement in human patients. This uncertainty is compounded by the lack of homology between most of the behavioral changes seen in the animal model and the human disease. Thus, a behavior that is affected by transplants in an animal model may not be "the same," from a neural circuit standpoint, as the clinical manifestations of Huntington's disease.

Is it possible, on the other hand, that the assumption that grafts in Huntington's disease would have to perform a complex integrating function is wrong? Could improvement in Huntington's disease and the corresponding animal models—even a little improvement—be obtained by grafts that release a neurotransmitter? Perhaps grafts that release GABA (one of the major neurotransmitters of the medium spiny neurons) into the striatum, or into the globus pallidus, would somehow alleviate the motor dysfunction, or produce other, even minor, beneficial effects. Perhaps some damaged circuits could be made more functional by administering GABA-producing cells into the region, or by some similar manipulation. This possibility cannot yet be discounted.

Experiments in Rodents

The first experiment on transplanting tissue into the brain in an animal model of Huntington's disease (Deckel et al. 1983) employed the following scheme. First, adult rats received bilateral lesions of the neostriatum with kainic acid. Such animals are somewhat hyperactive; that is, when placed into devices which measure their locomotor activity (how much walking around they do), lesioned animals are more active than animals without lesions. The measure of activity used in the first study was the number of movement episodes rather than the total amount of movement. During the hour interval from 30 to 90 minutes after the animals were placed in activity-measuring boxes, the lesioned animals were hyperactive. Normal ("sham" lesioned) animals showed approximately 140 movement episodes, while the rats with kainic acid lesions showed about 225 movement episodes.

There were three groups of animals: (1) three basically normal rats that received sham lesions and, one week later, sham transplantation; (2) six rats that received lesions of the striatum and sham transplantation; and

Table 17.1
Approximate activity episodes per 30 minutes

	Time after start of activity testing		
Group	30–60 Min	60–90 Min	90–120 Min
Control (no lesion)	80	59	60
Lesioned (no transplant)	129	96	56
Lesioned plus transplant	63	32	71

Adapted from Deckel et al. 1983.

(3) six rats that received transplants one week after receiving lesions of the striatum. The last group of animals received striatal tissue transplants from 18-day gestational rat fetuses, in solid form, into the lesioned striatum.

The animals were tested 12 weeks after transplantation. The animals with striatal transplants did not show hyperactivity but were similar to the controls; actually, they were slightly less active, although this difference was not statistically significant. Thus, the animals with kainic acid lesions of the striatum and sham transplants showed a behavioral abnormality that was not seen in animals that had received transplants. Activity was measured in this study when the animals were first placed in activity-measuring chambers, which indicates activity related to exploration. After 90 minutes, when the animals presumably were finished with their exploration, the groups were not statistically different (see table 17.1).

Limitations of this first experiment (which was quite preliminary) include the facts that no tissue was implanted in the control group, that the number of animals was small, and that behavioral testing was limited. Also, the tendency for the transplanted animals to be less active than the controls suggests that there probably should have been a group that received transplants but no lesions, in order to determine whether the transplants themselves decreased activity. Most of these questions have been addressed in later experiments, for example, the studies by Deckel et al. (1986) and Deckel and Robinson (1987). The latter study showed that transplantation reduced spontaneous locomotor activity by several measures, but transplants did not alter hyperactivity induced by amphetamine. Transplants also did not improve deficits that were measured by a neurological examination designed to test sensorimotor function.

There have been many subsequent experiments on the reversal of behavioral and motor function deficits by transplantation of fetal tissue into the striatum. There is a consensus that striatal transplants can, at least to some degree, reverse some of the behavioral abnormalities in animals with striatal injury. The hyperactivity test that has been most frequently employed has, however, proved to be an inconsistent indicator of striatal injury (see Koutouzis et al. 1994). It is not clear to what degree animals are generally hyperactive after striatal lesions. In some studies, persistent hyperactivity has been found (Giordano et al. 1988; Isacson et al. 1986; Sanberg, Giordano et al. 1989). In some cases, however, animals may show hyperactivity only at certain times (Giordano et al. 1988). Giordano and coworkers (1990) found that in some animals, kainic acid lesions of the striatum did not produce hyperactivity in response to amphetamine. Deckel and Robinson (1987) found that the hyperactivity gradually disappeared in male rats, but persisted for long periods of time in female rats. Nevertheless, the important point is that when hyperactivity is found after striatal injury (as it usually is, at least to some degree), it generally is eliminated almost entirely by striatal grafts.

A variety of additional tests have been used. Giordano and coworkers (1990) found improvements in tests of catalepsy (a trancelike state, induced by haloperidol, in which animals do not respond to their environment) and in some measures of motor coordination. Isacson et al. (1986) employed measures of learning.

Interestingly, control grafts of tissue from cerebral cortex and tectum also produce some behavioral improvements (Giordano et al. 1990). This clearly suggests that some effects of striatal transplants may depend on the release of chemical substances from grafts rather than on reintegration of the striatal neural circuitry. By comparison, very similar experiments were performed in animals with substantia nigra lesions (the Parkinson's disease model), using the same two tissues (cerebral cortex and tectum) as controls (W. J. Freed 1983; W. J. Freed, Ko et al. 1983). In this case, improvements were produced only by the substantia nigra grafts; the control grafts of tectal and cortical tissue had no effect. This suggests that improvement in the substantia nigra lesion model depends on release of a specific neurotransmitter, while improvement in the Huntington's disease model may depend in part on the release of trophic factors or other effects that are more general properties of neural tissue function.

As mentioned, most of the earlier tests that were used to measure functional impairment associated with excitotoxic lesions do not have very good face validity; that is, the deficits do not appear very similar to the motor symptoms of Huntington's disease. More recently, more sophisticated tests of motor function have been used (Dunnett, Isacson et al. 1988; Montoya et al. 1990). One rodent model that seems quite analogous to measurement of impaired human motor function was reported by Dunnett and coworkers in 1988 and by Montoya and coworkers in 1990. These investigators employed a test of animals' ability to retrieve food pellets by reaching through a narrow opening in the floor, using each paw separately (see figure 10.4). Impairments in performance of this test are induced both by lesions of the striatum and by lesions of the substantia nigra, using 6-hydroxydopamine (see chapter 10, section "Behavioral Tests"). Two sets of animals received either type of lesion, and also received either no graft, substantia nigra grafts, or striatal tissue grafts. The tissue used for transplantation was obtained from embryonic day 14 donors. This is somewhat more immature than the tissue used for most of the earlier experiments on hyperactivity. It was found that improvements in paw-reaching were obtained only in animals that had striatal lesions and received striatal grafts (see table 17. 2). Control grafts of substantia nigra did not produce improvement, and even substantia nigra grafts in animals with substantia nigra lesions did not produce improvement.

Even here, however, the improvement seen was fairly small. Nonetheless, this is definitely one of the most convincing studies. An especially important fact is that the paw-reaching is obviously a test of a deficit, as opposed to tests such as locomotion, where hyperactivity may be a very indirect indicator of a deficit state. Especially, decreases in hyperactivity are not necessarily an indication that the deficit has been corrected. On the other hand, it is still possible that paw-reaching is indicative of deficits in processes other than motor coordination per se; particularly, changes

Table 17.2
Effects of striatal grafts on deficits in paw-reaching behavior

Type of Lesion	Type of Graft	Result after 3 Months (number of pellets retrieved*)
none	none	11–12
substantia nigra	none	7–8
substantia nigra	substantia nigra	7–8
substantia nigra	striatum	6–7
striatum	none	6
striatum	substantia nigra	6
striatum	striatum	8–9

From Montoya et al. 1990.
* Retrieval of 14 pellets represents perfect performance.

in motivation to obtain the pellets could be involved. Nevertheless, it is clear that (1) inability to reach the pellets is an indication of a deficit state, and (2) correction of this deficit by transplants indicates that transplants are producing an effect which is relatively specific, and cannot be explained in terms of additional injury or impairment.

Connections of Striatal Grafts

Transplantation of fetal striatum into the striatum of animals with excitotoxic lesions of the striatum results in formation of a graft having a fairly well integrated structure with many striatal properties. The grafts contain neurotransmitters and neurotransmitter receptors characteristic of the normal striatum. Grafts generally contain these normal components irrespective of the graft location or surrounding environment, although sometimes they have a patchy distribution that is not typical of the normal striatum.

It is generally presumed, as has been discussed above, that striatal tissue grafts could not be entirely effective if they simply released a neurotransmitter. The principal neurons that must be replaced are the medium spiny neurons, and as has already been described, these neurons make a number of important connections with widely dispersed nuclei. Although it may not be essential to re-form all of the connections of striatal neurons to obtain a partial restitution of function, it is thought that some degree of reconnection is required.

A series of very thorough studies of the connections formed by striatal tissue grafts has been performed by Wictorin and coworkers (e.g., Wictorin et al. 1989). Generally, striatal tissue transplants form connections with most of the regions that normally connect with the striatum, although the connections formed by grafts are much less extensive than normal. The major efferent projection from striatal grafts appears to be the globus pallidus. Striatal grafts receive inputs from a number of brain regions, including cortex, thalamus, dopaminergic projections from the SN, and serotonergic projections from the raphe nucleus. Compared with the normal connections of the striatum, the connections of striatal grafts are quite minor, and it is not clear whether they are sufficient to mediate behavioral restoration.

It might be suspected that the degree to which connections form with striatal grafts depend upon the circumstances, in relation to the host brain, under which the grafts are made. In other words, a graft implanted shortly after a striatal lesion might form extensive connections, while a graft implanted long after a lesion occurs might form less extensive connections. It is possible that a graft implanted *prior* to a lesion would be even more effective in forming new connections. It is also probable that grafts would develop more extensive connections when transplanted into relatively immature hosts. Because genetic testing can be used to predict who will develop Huntington's disease, these possibilities have implications for potential clinical studies. This is discussed further at the end of this chapter.

Possibilities for Transplantation to Produce Trophic Effects and Prevent Neuronal Loss

The degeneration of striatal neurons in Huntington's disease may be caused by a toxic agent, or by the lack of a necessary trophic or supporting agent of some type, or by some injury that could be mitigated by the presence of a trophic factor. It might be reasonable to attempt to alter the degenerative course of the disease by providing a trophic agent, through secretion from a transplant or by some other means. Although this possi-

bility cannot be pursued systematically unless the biochemical events that precipitate the disease are better understood, there have been studies that suggest trophic factors can mitigate or decrease the excitotoxic brain injury in animal models (e.g., Aloe 1987).

Some data suggest that at least some part of the behavioral improvement induced by striatal transplants may involve trophic effects. For example, behavioral recovery may begin prior to the development of new connections of the grafts, and the connections of striatal grafts are not very extensive. Moreover, behavioral improvement can be produced by grafts of several tissues other than striatum; for example, tectal tissue and cortical tissue, as in the experiment by Giordano discussed above.

The possibility of alleviating striatal injury with trophic factors has been explored systematically by Frim and coworkers, using cells that have been genetically engineered to produce growth factors (figure 17.2). The technology for altering cells to produce growth factors is discussed in detail in chapter 23. For the moment, it is enough for the reader to know that cells can be altered so that they produce nerve growth factor (NGF) or any similar growth factor, but often the production of growth factors decreases gradually when the cells are transplanted into the brain.

Frim, Short, et al. (1993) employed a Huntington's disease model in which striatal neurons were destroyed by the excitatory toxin quinolinic acid. For this study, rat fibroblasts that can be grown in tissue culture (Rat 1 cells) were modified to produce NGF. These cells were transplanted into the corpus callosum of rats, just above the striatum, and cells that had not been modified were used as a control. Seven days after the cells had been implanted, quinolinic acid was infused to lesion the striatum. When the animals were examined after 18 days, it was found that the NGF-producing cell grafts had decreased the size of the lesions markedly, and in particular resulted in an increase in the numbers of acetylcholine-producing neurons that survived the lesioning. By comparison with animals that had not received grafts, or that had received grafts of the original Rat 1 cells, the size of the lesions had been reduced by about 80 percent. Interestingly, the NGF-producing grafts did not decrease the size of the lesions on the opposite side of the brain. Thus, it appeared that the distance over which the secretion of NGF was effective was limited to a few millimeters.

1. Insert gene for nerve growth factor (NGF) or ciliary neurotrophic factor (CNTF) into rat fibroblasts or other cells

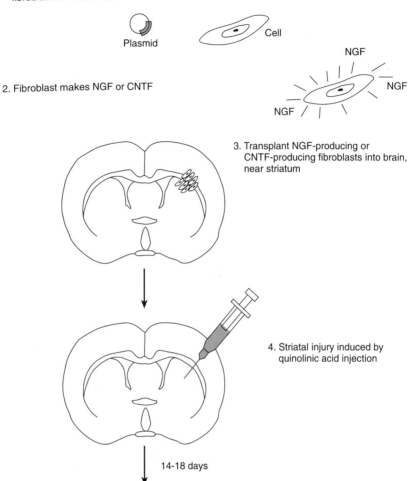

2. Fibroblast makes NGF or CNTF

3. Transplant NGF-producing or CNTF-producing fibroblasts into brain, near striatum

4. Striatal injury induced by quinolinic acid injection

14-18 days

5. Animals with NGF or CNTF-producing grafts show on the order of 80% less damage than controls

Figure 17.2
Experimental scheme for studies by Frim, Short, et al. (1993) and by Emerich, Hammang, et al. (1994), Emerich, Lidner, et al. (1996), and Emerich, Winn, et al. (1997) showing that transplants which secrete growth factors can protect against chemically induced striatal degeneration.

In the Frim et al. experiment, the NGF-producing cells were for the most part found to have stopped producing NGF by 7 to 18 days after transplantation, even though the cells had survived and remained healthy. A few NGF-positive cells were found, generally at the edge of the grafts. Thus, the procedure was effective, because the trauma occurred all at once, a few days after transplantation, when the effect of NGF produced by the cells shortly after implantation was still being exerted. Presumably, such a procedure would not be effective in a chronic illness, where the loss of cells occurs gradually, over an extended period of time. The cessation of expression of transferred genes therefore continues to be a major problem for this area of study.

Frim, Simpson, et al. (1993) studied the possibility that neuronal damage caused by inhibition of energy metabolism could be prevented by NGF-producing cell grafts. A drug that inhibits mitochondrial energy metabolism, 3-nitropropionic acid, was used. This drug causes a pattern of striatal injury resembling that seen in Huntington's disease. Administration of NGF via grafts greatly diminished the severity of striatal lesions induced by this agent, similar to the effect seen with excitotoxic lesions.

A follow-up of this study, using a different kind of transplantation technique, was reported in 1994 by Emerich and coworkers, in which human NGF was delivered from genetically modified cells that had been contained within polymer capsules prior to being transplanted. Before animals were lesioned with quinolinic acid, capsules containing cells that produce NGF were implanted into the lateral ventricles. This procedure was also effective in decreasing the severity of the striatal lesions. In this experiment, NGF production was more sustained, in that NGF was found in the capsules following their removal from the brain after about one month. Other trophic factors, especially BDNF and NT–3, may also be effective in protecting striatal neurons from injury (Nakao et al. 1995; Frim, Simpson, et al. 1993). Further developments in this area can be expected.

In the most recent such studies, by Dwaine Emerich and coworkers (Emerich, Lidner, et al. 1996; Emerich, Winn, et al. 1997; Emerich, Cain, et al. 1997), human ciliary neurotrophic factor (hCNTF) has been used. Fibroblasts that produced hCNTF were transplanted into the striatum of rats or monkeys, followed after a few days by the induction of striatal lesions with quinolinic acid. In each of these experiments, the cells were transplanted in polymer capsules, a strategy developed by a private company in Rhode Island, Cytotherapeutics. The basic principle of this method is to seal cells inside the small polymer capsules, thereby allowing nutrients to enter and therapeutic substances to escape; in this case, the therapeutic substance is hCNTF. In addition to containing the cells, so that they do not overgrow or spread around, the capsules protect the cells from rejection by the immune system.

One of these experiments will be described here (Emerich, Cain, et al. 1997). In this study, rats received transplants of fibroblasts (derived from hamster kidney) in polymer capsules. Fibroblasts genetically engineered to produce hCNTF were used for transplantation in one group of animals, and a second group of animals received transplants of unaltered fibroblasts (i.e., they did not produce hCNTF). One to three weeks after lesioning, the animals were tested for deficits in motor functioning, using a range of tests. By most of the tests, animals receiving hCNTF-producing grafts not only were improved, but were virtually indistinguishable from normal animals that had not received lesions. Measures of lesion severity included loss of body weight, decreased spontaneous activity, ability to resist being pushed sideways, responses to tactile stimuli, grip strength, and maze learning.

One of the tests used was the forepaw-reaching task developed by Montoya et al. in 1990, and described earlier in this chapter. By this measurement, normal animals were able to retrieve an average of about 18 pellets after seven testing trials, while the quinolinic acid-lesioned animals were able to retrieve only four. The animals that received quinolinic acid and hCNTF-producing transplants retrieved an average of about 17 pellets, performing only slightly, and not significantly, worse than the animals that had not been lesioned. The remarkable extent of protection shown to be afforded by hCNTF is very encouraging for future human use. Protection of striatal neurons has also been observed in monkeys, using a similar experimental paradigm (Emerich, Winn, et al. 1997). Perhaps the two major caveats are that (1) the degree to which improvement in this model (quinolinic acid lesions) is predictive of improvement in

Huntington's disease is unknown, and that (2) in this model, the lesions are made over a short time span, whereas it presumably would be necessary to obtain hCNTF production in human patients with Huntington's disease for many years, not just a few days.

Nonhuman Primate Models

There is no question that the ultimate intent of transplantation studies in animal models of Huntington's disease is to develop a procedure that might be useful for human patients. Since Huntington's disease invariably and inexorably progresses, leading to death within a few years, there is every reason to attempt any transplantation procedure that has a reasonable expectation of success. As in Parkinson's disease, the first human clinical trials did not precisely follow procedures that had been developed and used in animal models. The most important experiments for development of human clinical procedures are those performed in primates, and there is only one significant study of transplantation in a primate model of Huntington's disease.

Isacson and coworkers (1990, 1991) developed a model of Huntington's disease in baboons (*Papio papio*), using intrastriatal injections of the excitotoxin ibotenic acid. In primates, the ibotenic acid is injected into seven sites in the caudate putamen. Depending on the amount of ibotenic acid used, between 20 and 80 percent of the caudate and putamen is lesioned, resulting in a general neuronal depletion.

When lesioned in this manner, the baboons (amazingly) did not show clear spontaneous abnormalities. However, when injected with the dopamine agonist apomorphine, a series of distinct abnormalities developed. However, other primates (cynomolgus monkeys) did not develop clear behavioral abnormalities following similar lesions. The requirement for the use of apomorphine (a dopamine agonist) to elicit abnormal function following these lesions, although certainly a limitation of the model, is not inconsistent with Huntington's disease, since dopamine agonists may stimulate or elicit symptoms in Huntington's disease patients prior to the appearance of spontaneous motor dysfunction. Apomorphine doses of 1 to 1.5 mg/kg caused marked stimulation of locomotor activity in animals with ibotenic acid lesions of the striatum. In addition to general increases in activity, there were postural asymmetries, dystonic movements of the hands and head, circling behavior, orofacial dyskinesias, stereotyped jaw movements, and sometimes periods of explosive movement including jumps and random ballistic (large-amplitude flinging or flailing) movements of the limbs.

Hantraye and coworkers (1992) examined effects of striatal tissue grafts in this model. Donor tissue was fetal rat striatum, so that the grafts were xenogeneic. To prevent graft rejection, the hosts were immunosuppressed with cyclosporine. The tissue was transplanted into baboon striatum in the form of dissociated cells. The severity of apomorphine-induced abnormal movements was reduced markedly by the rat tissue transplants, with reductions in severity of more than 75 percent occurring over the course of seven to nine weeks.

When cyclosporine treatment was discontinued, presumably ending the protection of the grafts from immune rejection, the dyskinesias became more severe but the reversion was incomplete, increasing in severity by about 67 percent. Thus, transplantation of rat striatal tissue into the baboon striatum was able to decrease the deficits seen after striatal injury.

Although the effects of grafts in this model were indeed remarkable, a few questions remain. First, why did rejection of the grafts result in loss of beneficial effect of the transplants? Presuming that the beneficial effect of the transplants was due to integration with the host brain, when the graft and its associated functional connections were rejected, the functional improvements would be lost. This model, exploiting the species difference to provoke graft rejection, is a very powerful one, and the results indeed suggest that the behavioral improvements were due to integration of the grafts into the host brain's neural circuitry.

On the other hand, there are alternative interpretations. Perhaps, for example, invasion of cells and secretion of chemical mediators (cytokines) into the area of the transplant during induced graft rejection caused further "bystander" damage to the host striatum, thereby making the lesion worse. The fact that the degree of worsening when cyclosporine was discontinued was similar to the overall improvement after transplants tends to argue against this possibility. However, this was not true for all of the animals, and in at least one case only about 20 percent of the improvement was lost after cyclosporine was stopped (Isacson et al. 1991). In addition, it is possible that the cyclosporine itself contributed to the improvement, since it has been found to have trophic effects on the brain (Snyder et al. 1998).

The fact that fetal rat tissue is effective in this model is, in itself, interesting. Generally, it appears likely that fetal rat dopaminergic neurons are capable of extending neurites for shorter distances than are human dopaminergic neurons. If the same is true of striatum, it is surprising that the grafts from rats are behaviorally efficacious in baboons. There was some growth of processes from the rat grafts into the host baboon brain, but the extent of this growth probably was relatively minor. Such an observation is consistent with the possibility that grafts work in Huntington's disease through mechanisms other than development of connectivity between graft and host brain. These mechanisms might be interesting ones—such as the release of a peptide or a neurotrophic substance—or relatively trivial mechanisms—such as the provoking of host gliosis, a host tissue reaction to injury induced by the tissue implantation, or even mechanical pressure on the surrounding tissue induced by the growing fetal tissue graft.

Appropriate controls could largely resolve this issue, as well as the question of why graft rejection was accompanied by only a partial loss of the functional benefit. The experiment of Hantraye and colleagues (1992) did include one control animal that received transplants of brain stem tissue. In another study, one animal received a lesion only, but no transplant (Isacson et al. 1991). Neither of these two animals improved. A more substantial control group would have made this study more convincing.

Very little work has been done on grafts in Huntington's disease models using subhuman primates, and because of the great effort and cost of such studies, this probably will be a continuing problem. Although the improvement that was seen was very substantial, and provides some justification for human trials, several questions remain. Additional primate studies that include controls and use allografts would be highly desirable prior to human clinical studies.

Prospects for Clinical Studies

Huntington's disease is likely to ultimately be an excellent candidate for clinical trials of neural transplantation. First, the disease is inevitably fatal and there is no available therapy. There is little to be lost and much potential gain from even a small therapeutic benefit of neural transplantation. Moreover, procedures similar to those that would be used in patients with Huntington's disease have been used in many human patients with Parkinson's disease, with few adverse effects.

Notwithstanding, there are several issues that should at least be considered. One is discriminating truly beneficial effects of the transplant from minor improvements due to injury of the host brain. Another possible problem is whether the disease itself might cause degeneration of the transplant in addition to causing degeneration of the host striatum. This is not known, but the answer to this question may emerge if the cell biology of the disease becomes better understood. The issue of number of transplants to be performed will be an important issue: Should it be tried first on one or two people? How will we know whether or not they have improved? When should larger trials be initiated? For any large-scale trials (say, more than two or three patients), inclusion of controls is a complex problem. Should controls receive no surgery—just parallel evaluation—or sham transplants, or nonstriatal tissue grafts? The animal data on whether the effect of striatal grafts are specific is equivocal at present—it may be that grafts from other brain regions works nearly as well.

There have already been a few very minor attempts at neural transplantation in Huntington's disease, none of which has been a thorough or optimal test. In 1988 Allen and coworkers attempted transplants of adrenal medulla in patients with Huntington's disease (Sanberg and Norman 1988). The reasoning for this study was not explicitly stated, but apparently was the following. Adrenal medulla transplants appeared to produce some improvement in Parkinson's disease, and at the time, it seemed that this improvement might be due to the production of a trophic factor by the transplanted adrenal chromaffin cells (or other cells in the graft). This trophic factor might also have a favorable effect on the survival or function of intrinsic striatal cells.

There is no indication that the patients improved. The procedure was not tested in animals at all, and certainly was ill-considered, but it *could* have worked. Adrenal chromaffin cells produce a variety of trophic factors, as subsequently demonstrated by Unsicker and his coworkers (Unsicker 1993), and one or more of these trophic factors might very well promote survival of striatal neurons. Subsequent studies have shown very substantial beneficial effects of trophic factors on survival of striatal neurons in animals. What would be our current perspective on this clinical trial if it had worked very well?

There was also a trial of adrenal medulla transplantation for another severe degenerative disorder, progressive supranuclear palsy (Koller et al. 1989). The reasoning was similar to that for trying adrenal medulla grafts in Huntington's disease, but again no improvement occurred.

Actually, the transplanted chromaffin cells probably did not survive well in either case; as it turned out, they did not survive well in the autopsy cases from the trials in Parkinson's disease. Is the possibility of transplanting adrenal chromaffin cells in Huntington's disease worth exploring even now, especially using methods that will result in survival of the transplanted chromaffin cells? There might be sufficient reason to perform an animal experiment or two, although, as discussed in chapter 11, adrenal medulla transplantation is associated with a high frequency of fairly serious side effects.

A second clinical trial of fetal tissue transplantation in human patients with Huntington's disease was reported by Madrazo and coworkers, in this case using fetal tissue (Madrazo, Franco-Bourland, Cuevas et al. 1991; Madrazo, Franco-Bourland, Castrejon et al. 1993). This trial has not yet been reported in the scientific literature in a complete form, but is discussed in more detail by Sanberg et al. (1993). Two patients received transplants. No major improvement was found, although there were some subjective signs of improved function in both subjects. In this trial, the fetal tissue was transplanted into cavities created in the wall of the lateral ventricle, so that the transplants were partially embedded into the substance of the striatum but also in contact with the cerebrospinal fluid.

A significant problem regarding the reports by Madrazo and coworkers has been the method of tissue transplantation. The procedure used was identical to that employed in Parkinson's disease patients. In animal studies of striatal transplantation, transplants placed into the lateral ventricle have been ineffective (Sanberg, Giordano et al. 1989). It appears to be necessary to implant tissue directly into the striatum. Thus, based on the animal data, it has been argued that the procedure would probably be ineffective. The method employed, however, did not exactly involve transplanting tissue into the ventricle; nevertheless, the procedure was not tested in appropriate animal models.

A third clinical study, reported by Kopov and coworkers (1998), included three patients with advanced Huntington's disease. For these patients, the methods used resembled techniques employed in animal models of Huntington's disease. It appeared, from magnetic resonance imaging (a brain-scanning technique), that the grafts had survived one year after transplantation without apparent adverse effects. Complete results regarding clinical outcome have not yet been reported.

A current trial of fetal tissue transplantation for patients with Huntington's disease is also under way at the University of South Florida. One patient in this study died about 18 months after transplantation, and was found to have surviving striatal grafts and evidence of integration of the graft with the host brain (Freeman et al., 1999).

Ultimately, additional clinical trials of transplantation in Huntington's disease are almost inevitable. If one compares earliest trials in Parkinson's disease with the present state of affairs regarding Huntington's disease, there are already more animal data on Huntington's disease (compared with when Parkinson's disease trials were started), the data are about as convincing, and the risk-benefit ratio is much better than for Parkinson's disease, where there are many alternative treatments.

Speculation

If any beneficial effects of transplants are obtained in humans, there are some interesting extensions. Although this possibility has not yet been studied directly, in other models, transplants are usually (in fact, almost always) more effective when immature host animals are used. Thus, the use of fetal brain tissue transplants for Huntington's disease, in a preemptive manner, is a distinct possibility. In other words, if grafts are found to be effective, they could be implanted prior to the development of Huntington's disease symptoms. Since it is now possible to test for Huntington's disease, using genetic techniques, prior to the development of overt symptoms, one might consider transplanting fetal striatum into the striatum of patients who are destined to develop the disease.

In fact, striatal tissue could be transplanted into these patients shortly after birth. Or, to carry this still further, grafts could be implanted before birth. In this way, a graft would have the maximum possible opportunity to become integrated into the host brain. Studies by Olsson and coworkers (1997) have shown that transplants of striatal neurons into the striatum have an increased ability to become integrated into the host brain circuitry when transplanted at early stages of development. Thus, it seems probable that striatal transplants would be more effective the earlier they are implanted.

Suppose that some such preemptive transplantation procedure became routine, as it conceivably might. Yet, suppose that under these circumstances transplantation was still found to be only moderately effective. It might turn out that transplants made in utero were capable of replacing part of the host circuitry, but some host neurons and their connections remained, resulting in degeneration as the disease progressed. Then what could be done to improve matters still further? Suppose that we found a means of lesioning the host system in utero. One could then imagine destroying the patient's own striatal neurons in utero, and replacing them by transplantation *in anticipation* of their eventual degeneration.

This is starting to become almost frighteningly intrusive, but in a way it can be carried still farther. We are hypothesizing that one fetus (the donor) is being used to replace tissue from a second, defective fetus (the host, which is destined to develop Huntington's disease as an adult). In that case, might it not be better to replace the entire fetus, intact? For that matter, why not terminate the pregnancy and initiate a second pregnancy? The host fetus will not be completely repaired by transplantation of tissue fragments or cells, no matter how good our surgery becomes. To make a perfect fetus, the only possibility is to depend on biology, or nature, to do it for us.

This raises difficult ethical issues and quandaries. Where do we draw the line? The reason that Huntington's disease tends to raise such issues is largely because of the possibility of performing a reliable genetic test to predict who will develop Huntington's disease. Yet, the disease may not be unique, and sooner or later similar ethical difficulties may develop for other disorders as well.

Further Reading

Bjorklund, A., Campbell, K., Sirinathsinghji, D. J., Fricker, R. A., and Dunnett, S. B. (1994). Functional capacity of striatal transplants in the rat Huntington model. In *Functional Neural Transplantation,* S. B. Dunnett and A. Bjorklund (eds.), pp. 157–195. Raven Press, New York.

Bjorklund, A., Lindvall, O., Isacson, O., Brundin, P., Wictorin, K., Strecker, R. E., Clarke, D. J., and Dunnett, S. B. (1987). Mechanisms of action of intracerebral neural implants: Studies on nigral and striatal grafts to the lesioned striatum. *Trends Neurosci.* 10: 509–516.

Koutouzis, T. K., Emerich, D. F., Borlongan, C. V., Freeman, T. B., Cahill, D. W., and Sanberg, P. R. (1994). Cell transplantation for central nervous system disorders. *Crit. Rev. Neurobiol.* 8: 125–162.

Norman, A. B., Giordano, M., and Sanberg, P. R. (1989). Fetal striatal tissue grafts into excitotoxin-lesioned striatum: Pharmacological and behavioral aspects. *Pharmacol., Biochem., Behav.* 34: 139–147.

Sanberg, P. R., Koutouzis, T. K., Freeman, T. B., Cahill, D. W., and Norman, A. B. (1993). Behavioral effects of fetal neural transplants: Relevance to Huntington's disease. *Brain Res. Bull.* 32: 493–496.

Sanberg, P. R., Wictorin, K., and Isacson, O. (eds.). (1994). *Neural Transplantation for Huntington's Disease.* CRC Press, Boca Raton, Fla.

Shannon, K. M., and Kordower, J. H. (1996). Neural transplantation for Huntington's disease: Experimental rationale and recommendations for clinical trials. *Cell Transplant.* 5: 339–352.

Sharp, A. H., and Ross, C. A. (1996). Neurobiology of Huntington's disease. *Neurobiol. Disease* 3: 3–15.

Young, A. B. (1994). Huntington's disease: Lessons from and for molecular neuroscience. *Neuroscientist* 1: 30–37.

18

Spinal Cord

The spinal cord is the structure that carries the connections between brain and skeletal muscles, including the sensory, sympathetic, and parasympathetic nerve connections to most of the body (figure 18.1). Repairing the spinal cord presents a number of special problems. Scarring after spinal cord injury is extensive, and large cavities tend to form. The spinal cord is a very delicate structure, so that even minor manipulations can cause damage. Furthermore, its circuitry is complex and precise, so that ultimately it may not be sufficient simply to induce some sort of connection across the site of an injury.

Peripheral nerve regenerates readily, but when it does so, abnormal connections often form. Functional recovery after proximal peripheral nerve injury (injury close to the spinal cord) is often poor *even though* the nerve regenerates. The situation may be similar (or even worse!) in the spinal cord. That is, even if we can get the spinal cord to regenerate, there may be problems in obtaining functional recovery related to the formation of inaccurate connections. Despite these problems, however, there is ample reason to hope that some form of spinal cord repair, even if it is only partial, may eventually be achieved.

Attempts to repair the spinal cord have a long history; until the recent emphasis on Parkinson's disease, in fact, spinal cord injury had been the disorder engendering most research on promoting CNS regeneration and repair. There are obvious reasons for this emphasis on spinal cord research: the functional deficits following spinal cord injury are clearly related to the localized trauma, and to the failure of spinal cord axons to regenerate. The failure of the severed spinal cord to form reconnections

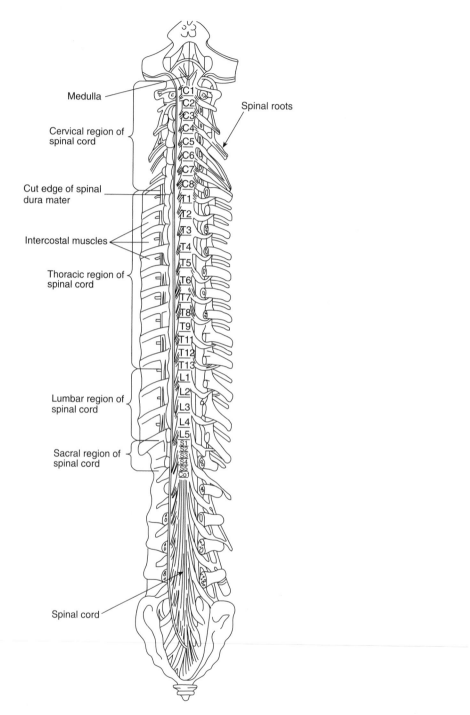

Figure 18.1
General anatomy of the spinal cord. (Adapted from Everett et al. 1971)

between proximal and distal stumps is a clearly defined deficit seemingly amenable to correction by scientific enterprise.

Imagine yourself as a neuroscientist (although the term did not yet exist) in, say, 1940. At that time, the general organization of the brain and spinal cord was quite well known. Neurons had been classified into types according to shape and location, and the general organization of the brain seemed to be clearly understood. The current understanding of the complex biochemistry of the brain and specialization of neurons was hardly suspected; however, the absence of this knowledge was not known to be an impediment. Much of the relevant knowledge we have now—such as the biochemistry of the molecules that control cell–cell contacts—was not known to be lacking.

In contrast to most degenerative disorders and even traumatic disorders of the CNS, in spinal cord injury it was both quite clear what was wrong and apparent that there was a great deal of scar formation. The classic work of Ramón y Cajal, translated and published in English in 1928, showed that some growth of fibers does occur following spinal cord injury. Ramón y Cajal described this abortive fiber growth after spinal cord injury in considerable detail, showing that growth occurs early after injury but fails to cross the scar tissue and coalesce to form new tracts.

At the time of Ramón y Cajal's work, there had already been a considerable number of investigations into the pathology of spinal cord injury. He concluded that

These investigations . . . have also confirmed the old concept of the essential impossibility of regeneration, showing that, after a more or less considerable period of progress, the restoration is paralyzed, giving place to a process of atrophy and definitive break-down of the nerve sprouts. (Ramón y Cajal 1928, 509)

On a more positive note, he concluded the chapter by stating:

It thus seems natural to conjecture that the regenerative process of the white matter, which is so remarkably faint and sluggish under ordinary conditions, *can be powerfully stimulated by means of active or trophic substances liberated by the mesodermal scar and diffused in the spinal wounds and their edges.* (Ramón y Cajal 1928, 530; italics in original)

A considerable effort was made to find substances that would inhibit the extensive scar formation which occurs following spinal cord injury, in the hope that this would increase regenerative growth of fibers. A number of things were tried in animals, including curiosities such as wrapping a gall bladder around the severed stumps (an unusual kind of transplant!) in the hope that digestive enzymes would inhibit the formation of scar tissue (Davidoff and Ransohoff 1948). It didn't work, but the researchers were on the right track, since later investigations showed that a number of substances which inhibited scar formation following spinal cord injury were effective in enhancing the growth of fibers. These substances included the proteolytic enzyme trypsin and inflammatory substances isolated from bacterial cell walls. The most thoroughly studied of the latter were piromen, a bacterial polysaccharide, and pyrogenal, a bacterial lipopolysaccharide (for review, see W. J. Freed, de Medinaceli, and Wyatt 1985 or Nesmeyanova 1977). Although these substances were effective in increasing fiber growth after spinal cord injury, they did not increase it to the point that fibers regenerated across the gap. There were also claims that these substances induced some functional recovery in animals, but it was lost approximately 12–18 months later. In addition, there were trials of piromen in human patients (for details, see Nesmeyanova 1977).

There is an interesting sequel: progesterone, a steroid hormone, is now routinely administered to patients with spinal cord injury. This treatment is not given to promote regeneration, but instead to prevent secondary damage through inflammation (Young 1993). The experiments that led to this usage of progesterone can be traced back to the early studies of attempts to increase spinal cord regeneration. Thus, although these early experiments did not achieve their original goal, they were still useful, but in a different manner.

From the perspective of today's knowledge, we might feel that the neuroscientist (including in that term "neurosurgeon") of 1940 did not have a great deal of knowledge about the functions of the CNS. Yet, neuroscientists of the time almost certainly did not feel that way. In fact, the general anatomical and histological organization of the CNS had been quite thoroughly studied. Traumatic spinal cord injury presented to the neuroscientist-clinician (generally, neurosurgeons) a disorder—in fact, nearly the only disorder—where the cause of the deficit was known and could be pinpointed. Yet, science and medicine could do nothing. This helps to explain the great concentration of research, some of it primitive by today's standards, on spinal cord injury between 1940 and 1980. It probably also explains the relatively frequent attempts to repair spinal cord injury in human patients by surgical manipulation (e.g., Street 1967). Before going on to discuss the basic information on spinal cord repair, we will describe several of the attempts to treat spinal cord injury in human patients by transplantation. These attempts have usually been premature in that they have been based on insufficient animal data. At best, they have been harmless and may even have succeeded—but by chance rather than by design. At worst, they have been entirely worthless and occasionally harmful.

The first of these, reported in the scientific literature in 1944 by Woolsey and coworkers, involved implantation of a piece of spinal cord tissue, which had been fixed in formaldehyde, into a region of spinal cord injury. Formaldehyde, which is commonly used as a fixative, an agent that hardens and preserves tissue largely by linking together protein molecules, completely destroys the biological structure of the tissue: the proteins that make up the tissue lose their biological functionality. Thus, in this case the implanted tissue was dead, and nearly all of the proteins that might (conceivably) have been able to promote neuronal growth would have been destroyed. Fortunately, although the patient did not improve, there was no serious adverse reaction. The patient, a 16-year-old boy, died four months after the operation, from other causes.

Another misguided transplantation surgery episode that took place relatively recently was described by Nicholas and Arnason (1989). Although directed at multiple sclerosis (not spinal cord repair), and thus aimed at altering autoimmune processes, it is useful to consider as an illustration of the fact that doing something useless can be worse than doing nothing. Twenty-four patients with multiple sclerosis received transplants of fragments of pig brain to the subcutaneous abdominal fat. No cogent rationale for this procedure was evident. None of the patients improved, and complications developed in at least five cases. In one case, the patient developed an immune response to the graft. This response, directed to a molecule present in both the implanted pig brain and the host brain (gangliosides), led to the patient's death (Knorr-Held et al. 1986).

The above is reminiscent of an earlier episode in which freeze-dried fetal calf tissue was implanted subcutaneously in a patient with

Parkinson's disease, leading to death of the patient following an auto-immune reaction some months later (Jellinger and Seitelberger 1958). It should be emphasized that both of the episodes in which brain tissue implantation led to autoimmune reactions and death involved *peripheral* implantation of *animal* brain tissue. Very vigorous immune reactions can be induced by peripheral implants (compared with implants into the brain or spinal cord), and animal tissue is a very strong immune stimulus in human patients. There are no known examples of adverse systemic immu-nological events following transplantation of human tissue into the brain or spinal cord. Nevertheless, the potential for such an occurrence cannot be entirely dismissed.

Another surgical technique that has recently been employed in patients with spinal cord injury is "omental transposition." Although this is not transplantation per se, it does involve relocation of tissue to a site other than its normal position. The omentum is a folded, sheetlike membranous structure connected to the stomach and abdominal viscera. It has a very extensive blood supply, secretes a serumlike fluid that surrounds the vis-cera, and can easily be stretched and elongated. The technique, developed by Harry Goldsmith of Boston University Hospital, involves moving and stretching an end of the omentum, and tunneling through surrounding tissues to bring the omentum into contact with the spinal cord (Gold-smith et al. 1983). The principle is that this may improve the blood supply of injured tissues, and carry blood-borne growth factors to the site of injury.

Although there is nothing inherently unreasonable about this idea, its use for treatment of spinal cord injury is not well founded in animal re-search. There is no evidence that omental transposition can promote re-generation or induce any kind of functional improvement of injured spinal cord. Recently, financial reimbursement for costs of the proce-dure was awarded to patients with spinal cord injury who were involved in a trial of this technique, based on the conclusion that the benefits of the procedure were overrepresented to the patients (Money Offered in Spinal Surgical Trial 1994). The fundamental problem with this proce-dure was not that it was inherently unreasonable; rather, it seems that the animal experimentation performed prior to initiation of human trials was insufficient.

Probably the most extensive series of experiments on spinal cord injury treatment by transplantation in humans has been conducted by Dr. Pogos Katunian, at the Brain Research Institute of the Moscow Academy of Medicine (cf. Reier et al. 1994). The basic approach involved transplantation of tissue from the cerebral cortex of eight- to nine-week-old fetuses into the spinal cord. Although this approach is generally consistent with recent ideas in this area, animal research on this particular approach has been minimal. Most animal work has concentrated on implantation of fetal spinal cord, rather than cerebral cortex, into the spinal cord. There has been no demonstration in animals that implantation of fetal cerebral cortex into the injured spinal cord promotes functional recovery, and the few experiments that have implanted cerebral cortex into the spinal cord are certainly not sufficient to provide a basis for doing this in human patients.

Results of these studies were reported by Katunian at a workshop on spinal cord transplantation in August 1993 (cf. Reier et al. 1994). Human fetal neocortex was transplanted into 41 patients with spinal cord injury beginning in 1986. These patients all had severe injury of the spinal cord at least six months, and in a few cases two to three years, earlier. The cord injury was at a high level (thoracic) and judged clinically to be complete (i.e., the spinal cord was completely interrupted), so that the degree of impairment was severe.

Tissue used for transplantation was obtained from human fetal neocortex of eight to nine weeks' gestational age. The tissue was mechanically dissociated into small aggregates of cells, and these cells were transplanted under the pia mater at a number of locations around (but not within) the injury site. This again differs from most recent animal studies, in which tissue is usually transplanted directly into the site of injury.

What was the outcome? As judged against a number of earlier patients that had received other spinal cord procedures, there was slight evidence of neurological improvement extending slightly beyond the level of the injury. These assessments were not judged, however, to be sufficiently rigorous or quantitative to be reliable (Reier et al. 1994). Nevertheless, a positive aspect of this study was that there was no evidence of side effects, worsening of neurological function, or increased pain, and there were no deaths. The patients were not immunosuppressed, and it is not certain that the transplanted tissue survived. Although there is no compelling reason to believe that this procedure is likely to have produced clinical benefit, the lack of adverse effects is encouraging for possible future applications of tissue transplantation procedures to human patients with spinal cord injury.

Most of the early transplantation episodes described above were essentially scientific dead ends, more or less isolated from the mainstream of scientific study of spinal cord injury and repair. One series of experiments that had quite different consequences is the studies by C. C. Kao on peripheral nerve implants into the spinal cord. These experiments were certainly more systematic and better founded than those described above, although there was also a human trial that was equally unsuccessful. Whereas the other human transplantation misadventures were more or less dead ends, this story has an interesting series of sequelae that continue to reverberate in neuroscience and spinal cord research. The finding that engendered these studies was that in 1977, Kao and coworkers reported that lengths of peripheral nerve transplanted to the spinal cord were invaded by numerous growing neurites. This phenomenon was shown by using silver staining, which highlights neurofilaments, the filamentous proteins that provide a part of the structure of neuronal fibers (neurites).

This story actually begins earlier, with experiments by Tello (1911), who found that peripheral nerve fragments transplanted into the brain were invaded by growing axons. There were several experiments on this topic that engendered some controversy about whether these growing axons originated in the brain or from peripheral nerves. In the spinal cord, the story begins with studies by Sugar and Gerard (1940), who showed that growing neurites invaded peripheral nerve implants in the spinal cord. R. May (1955) transplanted cerebral cortex combined with pieces of peripheral nerve into the anterior chamber of the eye, and showed that the peripheral nerve grafts were invaded by growing fibers. These experiments, as well as those by Kao and coworkers, were able to demonstrate the presence of new fibers, but not their origin.

For the spinal cord especially, this is an important distinction, as these fibers might have originated from the peripheral nervous system rather than from the spinal cord. Under normal circumstances, peripheral nerve fibers regenerate much more readily than CNS axons in the brain and spinal cord. In fact, fibers in peripheral nerve grow very vigorously, even forming a clumped collection of fibers called a neuroma if there is no suitable terrain over which they can elongate. Thus, a possible explanation for the presence of these fibers growing into the peripheral nerve grafts (located in spinal cord) is that they originated from peripheral nerves.

Also, we should note that even if axons regenerate very enthusiastically into such peripheral nerve grafts, one might expect that they would encounter conditions similar to the original spinal cord (into which they cannot grow) at the distal (farthest from the brain) end of the graft, and that growth might therefore cease before these axons reached any useful target. As will be seen, this suspected impediment turns out to be the case.

This observation, made by Kao and coworkers, engendered a great deal of basic research related to this observation. Basic research on the subject continues, and a number of investigators, especially Albert Aguayo, Martin Schwab, Richard and Mary Bunge, and their coworkers, have continued to investigate the growth-stimulating property of peripheral nerve and peripheral nerve components, resulting in a line of study that has shed light on the processes which are responsible for controlling and limiting CNS axonal regeneration This research will be discussed in more detail below.

If scientists have not become more successful in restoring spinal cord function in the past 10 or 20 years, at least as a group we are more sensible and more realistic. The most recent episode of transplantation in spinal cord injury has involved patients with syringomyelia, a serious degenerative disorder in which a gradually expanding cavity forms within the spinal cord (Thompson et al. 1998; Wirth et al. 1998). Syringomyelia occurs in approximately 10 percent of patients with serious spinal cord injury, can cause progressive loss of function and is a serious, painful, and crippling condition. Fetal spinal cord cells were transplanted into the cavity in an attempt to stabilize the condition and prevent or slow the rate of deterioration. Initial results are quite promising (Wirth et al. 1999). No claims or goals of restoring the prior damage were involved. This procedure, therefore, seems entirely reasonable, and given the seriousness of the condition, the risk-to-benefit ratio seems quite high. If transplantation is effective in arresting the progression of syringomyelia, it would indeed be a very useful and exciting development.

More Details on Basic Research: Experiments by Kao and Coworkers

Since scar tissue was thought to be a major impediment to spinal cord regeneration, Kao first investigated reduction of this scarring. His initial efforts, in fact, reported in 1970 (Kao et al. 1970), involved implanting brain tissue into the spinal cord to inhibit scarring. To put this finding into perspective, imagine that a procedure which substantially reduced scar formation, but accomplished no more than that, was found. Scar formation after spinal cord injury can be very extensive and result in progressive impediments, related especially to progressive cavitation in uninjured parts of the spinal cord. It might very well be considered desirable, and worthwhile enough to warrant performing the surgery, to implant brain tissue into the sites of spinal cord injury in human patients for that reason alone. Between the time that I initially wrote this paragraph and the final draft of this book, a procedure of this type was, in fact, tried in human subjects with syringomyelia (see above).

In a later experiment, the results of which were published in 1974, Kao transplanted brain tissue, peripheral (sciatic) nerve fragments, and peripheral ganglia fragments into the transected spinal cord. In this experiment, rather than just decreasing scar formation, the peripheral nerve grafts engendered an apparent growth of new neurites into the graft. These neurites were detected by using silver staining, the best method available to Kao at that time. The method stained more or less all axons nonselectively. In this 1974 experiment, Kao was, of course, hoping that a reduction in scar formation would permit some new axons to grow, and so, quite naturally, stained for these axons, using the Bodian silver staining method, which had often been used for the same purpose. Kao was, we can be quite sure, both surprised and delighted to find not only some increased growth of axons but also some axons growing into the peripheral nerve for considerable distances, far exceeding what had been accomplished by any previous scar-reduction effort.

Moreover, similar growth did not take place in the spinal cords of animals that had received the brain or peripheral ganglia implants. Kao followed up these experiments with studies to show that these growing fibers, in rats with peripheral nerve implants, were in fact axons, by using electron microscopy (Kao, Chang et al. 1977). In an experiment published in 1982, Jean Wrathall and coworkers (1982) showed a similar enhancement of growth by peripheral nerve implants into the spinal cord of cats, and that the spinal cord could to a degree be (using their term) "reconstructed" by the grafts, insofar as the newly growing axons penetrated for considerable distances into the grafts. In this latter experiment, too, it was shown that axonal growth could be stimulated even if there was a considerable delay between spinal cord injury and graft implantation. Kao and coworkers also reported evidence of functional recovery following peripheral nerve grafting that, to my knowledge, has never been fully published (cf. Kao, Chang et al. 1977).

At this point in the narrative, Kao reportedly implanted peripheral nerve into the spinal cord of a group of patients with spinal cord injury (see Schwab 1996; Kao et al. 1983). On the one hand, at that time he had shown that peripheral nerve grafts could induce a quite vigorous growth of axons in the transected spinal cord of the rat. He also had completed similar experiments in larger animals. What he had not shown, however, is that these growing axons would emerge from the distal end of the transplant and perform any useful function there—such as making connections with neurons distal to the graft. Moreover, he had not shown in animals that the procedure was capable of inducing any sort of functional recovery. Clearly, this attempt was ill-considered.

On the other hand, to be fair, Kao and his colleagues had shown a remarkable degree of anatomical recovery, including axonal growth to a much greater extent than in any prior procedure. Other methods, notably administration of piromen, a pyrogenic extract that caused fever and produced a relatively modest increase in the growth of severed spinal cord axons, had already been used in humans, with little benefit. Moreover, since the spinal cord was essentially destroyed anyway, and susceptible to further long-term deterioration with no prospect of functional recovery, experimental surgery in the area could hardly make matters worse. Finally, even if the growing axons were to grow only a very short distance into the distal part of the spinal cord, it might be sufficient to allow them to make useful contacts with spinal cord neurons, thus bridging the gap without fully re-forming spinal cord circuits. Thus, although we now know that this did not work, at the time, who could have predicted with certainty that it would fail?

Although Kao's last scientific paper on this topic (to my knowledge) was published in 1984 with Wrathall, his work has played a large part in revitalizing the study of spinal cord regeneration and reconstruction, which is still unfolding. Subsequent experiments by Albert Aguayo, Martin Schwab, and Richard Bunge, and even the recent studies by Cheng, Cao, and Olson, discussed later in this chapter, among others, owe a debt to the studies by Kao.

Albert Aguayo

Kao's studies, although intriguing, left many questions unanswered. Foremost among them was the source of the fibers invading the peripheral nerve grafts: Were they simply peripheral fibers? An elegant series of experiments performed by Aguayo and coworkers, of McGill University in Quebec, clarified these issues (cf. Aguayo et al. 1983, 1991; Bray et al. 1981, 1987 for reviews).

Methods for tracing the origin and termination of neurites were, until the 1970s, quite primitive by present standards. Usually, damage was produced in a certain area, and connections with other areas of the brain were identified by stains that selectively marked degenerating fibers. A much more sophisticated method, developed more recently, involves exploitation of the phenomenon of retrograde axonal transport. Protein molecules and many other substances that are placed near nerve terminals will be taken up by those terminals, and slowly transported back along the axons to the neuronal cell bodies from which those axons come. Thus, if a molecule that can be seen through the microscope is injected in small amounts near a group of terminals, it will be transported back to the cell bodies, and the cell bodies that produced those axons and terminals can then be identified. The first retrograde tracing technique of this type employed the enzyme *horseradish peroxidase*. Horseradish peroxidase can be identified histochemically; that is, it can be stained, using any of several molecules that produce a dark substance from the enzymatic reaction it catalyzes.

Aguayo and his coworkers employed this horseradish peroxidase retrograde tracing technique to identify the cells that gave rise to the axons which project into peripheral nerve grafts. In a classic study by P. M. Richardson, U. M. McGuinness, and A. Aguayo (1980), peripheral nerve grafts were implanted into the completely transected spinal cord. After two to four months, horseradish peroxidase was injected into the spinal cord immediately adjacent to the graft, on either the distal or the proximal side (figure 18.2). The horseradish peroxidase was injected through a fine glass pipette in very small amounts, so that it did not spread to other sites. Labeled neurons, which had sent axons into the grafts, were found in the spinal cord both above and below the graft. Later experiments showed that peripheral nerve grafts into various other locations were able to induce the growth of axons of several types, with cell bodies located in the brain. When the growing axons reached the distal ends of the grafts, however, their growth ceased quite abruptly. Most axons entering the distal part of the spinal cord continued to grow for only very short distances. Even the most vigorous axons penetrated no more than 1 or 2 mm.

This lack of continued growth of axons after exiting the grafts clearly suggests that peripheral nerve grafting, as done in animals, would not produce recovery from spinal cord injury in humans in a simple or straightforward manner. Still, this research has produced a number of long-term benefits. First, research related to this topic is ongoing, and there is a distinct possibility that some related method will eventually become applicable to human patients. Second, this line of research has produced significant benefits related to understanding of the mechanisms that control and limit regeneration and axonal plasticity in the nervous system.

A question that should be considered is how reconstructions of the spinal cord might be achieved. Is it necessary to rebuild the spinal cord entirely, in the form in which it existed prior to being severed? Possibly not. Although the spinal cord is often considered just a bundle of very long axons, this is a greatly oversimplified conceptualization. The spinal cord, over its entire length, contains regions of gray matter (neuronal cell bodies) and white matter (areas of myelinated axons). The long fiber projections from the brain pass through the white matter. Direct control

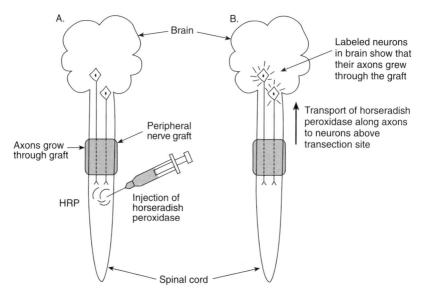

Figure 18.2

Illustration of the method employed by Richardson and coworkers (1980) to show that peripheral nerve grafts in the spinal cord stimulated the regeneration of axons from CNS neurons. Horseradish peroxidase, an enzyme, was used as a tracer. This substance was injected into the spinal cord distal to a peripheral nerve graft implanted in the spinal cord following complete transection of the cord. This tracer was then shown to be transported retrogradely to neurons in the brain.

of large muscle function is largely mediated by these long white matter projections.

Skeletal muscle can also, however, be influenced by reflex arcs that are contained entirely within the spinal cord. Although the gray matter of the spinal cord retains some of its connections with the musculature after spinal cord transection, interruption of the long projections means that all voluntary (brain-directed) control of the musculature is lost (figure 18.3). Afferentation of the musculature is thus retained, but can be activated only by reflex activity. This may be sufficient to cause fairly complex movements under certain conditions; for example, "spinal stepping," consisting of coordinated stepping movements, can sometimes be activated (in animals with transected spinal cords) by placing their limbs on a treadmill. In addition to voluntary control of the muscles, other functions, such as proprioceptive and sensory input to the brain and balance reflexes, are lost after spinal cord transection.

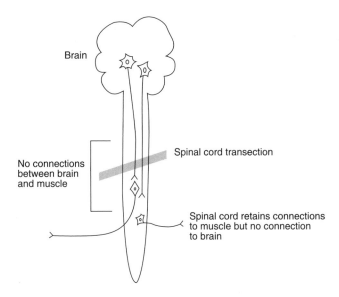

Figure 18.3
Illustration of the consequences of spinal cord transection. Even though neurons in the spinal cord remain connected to skeletal muscles after the spinal cord has been severed completely, there are no longer any connections between the distal part of the spinal cord and the brain. This means that there is no longer any voluntary control of motor function, nor sensory input from the periphery to the brain. In lower animals, circuits within the spinal cord may generate reflexive movements, even walking, but spinally generated reflexive walking is not often seen in human subjects with spinal cord injury.

Thus, it may be possible to induce functional recovery after spinal cord injury with peripheral nerve grafts or some analogous strategy, even if complete restoration of long fiber tracts does not occur. Possibly, fibers that grow short distances into intact segments of the spinal cord would be able to establish contacts which would permit them to activate motor control circuits (figure 18.4). Therefore, it is within the realm of possibility that some functional recovery could be induced by fibers which emerge from peripheral nerve grafts and grow into the spinal cord for only short distances (see discussion of Cheng, Cao, and Olson 1996 below).

Motor neurons, located in the spinal cord gray matter, project to skeletal muscles by way of the ventral spinal roots and peripheral nerves. Upon passing from spinal cord to ventral root, the axon continues to be myelinated. Regeneration can occur effectively in the peripheral portion, but

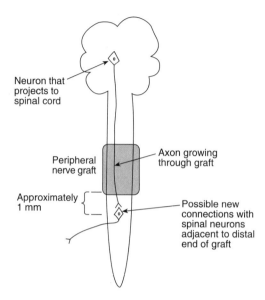

Neuron that projects to spinal cord

Peripheral nerve graft

Axon growing through graft

Approximately 1 mm

Possible new connections with spinal neurons adjacent to distal end of graft

Figure 18.4
One possible means by which axons regenerating through a peripheral nerve graft in the spinal cord might restore movement. Even though these regenerating axons do not continue to grow once they have reached the distal part of the spinal cord, they could form connections with neurons adjacent to the site of injury, thereby restoring some limited connectivity between the proximal and distal segments of the spinal cord. Since these axons grow only about 1 millimeter into the distal segment of the spinal cord, the possibilities for such connections are quite limited.

not within the spinal cord white matter. Thus, each corticospinal axon passes from a region where it cannot regenerate (spinal cord white matter) into a region where regeneration is vigorous (the peripheral nerve) quite abruptly (figure 18.5). Since the axon apparently does not change, researchers have focused upon the surrounding material—the myelin sheath and basal lamina of peripheral nerve (figure 2.6)—as a major influence on axonal regeneration. The physiological reasons for this difference will be discussed later in this chapter, in "Studies by Richard Bunge and Mary Bunge."

In essence, the experiments by Aguayo and coworkers have exploited this difference between peripheral nerve and CNS environment by changing the local environment, so that a part of the axon that is normally in the CNS is instead in a peripheral nerve environment. The trans-

ons, was added to the cultures in a relatively high concentration, the axons grew vigorously, but still did not grow into the optic nerve. Thus, even though axonal growth was stimulated, and growth into the peripheral nerve was increased, the axons avoided the optic nerve. Thus, stimulation of growth by the peripheral nerve did not appear to explain the lack of axonal growth into optic nerve. It therefore appeared that optic nerve tissue inhibited axonal growth, even when the growth was stimulated by other means (e.g., NGF).

Schwab and his associates then proceeded to isolate components of CNS tissue that were responsible for this inhibitory effect. The growth-inhibiting material was found to be present in oligodendrocytes, and was a component of CNS myelin. The inhibitory substance was present in the cell membranes, and consisted of a protein with molecular weights of 35 to 250 kDa. The 35 kDa form is a subunit, and can exist in complexes with the higher molecular weights of 60 and 250 kDa.

When purified, this protein can inhibit axonal growth in tissue culture in very low concentrations. It appears to work by contact rather than by diffusion through the culture medium. The mode of action is that growth cones collapse when they contact this protein molecule, and the collapse occurs in response to an increase in calcium in the growth cones. Antibodies to this inhibitory protein were developed.

Experiments were then designed to apply this information to an animal model. The method employed an entirely novel use of neural transplantation: to deliver antibodies to the surrounding tissue. This technique used hybridoma cells—hybrid cells that produce monoclonal antibodies—transplanted into the spinal cord. The purpose of these experiments was to block the effect of the growth-inhibiting material present on oligodendrocytes by continuously delivering antibodies to the area of spinal cord injury.

Before continuing, it would be worthwhile to describe the production of monoclonal antibodies. Monoclonal antibodies are produced by hybrid cells formed by fusion of antibody-producing cells obtained directly from an animal with tumor cells derived from bone marrow. This results in formation of hybrid cells that can produce antibodies but also can be grown indefinitely in tissue culture. In practice, mice are immunized with the material of interest—for now, let's call this antigen X. Antigen X can be present in material that contains the antigen in relatively impure form (e.g., mice can be immunized with brain that contains some antigen X), but the chances of success are better if purified antigen X is used. After the animal is immunized, an increased percentage of lymphocytes in the spleen will be devoted to producing antibodies that bind antigen X. Before immunization, perhaps only one B lymphocyte per 10^6 to 10^7 cells (or more, depending on the antigen) would have produced antibodies to antigen X, but after immunization, perhaps one of every 10^2 B lymphocytes might produce antibodies directed to antigen X. This increase occurs because immunization selectively stimulates the growth of those clones of B lymphocytes that produce antibodies specific for antigen X. After immunization, then, cells can be taken from the spleen, and a relatively high percentage will be producing antibodies that react to antigen X.

The next step is to fuse the spleen cells with myeloma cells obtained from a tumor that is predisposed to antibody production. Fusion involves the use of special techniques to combine two cells into a single cell. Cells that have successfully fused are selected by growth in "HAT" medium. This medium contains aminopterin (the A of HAT), which will kill cells by blocking a metabolic pathway needed for DNA synthesis. Normal cells contain an alternative pathway, which they can utilize (allowing them to survive even if aminopterin is present) if hypoxanthine (the H of HAT) and thymidine (the T of HAT) are added to the medium. The myeloma cells employed for fusion cannot use this pathway, so they are killed by the aminopterin in the medium. Cells that have been fused successfully will contain the alternative pathway, and thus will be able to survive in HAT medium. Cells that have not successfully fused contain only the metabolic resources of the original myeloma cells, and do not survive.

Once a collection of fused myeloma-lymphocyte cells (hybridoma cells) has been produced, it is necessary to select from this collection those cells which are producing an antibody of interest. Each cell produces only one type of antibody; thus, many individual clones of cells are grown in culture dishes containing many small wells, each colony starting from a single cell, and the clones are tested for production of antibody. In this way, a colony of identical cells (i.e., a clone) producing antibody to any particular antigen can be obtained.

Caroni and Schwab (1988) reported that they had employed this method to produce monoclonal antibodies to the growth-inhibiting protein from oligodendrocyte membranes. This antibody, called IN-1, was found to prevent the inhibitory effect of the oligodendrocyte membranes on the growth of neurites in tissue culture. Usually, these cells are used to produce antibody, either in tissue culture or extracted from animals with antibody-producing tumors. The antibody is then extracted and used for other purposes. In the experiments by Schnell and Schwab, the goal was to determine whether neurite growth in the spinal cord could be stimulated by this antibody.

To examine effects of the IN-1 antibody in animals with spinal cord lesions, Schnell and Schwab (1990) made partial lesions of the spinal cord in animals with the antibody-producing hybridoma cells transplanted into their brains. This experiment was done as follows. First, IN-1 antibody-producing cells, or control cells that produced an irrelevant antibody, were transplanted into the cortex of rats. Rejection of the transplanted tumor cells was prevented by the immunosuppressant drug cyclosporine. It appeared that the antibody was able to reach the spinal cord, via the cerebrospinal fluid, because IN-1 antibodies were present in the serum. After seven to ten days, the animals received spinal cord lesions. One effect of these lesions was that cerebrospinal fluid-filled cavities formed in the spinal cord tissue around the lesions, which may have facilitated access of antibodies to the spinal cord tissue. The lesions were made in the spinal cord by cutting the dorsal two-thirds of the spinal cord with scissors in order to completely transect the corticospinal tract, the pathway from cerebral cortex to spinal cord. This allowed some spinal cord tissue to remain intact.

When spinal cord lesions of this type are performed, some sprouting of spinal cord axons normally takes place. The injured axons generally begin to sprout just rostral (above) the lesion site, and may extend for slight distances below the lesion. In control animals, which are lesioned only, these sprouts extend for small distances, usually less than 1 mm. In the animals with the antibody-producing tumors, the growth of the sprouting axons was greatly stimulated; some axons grew as long as 5 to 11 mm, and in most animals the sprouts grew at least 2 or 3 mm. The control animals, with tumors producing an irrelevant antibody, were similar to animals with no antibody-producing tumor. The animals were evaluated "blindly," so that the observations were not biased by the experimenter's expectations.

It should be stressed, however, that this technique was successful in increasing axonal growth only in intact sections of the spinal cord, ventral and lateral to the lesioned area. In other words, the growing axons circumvented the lesion site, and did not grow through the gap. Moreover, only a few axons showed this extended growth; the majority did not show increased growth. Finally, only animals that had sprouts extending below the lesion site were evaluated. Some animals did not show such sprouts, and the number of such animals was not stated in the original study. Thus, although growth of axons was substantially stimulated by the IN-1 antibody (it was several times greater than what occurred without the antibody), the degree of stimulation was tiny in comparison with the total amount of fibers present in the spinal cord.

In 1990, Savio and Schwab explored another technique for preventing the inhibitory effect of myelin on spinal cord sprouting. In this experiment, rats were irradiated shortly after birth, when oligodendrocytes are developing. This resulted in a spinal cord that was essentially free of oligodendrocytes, and enhanced growth of axons was seen in these spinal cords.

One might place this in perspective by somewhat arbitrarily assigning numbers to the amount of growth. Say, perhaps, that the amount of sprouting seen after a lesion only is 1 unit. The IN-1 antibody might increase this growth severalfold, to perhaps 5 or 10 units. This amount of improvement is indeed substantial. The amount of growth required to completely restore the corticospinal tract, however, might be 1,000 or even 10,000 units, and to obtain any functional restitution, perhaps something like 500 or even 1,000 units might be needed. Thus, although the stimulation produced by the IN-1 antibody is indeed substantial, no one should feel that the problem of spinal cord injury was solved, at least not by this observation alone. Moreover, the fact that the sprouts do not cross the gap continues to be a major obstacle, as it had been for numerous prior studies of spinal cord regeneration. Indeed, techniques that are capable of increasing the growth of axons in the injured spinal cord, but do not succeed in promoting the growth of fibers across the site of an injury, have been available for many years.

As has already been mentioned, the spinal cord presents special problems for reconstruction and repair. The reaction of the spinal cord to injury is very severe. Scar formation and cavitation in the spinal cord are massive, and result in a large area with no infrastructure to support potential regeneration. Large fluid-filled cavities often develop, which can present a nearly impenetrable obstacle to regeneration. In fact, a number of techniques have been found to stimulate the sprouting of severed spinal cord fibers (e.g., protein synthesis inhibitors and piromen, discussed earlier in this chapter), but like the IN-1 antibody, these treatments have not been able to induce severed spinal cord fibers to cross a gap. In addition to simply crossing the gap, there may be obstacles, such as retaining an appropriate degree of organization, once the gap has been crossed. Nevertheless, understanding the importance of the myelin-associated inhibitory molecules is certainly an important step.

Schnell and coworkers (1994) went on to explore the possibility that the blocking of the myelin-associated growth inhibitory molecule by the IN-1 antibody not only allows growth per se, but also permits neurotrophic molecules to stimulate additional neurite growth in the spinal cord. Earlier in vitro experiments had shown that the optic nerve environment was nonpermissive to neurite growth, even when the growth was stimulated by NGF. By analogy to the in vitro experiments, therefore, blocking the myelin-associated inhibitory molecule would be expected to permit trophic factors to exert their stimulatory effect on the growth of spinal cord neurites. This possibility was explored by administering the neurotrophic molecules BDNF, NGF, and NT–3, then measuring neurite growth in the spinal cord following injury. In animals treated with the IN-1 antibody, NT–3 greatly increased, about fourfold, the number of sprouting axons. BDNF had no effect, and NGF produced about a twofold stimulation. To keep this in perspective, the total number of sprouting axons was increased from about 8 in the control animals to about 32 in the animals treated with NT–3, still a very small number.

The most recent development in this area is that treatment with the IN-1 antibody has been shown to promote functional recovery from spinal cord injury (Bregman et al. 1995). In this study, animals received spinal cord hemisection injury, as described below in the section "Kunkel-

Bagden and Bregman 1990 Study." The animals were then treated with the IN-1 antibody, by transplanting the antibody-producing hybridoma cells into the animals and allowing the cells to survive for two weeks. This limited duration of cell survival was achieved by immunosuppressing the animals with cyclosporine A for the two weeks in order to prevent graft rejection, and then discontinuing cyclosporine treatment so that the grafts were rejected. Controls received another antibody (to horseradish peroxidase) or no treatment at all. After an additional three to four weeks, recovery of motor function was assessed. The animals that had received the IN-1 antibody showed regenerative growth of a small percentage of corticospinal axons over a considerable distance, consistent with the previous experiments. The IN-1 antibody treatment also enhanced the recovery of locomotor function. One measure of the deficit induced by the spinal cord injury is that the animals make very short strides after injury; in the IN-1 antibody-treated rats, stride length recovered to normal. Other measures of locomotor function (for example, errors in foot placement) were not improved. The IN-1 antibody also caused recovery of some reflexive foot placement responses. Thus, the regeneration of spinal cord fibers produced by the IN-1 antibody can actually have functional consequences.

Further applications of this information are certainly possible. Most applications of neural transplantation, at least those where new axonal connections are formed, employ systems in which nonmyelinated axons grow and make connections over a relatively short range. Myelinated tracts may in certain circumstances form an impenetrable barrier to neurite extension from transplants, and the ability to block this inhibitory effect may permit applications of neural transplantation that would not otherwise be feasible. On the other hand, reconstruction of large myelinated tracts in the adult is a very difficult problem and may not be a realistic goal.

Studies by Richard Bunge and Mary Bunge

Whereas Schwab and his coworkers demonstrated that oligodendrocytes inhibit axonal growth, the corresponding cells from peripheral nerve are highly effective in promoting axonal growth. In fact, it has long been known that the structure and functions of central and peripheral myelin-producing cells are quite different (figure 2.6; Bunge 1968). Schwann cells, which produce myelin in the peripheral nervous system, are aligned in rows, and many are devoted to producing myelin for a single peripheral nerve fiber. When a peripheral nerve degenerates, the Schwann cells remain aligned within the basal lamina (a tubelike structure), ideally situated to provide a scaffold for axonal regeneration. Oligodendrocytes that produce myelin in the CNS, on the other hand, each have many processes which extend to produce myelin. When CNS myelinated fibers degenerate, no scaffolding—nor, in fact, any trace of the former structure—remains to guide regenerative growth. Regeneration through a field of oligodendrocytes would be, therefore, a chaotic process. Thus, it seems reasonable to expect that the biochemical properties of Schwann cells would promote regeneration, while oligodendrocytes would not. Indeed, this turns out to be the case.

While Schwab, Schnell, and coworkers have concentrated on blocking the inhibitory effects of oligodendrocytes, Bunge, Bunge, and coworkers have concentrated on further exploiting the growth-stimulating effects of peripheral nerve components. Schwann cells produce a number of factors that might be capable of stimulating spinal cord regeneration. These include neurotrophic substances as well as cell recognition molecules and extracellular matrix proteins, such as L1 and laminin, which can stimulate axonal growth.

Paino and Bunge (1991) studied the possibility of transplanting Schwann cells, the peripheral cells that produce myelin, into the spinal cord to promote regeneration. Schwann cells were obtained from rat fetuses, then grown on sheets of collagen. These sheets of collagen were rolled to form cylindrical structures, which were stabilized by coating them with rat plasma. Spinal cord lesions were produced with a laser-dye technique (discussed in detail in chapter 16, on cerebral cortex transplants). After 5 to 28 days the collagen-Schwann cell rolls were transplanted into the site of the lesions.

Numerous axons were found to grow into these Schwann cell grafts, while no axons grew into collagen tubes lacking Schwann cells. As might be expected, no evidence that the recruited axons were able to exit the graft and continue growing within the distal part of the spinal cord was reported. This observation is nevertheless significant because it suggests that Schwann cells alone are the significant component of peripheral nerve regarding stimulation of axonal growth. Since this study identifies a single cellular component for stimulation of axonal growth in the spinal cord, this might potentially become an avenue for use in combination with other techniques for spinal cord reconstruction.

The above discussion considers the possibility of promoting growth of neurites across the site of spinal cord injury by using peripheral nerve, Schwann cells, and manipulation of growth-inhibitory molecules. Earlier studies also had shown increases in growth of fibers by a number of drugs and locally administered substances, piromen being the prototypical example. These strategies have been, to varying degrees, somewhat successful in terms of increasing the growth of spinal cord fibers, but have not been successful in re-forming complete circuits that reconnect the proximal and distal segments of the spinal cord.

Improvements in, and variations of, these techniques might lead to improved results. However, simple incremental improvement might not have the desired effect, because there appear to be two different problems, both of which are not addressed by any single technique. There is the problem of growth of fibers across the site of an injury, and the problem of promoting continued growth (after the gap has been bridged) within uninjured parts of the adult spinal cord. So far, no single technique seems to be able to address both problems.

This, obviously, suggests that we might consider using a combination(s) of approaches. For example, one might imagine that we should use peripheral nerve grafts to induce the growth of fibers across the site of an injury, combined with blocking the growth-inhibitory properties of oligodendrocytes (as with the monoclonal antibody IN-1) to stimulate continued growth of fibers once they have crossed the gap and reentered the distal spinal cord. Other bridging techniques, as well as methods to augment axonal growth, such as administration of growth factors, may very well produce results that come closer to functional spinal cord reconstruction. It is conceivable that some combination of the techniques already at hand is all that is required to produce functional recovery after spinal cord injury.

Transplantation of Fetal CNS Tissues into the Spinal Cord

In addition to the possibilities for combining neurite growth-promoting techniques, several additional transplantation methods for spinal cord repair are being explored. These have generally fallen into two broad categories. The first is the transplantation, into or near the site of injury, of neurons (or, more properly, regions of the CNS that include both neurons and glia) the cell bodies of which are normally located in the brain, but which can send projections into the spinal cord. The second is the transplantation of fragments of tissue or cells from fetal spinal cord into the site of injury.

In both cases, the goal is generally to restore some form of communication between the proximal and distal segments of the spinal cord. It is important to emphasize that this does not necessarily mean a complete restoration of the spinal cord structure; rather, even a small degree of communication that leads to even a small degree of motor control could be of major significance. One scenario to achieve this communication would be—as with peripheral nerve grafts—to promote the growth of fibers across the gap. A second (and likely to be more readily achievable) idea is for the grafts to act as relays, so that neurons located above the gap would connect with transplanted neurons. The transplanted neurons would then send fibers into, and form connections with, distal parts of the spinal cord. This relay scenario could conceivably result in communication across the site of a transection, and hence some functional restoration.

Before discussing some of the recent experiments on repairing the spinal cord with fetal tissue transplants, it is necessary to consider the types of movement that can be mediated by the spinal cord. Located entirely within the spinal cord are circuits that can generate walking movements, at least in animals. In an animal with a spinal cord transection, when the front limbs are supported and the hind limbs are placed on a treadmill, the hind limbs may be able to (but cannot always) generate walking movements in response to the tactile stimulus from the treadmill. The neural circuits for activating these movements are contained entirely within the spinal cord, and are often referred to as "spinal pattern generators for locomotion" or "spinal generators of locomotion" (SGL). Of course, in an animal with a spinal cord transection, these SGL are not connected to the brain; and thus cannot generate purposive or intentional movements; at best, they can generate reflexive movement in response to tactile stimuli. In concrete terms, an animal with spinal cord injury may, under favorable circumstances, may be able to generate reflexive limb movements, but be unable walk across a room to obtain food. Thus signals from the brain cannot direct movement to occur, even when these movements can be generated reflexively. Moreover, even when SGL are structurally intact following spinal cord injury, their function may be impaired (e.g., as a result of disturbances in inputs to these circuits) due to abnormalities in spinal cord circuits generated by the injury.

There is some controversy regarding the presence of SGL in humans. In general, movement control is more subject to cortical influence, compared with subcortical control, in primates and especially in humans. In all probability, some element of SGL is present in humans, although the equivalent human circuits may be more sensitive to functional perturbation following spinal cord injury. Spinally generated movements in patients with spinal cord injury are not frequently seen. Therefore, one of the most readily achievable goals of neural transplantation in the human spinal cord may be to implant neurons that can activate SGL. Perhaps these transplants can be situated so that they can be influenced by circuits above the injury site (figure 18.6). In this way, a transplant may act as a relay to stimulate at least a partial return of motor function without producing a complete reconstruction of the spinal circuitry as it existed in the original intact state.

Transplants of Neurons from Above the Spinal Cord

Neurons from above the spinal cord are referred to as "supraspinal neurons." An example of a transplantation technique utilizing supraspinal neurons, from the earlier discussion on human trials, is the experiments conducted by Pogos Katunian, in which fetal neurons are transplanted into the site of a spinal cord injury (discussed earlier in this chapter). In a more conservative vein are several animal experiments which have

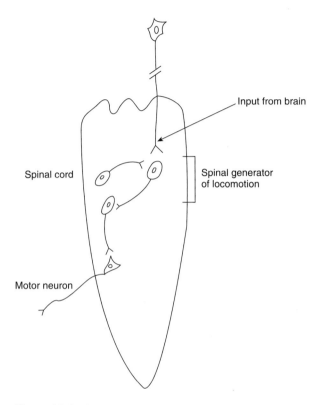

Figure 18.6
There are circuits within the spinal cord in lower animals, and probably in humans as well, that are capable of generating complete patterns of locomotion. This circuit is represented by the three oval-shaped neurons (spinal generators of locomotion). Under normal circumstances, these circuits are activated in response to signals from the brain. When the spinal cord is severed, these circuits generally remain silent. The possibility of finding ways to reactivate these circuits may be a key to achieving functional repair of injured spinal cords. Activation of spinal generators of locomotion may, for example, have played a role in the spinal cord repair method described by Cheng and coworkers (1996), illustrated in figure 18.7. (Adapted from Bregman 1994.)

shown that this approach can be partially effective, albeit under very restricted conditions.

The earliest experiments along these lines were reported by Kao and coworkers (1970), who transplanted cerebellar tissue into the spinal cord in order to inhibit scar formation. Aihara (1970) reported that a similar procedure led to functional recovery in some animals, although this result is now doubted. In 1983, Das examined the properties of embryonic neocortex transplanted into the spinal cord. A number of other experiments have examined the anatomical properties of tissue from various brain regions transplanted into the spinal cord; for the most part these will not be described here.

One series of experiments is based on the observation that stepping movements can be elicited in animals with transected spinal cords by application of norepinephrine agonists to the spinal cord below the injury site (Forssberg and Grillner 1973). This suggests that intrinsic spinal cord stepping generators, the SGL, can be activated by norepinephrine. Based on this idea, a number of experiments have been performed with the aim of transplanting norepinephrine-containing neurons to the spinal cord in order to activate these stepping circuits. In particular, one experiment examined transplants in animals with basically intact spinal cords, but with the catecholaminergic input destroyed by the catecholamine neurotoxin 6-hydroxydopamine (Buchanan and Nornes 1986). This experiment was able to demonstrate reactivation of stepping reflexes; however, this observation is relevant only to that specific circumstance, involving restricted and very selective lesions.

Another subsequent experiment that is somewhat more relevant to the aim of restoring function after spinal cord injury was reported by Yakovleff and coworkers in 1989. In this study, rats received spinal cord transections and after eight days received grafts of fetal locus ceruleus into the distal segment of the cord. As in other experiments on transplantation of fetal brain, only 1–2 percent of the transplanted cells were noradrenergic neurons. In three of the five rats that had received transplants, rhythmic stepping activity was elicited when the rats were held above a treadmill, with hind limbs and tail touching the moving belt. In two of these three rats, the frequency of stepping could be modulated by changing the speed of the treadmill. In these two animals, many surviving nor-adrenergic neurons were found, with processes extending in the vicinity of motor neurons. Although this is a rather small and somewhat prelimi-nary study, the results suggest that reflexive stepping can be facilitated by noradrenergic reafferentation of the distal spinal cord in animals with complete spinal cord transection.

In a similar vein, sexual reflexes (ejaculation) can be restored in rats by transplanting serotonergic neurons from the raphe nuclei into the dis-tal spinal cord (Privat et al. 1989). A number of addition experiments have examined transplants of other tissues, such as cortical tissue, into the spinal cord. Some of these latter experiments have shown that the tissue survives transplantation, but have not demonstrated any sort of functional recovery in animals with spinal cord injury that can be induced by the transplantation.

Fetal Spinal Cord Grafts

A major current research emphasis in spinal cord repair by transplanta-tion involves the transplantation of fetal spinal cord tissue into the spinal cord, usually into the site of injury. Compared with transplanting other tissues into the spinal cord, it is believed that a more complete restoration of function might ultimately be possible using this approach. In other words, fetal spinal cord grafts might be capable of restoring the structure and function of the spinal cord to a form most closely resembling the normal, uninjured spinal cord. The specifics of this approach have been described in detail by Bregman and coworkers (Bregman 1994; Bregman et al. 1997).

There are several specific structural goals of this kind of transplanta-tion. First, fetal spinal cord grafts may limit glial scarring, cavitation, and deterioration of the general structure of the spinal cord. Second, by providing an alternative target and/or trophic support, fetal spinal cord grafts may "rescue" neurons that would otherwise die after spinal cord transection. Third, spinal cord grafts might conceivably provide a "bridge" allowing fibers to grow across the gap, as is seen for peripheral nerve. Finally, and perhaps most important, fetal spinal cord grafts might perform a "relay" function. In other words, neurons within the transplant might receive inputs from above the injury site and send outputs into intact segments of the spinal cord below the injury site, thereby restoring a form of communication across the gap.

The ultimate goal is certainly to restore function, even if slight or partial, in cases of chronic and complete spinal cord injury. It is more feasible, however, to approach this goal incrementally; that is, by using models that involve immature host animals, short-term injury, and less severe forms of injury. Although very encouraging results have been seen in several such experiments, obtaining some functional restoration in an immature rat with partial spinal cord injury is many steps removed from repairing spinal cord injury in human quadriplegic patients. This is an important point to remember the next time one sees a headline about some recent breakthrough in the repair of injured spinal cords!

Anatomical Observations of Spinal Cord Grafts

Spinal cord transplants can certainly survive well and become integrated with the host spinal cord. Such transplants also may diminish glial scarring and reduce the death of neurons that have been axotomized by spinal cord injury (for reviews, cf. Bregman 1994; Bregman et al. 1997; Tessler 1991). In some cases, improvements seen after spinal cord transplants are simply due to reductions in adverse secondary consequences of injury.

As discussed above, potential functional restoration might take place via two major mechanisms: the grafts may provide a bridge for fiber regrowth, or they may relay information from above the injury site to below it. When grafts are placed into neonatal animals, fibers do grow through the transplants. This is thought to be related to the fact that the corticospinal tract is still growing in neonatal animals. Some of these not-yet-formed fibers are able to grow through the spinal cord graft, just as they would have grown through the normal spinal cord. Such fibers have also been found to make contacts with appropriate targets below the injury site. In adult hosts, however, fibers do not traverse spinal cord grafts to reemerge from the distal side.

Not only do these fibers fail to grow through the grafts in adult hosts (they do grow through peripheral nerve grafts), but even if they did grow through the grafts, they presumably would stop growing when they reentered the normal distal part of the adult spinal cord. Thus, this strategy does not, in itself, seem likely to result in functional improvement.

The relay mode of function, in contrast, might be viable in adult as well as in neonatal animals. To show that grafts actually cause functional recovery through a relay mode is a difficult task. What has been possible, however, is to show that grafts receive inputs from above and send outputs to below. This would demonstrate that relay function is possible.

In newborn animals, transplants "rescue" neurons above the injury site that would otherwise die, and some of these neurons send axons into, as well as through, the graft (Bregman 1994). Axons of neurons within the graft also project into the host spinal cord. Thus, assuming that the receiving neurons within the graft are in communication with the sending neurons, communication across the injury site may be reestablished in young animals.

A considerable number of studies have examined the connections of spinal cord grafts in adult animals. Host neurons have been found both to send axons into spinal cord grafts and to form synapses within the transplants (Itoh et al. 1996; Shibayama et al. 1998). Host neurons that send axons into transplants include neurons located in the cerebral cortex, raphe nucleus (the source of most serotonergic neurons), locus coeruleus (the region containing norepinephrine neurons), and neurons within the spinal cord. Thus, in the adult animal, there are connections of spinal cord grafts that could support communication across the site of an injury. Note, however, that these experiments have generally involved implantation of grafts immediately or shortly following injury.

Five major studies that have shown functional recovery induced by transplants in animals with spinal cord injury will be discussed below.

Kunkel-Bagden and Bregman 1990 Study

This study is especially noteworthy for several reasons; mainly, because it was the first to demonstrate functional recovery following transplants of spinal cord into the lesioned spinal cord, and second, because accurate, quantitative tests were employed to assess motor function. Additional refinements of this technique have been developed (e.g., Diener and Bregman 1998).

The animals used for this experiment were newborn rats. The model of spinal cord injury employed was "overhemisection," in which somewhat more than half of the spinal cord is severed. The lesions are made by cutting with scissors, a procedure which ensures that the transection on one side will be complete, with some overlap to the other side. Following such overhemisections, the animals remain relatively healthy and are able to walk, but show deficits in coordination. Fragments of fetal spinal cord were placed into the site of the lesions immediately after the overhemisections.

Two of the analyses that were done involved measurements of the animals' gait from walking tracks, and measurements of errors made in walking across a wire mesh grid. The animals with spinal cord lesions, compared with normal controls, walked with feet farther apart and held outward at an angle, and made many more errors in placing their feet on the wire grid. The transplants improved the angle and spacing of the feet, and slightly decreased the number or errors made in walking across the grid. The length of the animals' stride was decreased by the spinal cord lesions, but this deficit was not improved by the transplants.

Although this study was partially successful in producing functional restoration, two conditions were quite different from the circumstances expected in human spinal cord injury: first, the transplants were made immediately after injury, and second, the animals were very immature (newborn).

Iwashita et al. 1994 Study
This study was the first to report functional recovery following complete transection. The animals used were newborn rats. In this experiment, lesions were made in a lower part of the thoracic region, so that the functional impairment was relatively mild.

The spinal cord was exposed and completely severed. At the same time, intact segments of embryonic spinal cord were transplanted into the injury site. Control animals received grafts of spinal cord that were inverted (with the incorrect orientation), sciatic nerve, or no graft. The inverted grafts (surprisingly) did not survive. Of 22 rats with grafts in the correct orientation, the graft "united with the recipient spinal cord at both the rostral and caudal stumps and formed a seamless spinal cord" in 14 cases (Iwashita et al. 1994, 167). There was evidence from anatomical tracing studies for growth of fibers across the graft.

These authors also noted evidence for functional recovery in animals with grafts, although evaluation of their findings is difficult. First, the degree of functional impairment seen under these conditions, with the type of lesion used, was relatively mild. Not all of the animals showed paralysis, and all of the animals were able to walk. Since motor function was not measured by objective tests (e.g., footprint analysis), it is difficult to be confident about the degree of motor improvement seen in the grafted rats.

As mentioned, all of the animals were able to walk to some degree. Some of the animals, however, showed abnormal walking, with an absence of normal hind limb-forelimb coordination. Other animals showed hind limb paralysis. In all animals with successful grafts, walking was normal. In contrast, some degree of abnormal walking was present in all of the control animals and in the animals with anatomically unsuccessful grafts. Animals with successful grafts also showed normal righting reflexes, whereas the controls did not. Again, however, these alterations in motor function were not measured quantitatively, with objective tests. Nevertheless, the improvement seen in this study is consistent with the general hypothesis that considerable regrowth through spinal grafts, and reorganization of motor functions, can occur in immature animals.

Stokes and Reier 1992 Study

Of the studies in this area published until 1992, this experiment came the closest to demonstrating functional recovery after spinal cord grafts under circumstances relevant to human spinal cord injury. It was the first published study in which grafts were found to have a positive effect in adult animals, and also the only such study with a delay between injury and transplantation.

The method employed was as follows. Adult rats were anesthetized and the spinal cord was exposed. A contusion injury was produced by an electromechanically driven impact device under carefully controlled conditions. This technique produces a severe lesion of the spinal cord that evolves for some time after the injury, with progressively increasing cavitation. This is similar to the kinds of injury seen in human spinal cord injury patients.

Deficits in walking are maximal a few days after the injury, but spontaneously recover, without any intervention, over the course of about one month. The reason that the lesion grossly appears worse at the same time that the animals recover motor function is probably that circuits damaged by the lesion continue to degenerate, while circuits that remain structurally intact are disrupted immediately after the lesion but gradually recover functionally or are reorganized over the course of several weeks.

After injury, the animals were allowed to recover for 10 days before receiving transplants. Fetal spinal cord pieces from 14-day gestational rats were dissociated, and transplanted by injection into three or four locations around the center of the lesioned area.

Motor function was measured using methods similar to those used in the Kunkel-Bagden and Bregman (1990) study. A series of tests was used that can be divided into two groups: (1) general observations of walking in an open space and walking across a mesh grid, and (2) analysis of footprints. In general, the transplants did not improve general locomotion. For example, using a scale to rate walking function in an open space (the Tarlov scale), the transplanted animals were slightly, but not significantly, worse than the controls.

On the other hand, the analysis of footprints revealed some significant improvements in animals with transplants. The three measurements used were (1) base of support—animals with lesions space their feet more widely; (2) stride length—animals with spinal cord injury make shorter strides; (3) angle of rotation—animals with spinal cord injury rotate their paws outward, at an angle away from the body axis.

The transplanted animals had very substantial improvements in base of support, moderate improvements in stride length, and no improvements in angle of rotation. By the base of support measurement, the transplanted animals improved to the point that they were almost similar to their performance prior to injury. Therefore, although improvements were seen only for certain very defined measures, the transplants did produce a distinct improvement in some aspects of motor function.

The mechanisms through which these transplants produced improvements in motor function are unclear. One definite possibility is that the transplants decreased progressive deterioration in spinal cord circuits that would otherwise occur after 10 days. A second possibility is that the transplants promoted reorganization of circuits that survived the injury but remained dysfunctional. A third possibility is that the transplants performed a "relay" function, conveying information from above the injury site to below it. At the present time, however, the mechanism of action is unknown.

The Stokes and Reier (1992) study represents a very significant development in spinal cord restoration research. Under conditions roughly analogous to these in human spinal cord injury, it was possible to promote functional recovery, albeit to a small degree, using transplantation. The study was a technological tour de force from an experimental standpoint: motor function was measured with precise quantitative and objective tests, and the lesioning procedure, statistics, surgery, and monitoring methods were state of the art.

Before getting too excited about making spinal cord transplants in human patients, however, there are a few caveats. The type of injury used allowed for considerable recovery, even without transplants, and the amount of additional recovery produced by transplants was small. Second, the 10-day interval between injury and transplantation might be an issue for human application. This might be enough time to determine whether an individual injury was of a type that additional benefit might be expected from a transplant, but there would certainly be difficulties. Remember that by some measures it seemed that the transplants actually made matters slightly worse. Deciding whether to make a transplant during this interval would require that a transplant be made (risking additional attendant damage) before the full extent of spontaneous recovery was known. Considering that the benefits of the transplants were small even in the rat, such a decision would be very difficult to make. This procedure was most emphatically not a demonstration that transplants could restore motor function in an animal model of complete quadriplegia. In summary, in all probability, major and perhaps even fundamental improvements will be necessary before a procedure applicable to humans is developed.

Cheng, Cao, and Olson 1996 Study

One of the most exciting recent developments in spinal cord repair research is a series of experiments that have used a combination of surgical techniques, grafting, and growth factors to repair the spinal cord. These studies are likely to play an important role in the future development of spinal cord repair methods. Since this technique had several components, each will be described separately.

One component involved the use of a surgical technique to shorten the spinal cord, allowing the stumps to be apposed more closely. When the spinal cord is completely severed, the stumps retract significantly. Thus, any regenerating fibers encounter a gap that, if not closed, becomes filled with scar tissue and other material that is very inhospitable to neural regeneration. To avoid this problem, several researchers have shortened the spinal cord by removing vertebrae. Cheng and Olson (1995) employed a method that involved removing one vertebra and wiring together the spinal cord stumps to compress and immobilize the vertebral column. This resulted in a much smaller gap between the severed stumps of the spinal cord, and resulted in a substantial increase in the regeneration of serotonergic fibers across the gap. The spinal column was also distorted slightly to further compress the spinal cord.

The second technique that was employed was the use of a fibrin glue containing a growth factor (acidic fibroblast growth factor). Fibrin is the fibrous component of plasma that forms blood clots. The cut ends of the cord were united with a fibrin glue, produced by catalyzing coagulation of fibrinogen from serum with thrombin (Cheng et al. 1995). This helped to further stabilize the cord, and the growth factor may have helped to promote regeneration.

Finally, segments of peripheral nerve were used to bridge the gap. For this study, 18 segments of peripheral nerve were transplanted into the site of spinal cord transection, to reconnect the stumps. These peripheral nerve segments were placed in the gap in an aligned fashion, so that each piece of peripheral nerve was in contact with a defined spot in the white matter of the proximal stump of the spinal cord. The peripheral nerve fragments were not, however, oriented directly parallel to the spinal cord, but instead were located so that fibers from white matter were redirected toward gray matter. Remember from the discussion above that white matter is highly restrictive to axonal growth, whereas gray matter is relatively permissive (see discussion of Martin Schwab and Lisa Schnell experiments earlier in this chapter). This allowed regrowing axons to regenerate through the relatively permissive substrate of gray matter, rather than through the growth-inhibiting white matter, once these growing fibers entered the distal stump of the spinal cord. (See figure 18.7.)

Thus, the approach involved shortening the spinal cord, using fibrin glue incorporating acidic fibroblast growth factor, and placing precisely aligned peripheral nerve grafts into the gap (Cheng 1996; Cheng et al. 1996). Remarkably, although this surgery was performed after a two-week delay, it still resulted in the regeneration of many fascicles of new growing fibers across the injury site. Furthermore, the animals regained considerable open space walking capacity (although after recovery their walking ability was still far from normal); some of the results are shown in figure 18.8. This is probably the most comprehensive and encouraging study of spinal cord repair methods so far completed. It is unique in that it began the process of combining several methods that may be needed to overcome the multiple obstacles to restoration of function following spinal cord injury. Even though future studies are likely to improve on their technique, or other combinations of approaches may be found to be more efficacious, the principle of combining several manipulations to deal with problems of spinal cord repair has been established.

Li, Field, and Raisman 1997 Study

The most recent development in spinal cord repair research is a study that employed "ensheathing cells," a specialized type of glial cells found in the olfactory epithelium and olfactory nerve, for transplantation into the spinal cord. Olfactory neurons have the ability to regenerate, and the ensheathing cells are therefore especially conducive to axonal growth. In this respect, ensheathing cells resemble Schwann cells, but in other respects they are more akin to CNS glia (astrocytes).

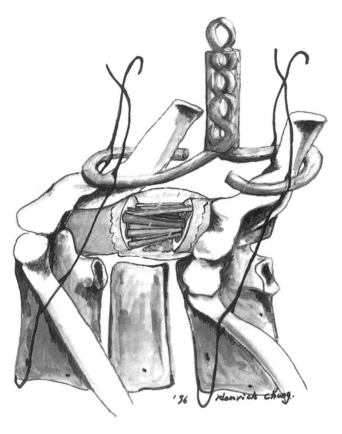

Figure 18.7
The method employed by Cheng and coworkers (1996) to reconstruct the severed
spinal cord. A 5-mm spinal cord segment is removed at the T8 level. The cut
stumps are brought into proximity by removing one vertebra, and stabilized by
wiring together the vertebrae on either side of the transection. Peripheral nerve
(intercostal nerve) fragments are used to bridge the gap because they can promote
axonal growth; however, when they are used in the normal manner, axonal
growth stops at the distal end of the peripheral nerve graft. In this experiment,
the peripheral nerve grafts were used to shunt axonal growth from white matter
tracts (where axonal growth is inhibited) to gray matter tracts in the distal stump,
since gray matter can permit at least some axonal growth. This may have allowed
regenerating fibers to grow far enough that they could make connections in the
distal part of the spinal cord. Finally, the spinal cord was further stabilized with
minced fragments of peripheral nerve and a fibrin-based glue containing acidic
fibroblast growth factor, which would stimulate axonal growth. (Drawing provided courtesy of Heinrich Cheng, formerly at the Department of Neuroscience,
Stockholm University, and currently of the Department of Neurosurgery, Veterans' General Hospital, Taipei, Republic of China.)

Adult rats were used in the study by Li and coworkers (1997). The corticospinal tract was severed on one side. Olfactory ensheathing cells were cultured from adult rats, and transplanted into the lesion site by simple injection. Extensive growth of corticospinal axons was induced. These axons not only grew through the implant area but also continued to elongate into the intact spinal cord distal to the graft. This regrowth was associated with recovery of directed paw-reaching behavior.

This study can be compared with that of Cheng, Cao, and Olson (1996), and shows a second set of conditions that can permit spinal cord regeneration. Although much remains to be done before this can be used as a clinical treatment, these experiments clearly show that the goal—developing at least a partial "cure" of spinal cord injury—is realistic.

Ensheathing cells, in fact, can be obtained from the olfactory epithelium of human subjects by biopsy, without serious adverse consequences, and then grown in culture (Vawter et al. 1996). This procedure might be entirely feasible in human subjects. A patient with spinal cord injury might receive a biopsy to obtain autologous olfactory epithelium, ensheathing cells might be cultured from the biopsy sample, and then transplanted into the same patient's spinal cord.

If this procedure of transplanting olfactory ensheathing cells, or something like it, turns out to be effective, there would be few real obstacles to developing a clinical treatment based on it. Human ensheathing cells can be obtained easily; the procedure does not, probably, require complete transection of the spinal cord; and it seems to work even in adult animals. Additional studies would be needed to verify that the procedure is functionally effective, especially in higher animals. Recovery was not observed in all animals, and even in the animals that showed some improvement, the degree of recovery was modest. Thus, some improvements of the method would probably be necessary. Studies of the kind of injury to which the method could be applied (complete or partial transection, contusion injury), and of the allowable interval between injury and transplantation, will also be needed. Nevertheless, since this procedure may not require invasive manipulation of the spinal cord, it or some related procedure derived from it may eventually become feasible for actual human use.

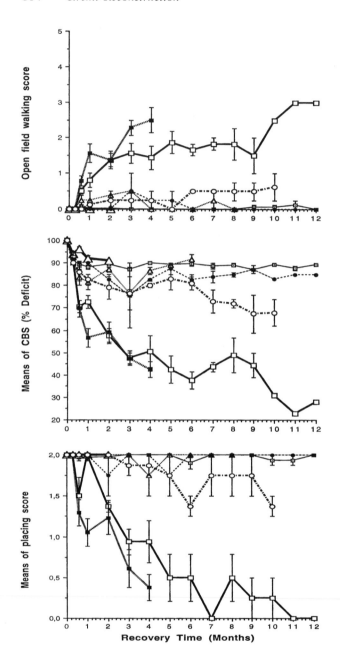

Recovery Time (Months)

Conclusions

We now have seen a considerable armamentarium of techniques that can be applied to spinal cord injury. What are the prospects for additional improvements in transplantation-related techniques for spinal cord repair? First, we will summarize what can be accomplished now. There are available, at the present time, several techniques that can be used to achieve different ends.

Bridging the Gap

In neonatal rats, spinal cord grafts can promote the growth of fibers across an injury site. In adults, spinal cord grafts are not effective in this regard, but peripheral nerve grafts are. In addition to peripheral nerve pieces, isolated Schwann cells (Paino and Bunge 1991) and olfactory ensheathing cells (Li et al. 1997) can stimulate fiber growth. In mature ani-

---

Figure 18.8
Limb function following spinal cord repair, as described by Cheng and coworkers (1996). Two groups of animals received the complete repair technique; one of these groups was repaired with autografts only (from the same animal), shown as black squares with dotted lines. These animals were studied for four months. A second group received a mixture of autografts and allografts (from other rats); these animals, shown as white squares with heavy solid lines, were studied for 12 months. A third group of animals, shown by white circles with dashed lines, received repair on one side only. These animals showed little improvement. The upper graph shows open field walking scores, in which a 5 represents normal walking and 0 indicates complete paralysis. The middle graph shows mean combined behavioral score ratings (includes evaluation of measures of climbing an inclined plane, swimming, motor skills, righting reflex, etc.), where 100 is complete impairment and 0 is normal function. In the lower graph, which shows ratings of paw placing, 0 represents normal function. The animals with the complete repair method showed substantial improvements, especially developing from three to six months after repair, by each of these measures. There were four control groups. Some animals received spinal cord transection only (small white squares), some received transection followed by removal of a 5 mm segment of the spinal cord (white triangles with heavy lines), others received repair but with omission of fibroblast growth factor from the fibrin glue (small circles and dotted lines), and some had nerve grafts connecting white matter to white matter, instead of white matter to gray matter (white triangles with dotted lines). No improvements were seen in any of these control groups. (From Cheng et al. 1996, with permission.)

mals, however, bridging the gap does not seem to be the only obstacle, since fibers usually grow poorly in the host spinal cord even after the gap has been crossed. Therefore, bridging the gap alone does not appear to be sufficient to produce functional recovery.

Growth Within the Spinal Cord

An injury site can be bridged in both immature animals (by spinal cord grafts) and adults (by peripheral nerve, Schwann cells, or ensheathing cells). Reconstruction, however, also requires continued growth within intact portions of the distal spinal cord. In the adult, growth within the spinal cord is poor. There are several potential methods for increasing this growth. First, monoclonal antibodies that block the growth-inhibitory function of oligodendrocytes have been shown to permit substantial growth of axons within the injured adult spinal cord. Additional growth can be stimulated by growth factors. In particular, growth of corticospinal axons can be markedly stimulated by NT–3 (Schnell et al. 1994), or by acidic FGF (Cheng et al. 1995).

It is curious that in the Li et al. (1997) study, ensheathing cells apparently produced growth of axons which continued after the axons reached the distal spinal cord. This suggests that, in some sense, corticospinal axons can be "conditioned" to continue to grow, or not grow, by the terrain they traverse. Exactly what "conditioned" means in this context is entirely speculative at this point.

In this connection, the older literature that showed increased sprouting of fibers following spinal cord injury by administration of substances that promote fever and inflammation, or influence scar formation, should be mentioned. These treatments were shown to increase fiber growth within regions of spinal cord injury, although not to the degree that the fibers transversed the gap.

Relay Function and Reorganization

It appears that some functional restoration can be attained by grafts of dissociated spinal cord cells into sites of spinal cord injury even in adults (Stokes and Reier 1992). At the present time, the mechanisms through which these grafts produce functional improvement are unclear, but it is probably not regeneration or regrowth of axons across the gap. The

within the spinal cord can be markedly increased, and functional reco\
can be stimulated, although only slightly, by grafts that appear to ﹅
neither of the above but probably operate via a third mechanism. Growtl.
can also be elicited by peripheral nerve grafts even in the chronically injured spinal cord (Houle 1991).

Whether these techniques, alone or in combination, can be employed
to obtain functional repair of spinal cord injury in humans is, of course,
not known. Moreover, complete reconstitution to a state of entirely normal function is probably an unrealistic goal, at least for the immediate
future. Nevertheless, there is every reason to be optimistic that at least
some partial functional repair, perhaps limited motor function, can eventually be obtained in patients with spinal cord injury.

Finally, a cautionary note is in order. It may not be sufficient simply
to stimulate axonal growth. Random growth, stimulated by, for example,
transplants of dissociated cells or by growth factors, could be so disorganized that it might be useless or nearly useless. Corticospinal axons certainly do not have an inherent degree of specificity that will allow them
to find their appropriate targets by themselves. Motor fibers can find their
way to muscles, but they may connect to the wrong muscles—for example, in such a way that when you try to move your arm, your thumb
moves instead. Or fibers may connect to opposing muscles in such a way
that nothing happens. In the adult, mechanisms that were present to guide
developing corticospinal axons to appropriate targets are no longer
present.

Let's try to imagine a situation in which growth of corticospinal axons
can be completely stimulated after injury, so that all of the severed axons
regrow until they find targets. Conditions at the injury site will almost
certainly be so chaotic that the axons will lose their way and become
completely disorganized in the process of crossing the gap, even if they
can be stimulated to find their way across. For this reason, the procedure
devised by Cheng and coworkers (1996) is particularly attractive, in
that it includes a means of maintaining some degree of organization of
the spinal cord at the injury site with an array of small pieces of peripheral nerve not only to stimulate growth but also to keep axonal
growth aligned in an appropriate columnar fashion. It is interesting and
fortuitous that a single method can be used for both purposes. For this

possibilities that were suggested include (1) alleviation of progress damage, (2) relaying information from above to below the injury si and (3) promotion of reorganization in remaining alternative netwo (Stokes and Reier 1992). Whichever of these mechanisms is, in fa operative, it might be exploited in the development of reconstructi strategies.

Combinations of Methods

There are several intriguing potential methods for improving spinal cor reconstruction by combining existing techniques. Most of these are prob ably obvious to the reader. For example, suppose grafts of periphera nerve or Schwann cells were used to induce growth of fibers across the site of a spinal cord injury. Under this circumstance, there is some, albeit very limited, growth of fibers once they reenter the intact distal spinal cord. If this growth could be increased from 1 mm to 10 or 20 mm, perhaps it would be sufficient to reestablish useful synaptic contacts. Would delivery of monoclonal IN-1 antibodies in combination with growth factors accomplish this goal? Or would grafts of olfactory en-sheathing cells, in combination with peripheral nerve grafts, produce im-proved results? It seems likely that this might occur. Another possibility would be the use of fetal spinal cord grafts in combination with the above approaches. Perhaps some combination of approaches would be capable of achieving significant functional restoration. It appears that a number of techniques are available which are capable of addressing vari-ous aspects of the reasons for the failure of spinal cord regeneration: scar formation, information transfer from above to below the injury site, fail-ure of axons to cross the gap, and failure of axons to grow within the intact spinal cord. Since, at least to some degree, each problem can be addressed in isolation, it may be that the overall problem of spinal cord repair can best be approached through the use of several techniques in combination.

Conclusions

One conclusion seems clear: it is certainly not the case that spinal cord injury is a final, immutable condition about which nothing can be done. Even in adults, growth across an injury site can be achieved, growth reason, even if other methods are employed, we may very well see the technique of Cheng and coworkers—or something very much like it— used as a component of any spinal cord repair strategy that is ultimately devised.

Spinal cord injury is no longer the hopeless situation that it once appeared to be. The available techniques that can stimulate regeneration or restructuring of the spinal cord are numerous: treatment with growth factors or growth-promoting antibodies; transplants of olfactory ensheathing cells, Schwann cells, peripheral nerve segments, and fetal spinal cord; and surgical techniques to assist in spinal cord reorganization. Each of these holds promise, and we can certainly expect further improvements. It is not at all unreasonable to believe that actual reconstructive treatment of spinal cord injury will become possible in the foreseeable future.

Further Reading

Anderson D. K., Howland, D. R., and Reier, P. J. (1995). Fetal neural grafts and repair of the injured spinal cord. *Brain Pathol.* 5: 451–457.

Bregman, B. S. (1994). Recovery of function after spinal cord injury: Transplantation strategies. In *Functional Neural Transplantation,* S. B. Dunnett and A. Bjorklund (eds.), pp. 489–529. Raven Press, New York.

Bregman, B. S., Diener, P. S., McAtee, M., Dai, H. N., and James, C. (1997). Intervention strategies to enhance anatomical plasticity and recovery of function after spinal cord injury. *Adv. Neurol.* 72: 257–275.

Cheng, H., Cao, Y., and Olson, L. (1996). Spinal cord repair in adult paraplegic rats: Partial restoration of hind limb function. *Science* 273: 510–513.

Fetal nerve cells transplanted into spinal cord. (1997). *Washington Post,* July 13, p. A7.

Freed, W. J., de Medinaceli, L., and Wyatt, R. J. (1985). Promoting functional plasticity in the damaged nervous system. *Science* 227: 1544–1552.

Nesmeyanova, T. (1977). *Experimental Studies of Regeneration of Spinal Neurons.* V. H. Winston and Sons, Washington, D.C.

Schwab, M. E. (1996). Bridging the gap in spinal cord regeneration. *Nature Medicine* 2: 976–977.

Tessler, A. (1991). Intraspinal transplants. *Ann. Neurol.* 29: 115–123.

Vrbova, G., Clowry, G., Nogradi, A., and Sieradzan, K. (1994). *Transplantation of Neural Tissue into Spinal Cord.* CRC Press, Boca Raton, Fla.

Young, W. (1996). Spinal cord regeneration. *Science* 273: 451.

19

Visual System

One of the initial models used for developing the techniques of neural tissue transplantation involved grafting of tissue to the anterior eye chamber (described in chapter 3). In these early experiments, the eye was simply a convenient vessel for the implantation and observation of tissue grafts. Thus, one would naturally think of the possibility of employing transplantation as a method for repairing the eye or in other ways influencing functions of the visual system. Would such a thing be possible? Could certain forms of damage to the visual system be repaired using transplantation? Or, to put it more bluntly, could transplantation be used to make blind people see again? To give a short answer, perhaps. But it would depend greatly on the cause of the blindness.

In animals, experiments on transplantation in the visual system have taken three distinct forms. First, there have been studies in which cells from the retina, or other visual system neurons, have been transplanted directly into the brain, usually near sites in which the axons of retinal ganglion cells terminate. This area has been investigated most extensively by Raymond Lund and coworkers, at the University of Pittsburgh and at Cambridge University. Second, a number of experiments have attempted direct repair of the retina itself, by transplanting cells into the eye. Manuel del Cerro, at the University of Rochester, James Turner, and others have investigated this approach, which has the greatest potential for human application. A third type of study has employed transplants of peripheral nerve to promote regeneration of retinal fibers. This topic has been investigated primarily by Albert Aguayo and associates in Montreal.

It might be useful first to consider the organization of the visual system in a rudimentary way. First, light is *optically* processed by nonneural components of the eye, for example, the lens and the cornea. The subsequent neural processing of light is, of course, crucial. Without the optical processing, however, perception of any sort of visual patterns is impossible. If you need glasses, think of how important glasses are for vision: without them, everything is blurred, but they do not impact the ability of light to reach the retina. In fact, an individual for whom neural processing of light is completely intact may be legally blind because of impaired optical processing of light. Glasses (or contact lenses) merely alter the optical processing of light. For any sort of visual system repair involving transplantation, both neural connections and optics need to be considered.

After optical processing, light is transduced into cellular signals in the retina. The photoreceptor cells (rods and cones) are directly stimulated by light. The second step in visual information processing is performed by a variety of other retinal cell types before the final output from the retina is organized. The optic nerve conveys information from the retina to the brain, via the axons of the retinal ganglion cells. The two optic nerves (one from each eye) meet in a structure called the optic chiasm. There, some of the axons cross to the other side of the brain, to varying degrees in different species. Most of the optic nerve axons terminate in two structures, the superior colliculus (tectum) and the lateral geniculate nucleus. The superior colliculus is relatively more important in lower animals, and the lateral geniculate assumes greater importance in higher animals and in humans. Further processing of visual information takes place in the cerebral cortex. In primates and especially in humans, cortical processing of visual information is of paramount importance. It occurs in rodents as well, but is relatively less important. Correspondingly, the relative importance of the lateral geniculate nucleus, which relays visual information to the cortex, is greater in higher animals, while the tectum is more important in lower animals.

Blindness, partial blindness, or visual impairment can occur as a result of interruption or damage to this pathway at any point. Cortical injury due to stroke, for example, can cause partial blindness. The most common causes of visual impairment are, however, damage or dysfunction in the eye itself, often at the level of the retina. Approaches to transplantation in the visual system with therapeutic intent (although in some cases this possibility may be remote) are mainly focused on transplantation of the retina or cells from the retina. Transplantation to alleviate visual impairment is already common practice, in the form of corneal transplantation for cataracts, and was one of the first forms of therapeutic transplantation to be used. However, transplantation of the neural components of the visual system (e.g., retina) for therapeutic purposes adds a great deal of complexity compared with transplantation of optic components (e.g., cornea), in that the neural components must make appropriate connections with other neural components in order to become functional.

First, let us assume a situation in which the entire retina must be replaced. Then a familiar problem arises: Does one attempt to transplant retina to the retina, or near the retina, where it can receive light input? If so, the transplanted cells face the problem of forming connections with cells in the brain, via the optic nerve—a virtually impassible terrain. On the other hand, transplanting retinal cells directly into the brain leaves the problem of how to convey optical information to the transplanted cells. If they are not within the eye, where the retina is normally located, an artificial device must be constructed to carry optical stimuli to the transplanted cells. Both kinds of transplants certainly are interesting in animals; whether either can be useful in humans, as clinical techniques to treat blindness, is a more complex question.

Intracerebral Grafts of Retinal Tissue

An extensive series of experiments on transplantation of retina into the brain has been performed by Raymond Lund and coworkers. The approach, generally, has involved removal of the connections from the host retina to the brain, by cutting the optic nerve, and transplanting a retina into one of the sites in the brain that receives retinal input.

Essentially all of the experiments in which functional connections have been shown to develop between transplanted retina and host brain have been performed in newborn animals. A few similar experiments using fetal retina and adult host animals have been tried; they have been unsuccessful. This lack of success obviously would impact any possibility of employing such transplants clinically. In addition to host maturity, a second factor that influences the degree of connectivity between retinal grafts and brain is the presence of the normal input from the host eye to the brain. Transplanted retinas have been shown to form more extensive connections with the host brain if the input from at least one eye is removed.

In one such experimental paradigm, Klassen and Lund (1987) employed the contraction of the pupils that occurs in response to light to test the possibility that transplants could convey visual information to the brain. This pupillary contraction is mediated by input from the retina to a nucleus called the olivary pretectal nucleus (OPN).

Fetal retinas were transplanted into the brain of newborn rats in such a way that they could provide input to the OPN and were near the surface of the brain. The animals were then allowed to mature for five months. An opening was then made in the skull, to expose the transplant and allow it to be illuminated directly. The grafts were observed, in most cases, to lie over the superior colliculus. Pupil contraction was tested by measuring the diameter of the pupils. Because visual input to this nucleus was removed by cutting the optic nerve (without damaging the eye itself), the ability of the pupils to contract in response to an appropriate signal from the brain was not impaired.

It was shown that the pupils contracted within a few seconds after the transplant-eye was illuminated. The pupillary contraction response obtained by illuminating the transplant developed over about 4–13 seconds after illuminating the transplant, much slower than the time course of normal pupil contraction (1 sec). In the initial tests, one optic nerve was allowed to remain intact, and moderate pupil contraction responses were observed. Removal of the intact eye greatly enhanced the magnitude of the pupillary contraction response. This may be related to competition between normal inputs and the relatively ineffective inputs from the transplanted retina.

Therefore, the transplanted retina was able to become integrated into the normal reflex circuit that controls pupillary diameter. Although this circuitry does not involve pattern perception, and does not even involve the conscious perception of light, it is one of the normal circuits that involve light input. Thus, a retinal transplant must form connections with the host brain, and these connections must be appropriate and quite precise in order for the pupillary contraction response to be restored.

A second kind of function of retinal transplants was investigated in a later experiment by Coffey, Lund, and Rawlins (1989). In this experiment, light input to the transplanted retina was used as a conditioned stimulus to mediate a learning response (described below). For this test, the transplant was not required to mediate a specific function (i.e., we do not know whether the animals perceived the illumination of the transplant as being light, or as something else). On the other hand, from the nature of the test, it appears that the input to the brain mediated by the retina would have been perceived (if this had been done in humans) as a conscious stimulus. To the degree that rats are "conscious," this study indicates that visual information conveyed to the animal by a transplant can mediate a sensory stimulus in the realm of conscious experience. These experiments are unique in that regard.

For these studies, Coffey and coworkers (1989) removed the right eye of newborn rats, and transplanted embryonic retina to the left tectum (superior colliculus). After the animals were allowed to mature for six weeks, the skull over the transplant was removed and replaced with a transparent plastic window.

The animals were then tested on a lever-pressing task designed to measure their ability to respond to a light stimulus. While the animals were in the process of pressing the lever to obtain food, an overhead light was turned on at random time points for 15 sec intervals. After the 15 sec of light, the animals received a mild foot shock. In normal animals, under these conditions, lever pressing decreased during the 15 sec intervals that the light was on, since the presence of the light indicated that shock was imminent, and thus distracted them from the lever-pressing activity. If the animals could "see" (or detect) the light via a transplant, presumably their lever pressing would decrease when the light was on.

The animals' intact eye was covered with an opaque patch. The animals were then tested for 10 days, to determine whether they were able to employ the light as a stimulus to decrease their responding. In fact, this did occur: The animals with transplants and with their normal eyes covered eventually learned to decrease their lever pressing when the light was on. Ultimately, compared with animals with their normal eye uncovered, the transplants were almost equally effective in conveying the light information to the animals. It took longer, however, for animals to learn via the transplants. When using the transplants, the animals required about three days of testing to learn to employ the light stimulus, while when using their normal eye, the animals learned this discrimination on the first day.

Finally, the testing was validated by covering the window over the transplant for one of the testing days, to block the light from reaching the transplant. This test was used to rule out the possibility—for example—that light was able to leak in around the eye patch, or that the animals were detecting heat from the light source. With the window uncovered, the animals responded at a rate of approximately 1–2 lever presses per minute, showing that they were using the light to suppress responding in anticipation of foot shock. The rate increased to about 8–10 responses per minute when the window was covered. Thus, it appears that the animals were able to use a transplant to convey light information to the brain, and were able to use this information to mediate a learned behavior.

In neural transplantation, this is the only case in which transplants have been used to provide sensory information directly to the brain. It is also unique in that the transplants must be integrated into the appropriate host neural circuitry. Still, the possibility of using this to "make blind people see" is quite remote. First of all, simply detecting the absence or presence of light is not sufficient for most people's definition of useful visual capacity. To make a useful difference in visual ability, a transplant would have to convey pattern-related information. The intrusive nature of the surgery, especially when the implantation of complex optic devices into the brain is considered (one could hardly have a simple plastic window in the skull of a human patient), probably would not be justified simply to allow someone to detect the presence or absence of light. Finally, current technology allows this degree of restoration to be accomplished in very immature animals only; however, even if this latter problem could be overcome, considerable obstacles to human use would remain.

Transplantation of Retinal Cells to the Damaged Retina

For several reasons, this procedure is more likely to lead to a clinical application than transplantation of eyes into the brain. First, although blindness is certainly a serious problem, it may not be serious enough to warrant implantation of both retina and optics into the brain. There would be considerable risk associated with such a procedure, which presumably would have to include the continued presence of artificial optical devices in the brain.

There are several disorders that involve retinal damage in humans. Especially in those cases which involve damage of the retinal photoreceptor cells, and the ganglion cells and their projections to the brain remain intact, there is the possibility of repairing the retina with grafts of retinal cells. Repairing or transplanting the entire retina would be much more difficult. In animals, the two main models are light-induced damage to photoreceptor cells and hereditary retinal degeneration. In humans, there are two fairly common disorders of the retina. One is age-related macular degeneration, a common condition in which photoreceptor cells in the macula (the center of the retina, where photoreceptor cells are found in the highest density) are lost. A second disorder is retinitis pigmentosa, a primary degenerative condition of the photoreceptor cells, or retinal pigment epithelium, that has its onset in early adulthood.

The basic principle of photoreceptor cell transplantation is to replace lost photoreceptors by transplanting new photoreceptors into the retina, and to allow these transplanted cells to establish connections with an otherwise intact retina. This strategy is entirely dependent on the remainder of the retina being intact; for example, if the photoreceptor cells degenerate consequent to an abnormality in another retinal cell type, this strategy will not work.

Transplantation of retinal cells into the retina, using the model of light-induced retinal injury, was first studied by del Cerro and coworkers in the 1980s (del Cerro et al. 1985; 1987), and by other groups as well. Numerous experiments have involved transplantation of retinal cells to both intact and injured retina, using various preparations of cells (Aramant and Seiler 1994; Berglin et al. 1990; DiLoreto et al. 1996; Gouras and Algvere 1996; Little et al. 1996; Lund et al. 1997; Lund and Hankin

1995; Seiler and Aramant 1995). The general conclusion is that it is possible to transplant retinal cells, and that they can become reasonably well integrated into the structure of the host retina, forming appropriate connections with other cell types. The photoreceptor cells are one of the most promising cell types for use in retinal transplantation, since they survive well and make connections with host cells, and there are several disorders that involve degeneration or damage of photoreceptor cells (see del Cerro 1990; del Cerro et al. 1997).

A model of retinal injury that has been used in many experimental studies of retinal transplantation involves light-induced damage to the retina. Albino rats are especially sensitive to retinal damage induced by continuous light. To induce this kind of injury, rats are exposed to fluorescent lights of moderate intensity (two 40 W bulbs) for several weeks. This procedure induces massive degeneration of the retina, with nearly complete loss of the photoreceptor cells. Transplantation of cells from immature retina has been studied extensively using this model (see del Cerro et al. 1997). Retinal receptor cells have been found to survive and repopulate the damaged host retina with cells of both neuronal and glial types, replacement of rod cells being particularly notable.

The most interesting question then becomes: Can transplanted photoreceptor cells restore visual capacity in animals with retinal injury? This possibility has been addressed in a particularly interesting experiment by del Cerro and colleagues (del Cerro et al. 1991). In their study, they used a model involving acoustic startle. This test involves measurement of the startle response of rats to the presentation of a sudden noise. In normal animals, a flash of light prior to the sound reduces the magnitude of the startle response. Light-blinded animals showed a lack of inhibition of startle by light—as might be expected; in addition, light paradoxically exaggerated the startle response to noise in these animals. In the light-blinded animals, retinal transplants reversed the paradoxical exaggeration of the startle response. The transplants did not, however, restore the normal suppression of startle responses by light. Counts of the number of viable photoreceptor cells in the host retina showed an increase to about one-third the normal number, whereas blinded animals without transplants showed only a few viable photoreceptor cells. Thus, it appears that photoreceptor cells transplanted to the retina can restore some degree of normal retinal function.

Recently there have been reports of studies on transplantation of photoreceptor cells in human patients with retinitis pigmentosa. In one study of two patients, no improvement was seen (Kaplan et al. 1997). In a second study, by Manuel del Cerro and coworkers at the University of Rochester, reported at the Society for Neuroscience meeting in November 1996, there was some improvement in visual perception. Eight patients received transplants of human fetal retinal photoreceptor cells, by injection of the cells into a small area under the existing retina. After at least one year, four and possibly five of the eight patients showed some signs of improvement. The patient with the most improvement was only able to distinguish light from darkness before the operation. After the surgery, this patient had a narrow "peephole" area of vision with a sharpness of 20/200, the ability to read the letters on the second-largest row of an optician's eye chart. With some improvements, it is easy to envision this procedure becoming a viable clinical treatment modality.

Conclusions

Some interesting possibilities are raised by the prospect of restoring vision by transplanting the entire, intact retina into the brain. Visual transplants are extraordinarily interesting, partly because of what they can tell us about how information can be relayed from transplanted cells to the brain. Let us think about transplanting entire retinas into the brain. First, we will assume that transplants can sense light information and transduce this light into neuronal signals. If these neuronal signals are relayed to the brain, it is not necessarily the case that they will be perceived as visual information. If, for example, signals from the retina were transmitted to the wrong place—such as auditory nuclei—the signals would probably be perceived as auditory information. Thus, the first possibility is that the signals from retinal transplants would be perceived, but not necessarily as light. Second, the signals from a transplant could be perceived as light, but not in organized patterns representing the outside world; rather, they might appear as random or vague flashes and patterns, or as a uniform haze. These first two possibilities are, for most purposes, equivalent. That is, in either case, the signals from the transplant are perceived, but not as visual patterns representing the outside world. Most tests of transplant function that could be devised for animals (especially lower animals) would not distinguish between these possibilities; however, because formation of synapses generally takes place only between appropriate pre- and postsynaptic elements, it is likely that transplant-mediated information received by the brain would be visual.

The second possibility is that light information transduced by a transplant could mediate specific reflex patterns—an example would be the pupillary reflex studied by Klassen and Lund in 1987 (described above). For a transplant to mediate such a function requires a more accurate integration of the transplant with the host brain than is required for simple transmission of sensation, since mediation of reflex activity requires that the transplant become integrated into appropriate visual circuits.

The third possibility is that retinal transplants could mediate the transfer to the brain of visual information which consists of patterned information that comprises an actual representation of the outside world. This is the most complex possibility, and is relatively unlikely to be achieved by transplanting entire retinas into the brain, for several reasons. First, the degree of patterning that is normally present in primary visual circuits probably cannot be duplicated by transplants. The specificity of visual circuits that results in pattern formation is formed during early development, under conditions that are not easily—and perhaps cannot under any conditions be—reproduced in adults. Transplantation of retinal tissue at very early developmental stages might circumvent this limitation to some degree, depending on how early in development transplants were performed. Also, the formation of a connection between visually perceived patterns and their representation in the outside world is probably to a considerable extent a learning and adaptational process that cannot easily be recapitulated later in development. Thus, even if a transplant were to become quite well integrated into visual circuits, the visual information perceived by the animal (or human patient) would not necessarily be usable in the normal manner. Finally, consider how minor aberrations in the visual system can result in severe visual impairment—cataracts and the need for glasses, for example—and that accurate pattern vision would require a transplant to function almost like a perfectly normal eye, not a retina alone.

It might be noted that the tests which have been used to show that transplants of retina or retinal cells restore visual capacity have invariably involved measurements of animals' ability to detect the presence or absence of light, rather than visual patterns or spatially organized information. For transplantation of the entire retina, this is probably a limitation that will not easily be overcome. As discussed in chapter 2, primary sensory circuits are often organized in a point-to-point manner so that particular cells send connections to other cells in a highly organized fashion. This degree of organization is essential for the transfer of patterned information, which in turn is responsible for the perception of patterns. Such a high degree of organization will not be easily duplicated by transplants.

In the foreseeable future will it become possible to employ transplants to restore vision to blind individuals? Transplants of retinal tissue into the brain are relatively unlikely to be employed clinically, at least not anytime soon. The risks of implanting tissue intracerebrally, in addition to the requirement for associated optic devices, would probably make any intracerebral procedure improbable. If the best possible outcome is only perception of light versus dark, this is not likely to be worth the risk. On the other hand, transplants into the retina are a distinct possibility. The risk of intraocular surgery is minimal. Any degree of return of visual function might be sufficient justification for a transplantation procedure involving the eye only. In addition, methods to enhance the regeneration of the optic nerve, or the development of connections between transplants in the retina and the brain, may also be possible.

Further Reading

del Cerro, M. (1990). Retinal transplants. *Prog. Retina Res.* 9: 229–272.

del Cerro, M., Lazar, E. S., and DiLoreto, D., Jr. (1997). The first decade of continuous progress in retinal transplantation. *Microsc. Res. Tech.* 36: 130–141.

Fetal retinal cell transplanted in search for eye disease cure. (1997). *Washington Post*, February 1, p. A2.

Josefson, D. (1996). Fetal retinal cells restore sight. *Brit. Med. J.* 313: 1353.

Kaplan, H. J., Tezel, T. H., and Del Priore, L. V. (1998). Retinal pigment epithelial transplantation in age-related macular degeneration. *Retina* 18: 99–102.

Litchfield, T. M., Whiteley, S. J., and Lund, R. D. (1997). Transplantation of retinal pigment epithelial, photoreceptor and other cells as treatment for retinal degeneration. *Exp. Eye Res.* 64: 655–666.

Lund, R. D., Coffey, P. J., Sauve, Y., and Lawrence, J. M. (1997). Intraretinal transplantation to prevent photoreceptor degeneration. *Ophthalmic Res.* 29: 305–319.

Lund, R. D., Radel, J. D., and Coffey, P. J. (1991). The impact of intracerebral retinal transplants on types of behavior exhibited by host rats. *Trends Neurosci.* 14: 358–362.

Qi Jiang, L., and del Cerro, M. (1992). Reciprocal retinal transplantation: A tool for the study of an inherited retinal degeneration. *Exp. Neurol.* 115:325–334.

Sharma, R. K., and Ehinger, B. (1997). Retinal cell transplants: How close to clinical application? *Acta Ophthalmol. Scand.* 75: 355–363.

Sheedlo, H. J., Gaur, V., Li, L., Seaton, A. D., and Turner, J. E. (1991). Transplantation to the diseased and damaged retina. *Trends Neurosci.* 14: 347–350.

VI

Genetic Engineering and Technology of the Future

20

Introduction to Genetic Engineering and Neural Transplantation

It is somewhat misleading to base a section on "future technology" on genetic engineering, since it is not really a technology of the future: it is here now. Nevertheless, the technologies of genetic engineering will continue to change, so we can expect that over the next 20 years, much of what is remarkable and new about neural transplantation will probably involve genetic engineering. For this reason, this section of the book is devoted to genetic engineering and technologies of the future.

What Can We Expect in the Future?

Until approximately 1990, the essence of neural transplantation was mainly removal of cells or pieces of tissue from one animal—a fetus in most cases—followed by reimplantation of the same cells, unaltered, into another organism.

Notwithstanding the fact that we will certainly see many additions to the ways that neural transplantation in that basic form can be used in the future, the most fundamental possibilities are likely to be based on the relatively new, and still developing, technology of altering cells through what is called genetic engineering. There are several quite different means of employing genetic engineering in relation to transplanting cells into and repairing the brain, but all have in common the goal of producing genetic alterations in cells.

Several fundamentally different approaches are being developed.

1. The use of existing cell types, altered so that they have some of the desired properties of neurons or neural support cells. Usually this involves

altering cells so that they produce a critical neurochemical. For example, glial cells might be altered in culture so that they produce nerve growth factor (NGF) or dopamine. This strategy will be discussed in chapter 23.

2. Another approach involves the generation of neurons or glia in tissue culture. This involves either of two strategies. In one, genetic engineering or other cell culture techniques are used to promote cell division. For example, viral genes, which code for the production of proteins that stimulate cell division, can be transferred into cells. The second strategy employs one or several clever "tricks" that can be used to induce neural cells, or their precursors, to propagate in culture. These methods will be discussed in chapters 21 and 22.

3. The first two approaches involve manipulation of cells in culture, followed by transplantation into the brain. An entirely different idea is the direct introduction of genes into *existing* brain cells, generally accomplished with the aid of viruses. Usually this method involves the use of viruses that have the ability to insert their genetic material into other cells, but are disabled (by removal of some parts of the viral genome) so that they cannot reproduce. Usually such viruses cannot incorporate these foreign genes into the host cell's genome, but the virus-carried DNA remains in the cell's cytoplasm. In addition, the possibility of inserting foreign genes into host cells by purely chemical means, using lipophilic reagents (a process called lipofection) cannot be entirely ruled out. This topic will be discussed in chapter 24.

These new strategies allow for many possibilities for repairing and restructuring the brain that would not otherwise be possible. Some of the most remarkable possibilities are opened up by the technology of molecular, or gene, transfer. Among the unique advantages of this approach are (1) the possibility of introducing genes into cells that could prevent degeneration, rather than only trying to repair cells after degeneration has occurred; (2) the possibility of enhancing the functions of neurons that already have intact and extensive connections with other neurons, which could help undamaged neurons to assume some of the functions of injured cells; and (3) the possibility of altering only single properties of neurons rather than introducing entire cells, which can produce a wide range of substances and exert numerous and often very complex (and perhaps deleterious) effects upon their neighbors.

Genetic Engineering

Most of this book has so far concentrated on the use of primary cells, that is, cells which have been taken directly from an animal or human. These cells are reimplanted directly into another organism. During the past 20 years, there has been a major revolution in biology that has touched nearly every aspect of biology and medicine. For our purposes, the most important aspect of this change is that it has become possible to produce permanent alterations in the genetic machinery of cells.

The "blueprint" for the workings of each cell is contained in its DNA, a long string of individual units (bases), several thousand or so of which comprise each gene. A single gene may encompass more than 100,000 bases. The linking of bases into chains requires additional components—sugar molecules and phosphates—that combine with the bases to form nucleotides. One gene dictates the structure of one or several related proteins (often a single gene is used in different ways to produce a group of related proteins). Genes are grouped together to form giant chains called chromosomes; each animal has a number of chromosomes.

Essentially, all of the cells in a particular individual have identical DNA. Depending upon developmental programs and extrinsic signals, a few genes (in each cell) are in operation at any one time while many remain inactive and unused. Genes that are "in operation" are transcribed (the process is transcription) to make messenger RNA (mRNA). Messenger RNA is an intermediary messenger molecule, similar in structure to DNA, that is used by the cell as a template to make proteins. The process of making proteins from mRNA is called translation (figure 20.1).

There are two kinds of DNA that can code for proteins (figure 20.2). Genomic DNA is the DNA contained within a normal, intact organism, and includes sections that code for protein, called exons, and large interruptions of (apparently) nonsense material called introns. For genetic engineering purposes, in most cases it is simpler to employ DNA that has the introns removed, since it is much smaller (the introns can comprise up to 90 percent of a gene). This kind of DNA, which contains the exons only, is called complementary DNA, or cDNA, because it is complementary to mRNA.

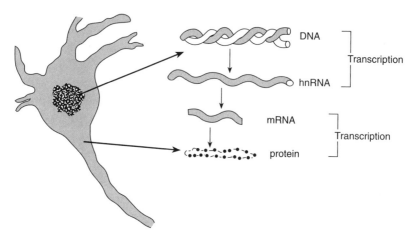

Figure 20.1
Illustration of the process through which genetic material directs the sequence of amino acids in proteins. The first step is the generation of heterogeneous nuclear RNA (hnRNA), which is copied from genomic DNA by the process known as transcription. Removal of intron sequences and processing of hnRNA yields messenger RNA, the template from which protein is synthesized.

The nature of any individual cell at a given moment is called its phenotype. In other words, is cell X a neuron or a liver cell? A dopaminergic neuron or an acetylcholine neuron? The phenotype of the cell depends not only upon the genes being transcribed at the moment when it is being observed, but also on the history of gene transcription by that cell. The process by which a cell becomes permanently committed to expressing a particular phenotype (a particular set of properties) is called terminal differentiation. This term implies that the differentiation is entirely irreversible; however, the terminal differentiation of at least some cell types can be at least partially reversed. The processes that control terminal differentiation are not well understood.

Molecular biology is the study of the molecular mechanisms that control the workings of the cell. Genetic engineering is a subdiscipline of molecular biology that seeks to alter cellular DNA, and gene therapy is a further subdiscipline that seeks to employ genetic engineering as a therapy for the treatment of disease. Genetic engineering employs strategies such as influencing cells within the body, altering cells in culture and then

Two Types of DNA that Can Code for Proteins

(a) Genomic DNA

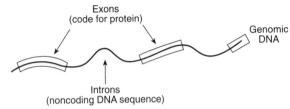

Exons
(code for protein)

Genomic
DNA

Introns
(noncoding DNA sequence)

(b) Complementary DNA (cDNA)

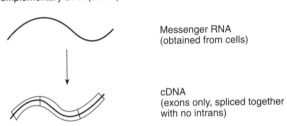

Messenger RNA
(obtained from cells)

cDNA
(exons only, spliced together
with no intrans)

Figure 20.2
Two types of DNA can code for proteins. Genomic DNA is the DNA present in the genome, and it codes for proteins under normal physiological circumstances. This type of DNA contains exons, which are the sequences that code for proteins, and introns (think "interruptions"), which are noncoding sequences interspersed between the exons. The introns apparently are mostly nonsense sequences, although some of them may perform functions such as regulating when genes are turned on and off. Introns usually are much longer than exons, generally comprising roughly 75 percent to 90 percent of genes. Complementary DNA, or cDNA, is made from messenger RNA, and has only the exons, spliced together, with the introns removed. cDNAs are much smaller than the corresponding genomic DNAs, and are used for gene therapy.

reimplanting them into the body, or reprogramming cells to adopt a new phenotype. These aims are accomplished either by inserting new or supplementary genes into cells, or by modifying existing genes (figure 20.3).

Let's look at an example. Imagine an individual who is unable to digest milk sugar, or lactose, because of a deficiency in the production of the enzyme lactase by mucosal cells in the small intestine. This disorder is called lactose intolerance. How might this problem be tackled by genetic

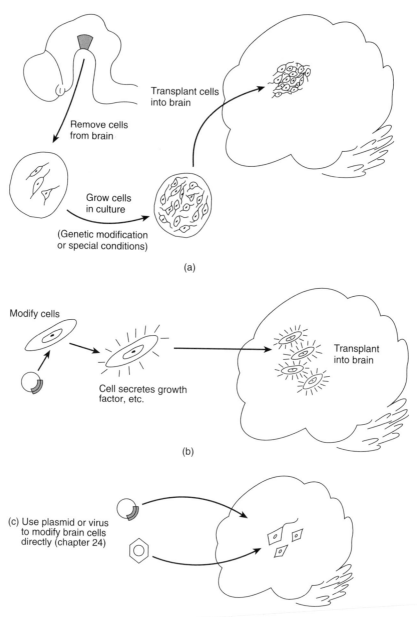

Transplant cells
into brain

Remove cells
from brain

Grow cells
in culture

(Genetic modification
or special conditions)

(a)

Modify cells

Cell secretes growth
factor, etc.

Transplant
into brain

(b)

(c) Use plasmid or virus
to modify brain cells
directly (chapter 24)

Figure 20.3

Three general categories of gene and cell therapy that can be applied to the brain.
A. Cells can be genetically altered or manipulated so that they can be grown in
culture prior to transplantation into the brain. These topics are discussed in chapters 21 and 22. B. Cells can be genetically modified so that they produce a particular desired protein prior to transplantation. This strategy is described in chapter
23. C. Disabled viruses or plasmids can be used as vectors to insert genes into,
and thus modify, cells within the brain (chapter 24).

engineering? There are at least three possibilities. First, cells might be altered in tissue culture, by removing intestinal mucosal cells, introducing into them the gene for the lactase enzyme, and then transplanting the same cells back into the small intestine. Cells to be used might be obtained from the small intestine of the individual receiving the transplant, they might be obtained from elsewhere in the body (muscle or skin), or they could be obtained from a donor (perhaps from a fetus). This strategy is discussed in chapter 23.

A second possibility is that intestinal mucosal cells from another individual, which have normal lactase activity, might be grown in tissue culture and then transplanted into the intestine of the individual with lactase insufficiency. Genetic engineering techniques or other culturing methods might be used to propagate the cells in culture. Being normal intestinal mucosal cells, they would produce lactase, and thus it would not be necessary to introduce a lactase gene into them. This second strategy is discussed in chapters 21 and 22.

The third strategy I will discuss would be to alter a virus—Herpes simplex virus and adeno-associated virus are often used for this purpose. Some of the functions of the virus that it normally uses for replication and that are responsible for injury to host cells are removed, and in their place cDNAs encoding for the enzyme lactase are inserted into the virus. The intestinal mucosa is then exposed to the altered virus. The virus enters into the host cells and confers upon them the ability to produce lactase. This third strategy, called molecular transfer, does not involve transplantation of cells per se. Rather DNA is transferred, so that existing cells are modified to have properties they did not have before. Although technically this approach does not involve transplantation, it is closely associated with transplantation and is discussed briefly in chapter 24.

Transferring DNA into Cells

Cells normally exclude any DNA that happens to be present in the medium surrounding them. This makes sense: cells cannot afford to randomly incorporate perhaps deleterious fragments of DNA that they encounter. There are exceptions, however, and it is also possible to force DNA into cells. There are several methods of inserting genes into cells,

GENE TRANSFER INTO MAMMALIAN CELLS

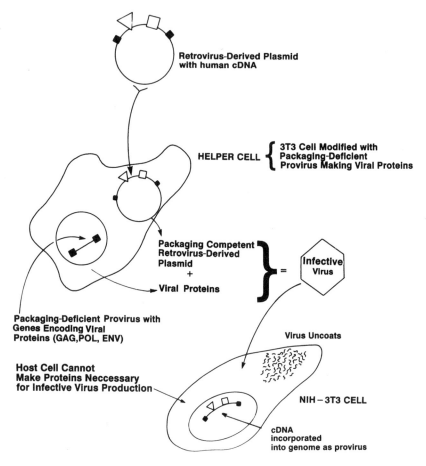

Figure 20.4
Illustration of the means by which retroviruses are subverted for use in gene therapy. The fundamental principle of all such schemes involves separation of the DNA-transfer functions from the structural and reproductive functions of the virus. The viral vector can then be made to contain the structures needed to insert its DNA into target cells, but essential elements needed for viral reproduction and structure are removed. In the case of retroviral vectors, a helper cell is employed to produce viral proteins GAG, POL, and ENV. Separately, a plasmid is constructed that contains the "packaging" signal, responsible for assembly of the virus, in addition to the genetic material to be transferred (let's call this the transgene). This plasmid is transfected into the helper cell (sometimes called a packaging cell

which are used routinely in vitro. Some of these are occasionally successful in living animals. Most are methods of penetrating cell walls or making small openings in cells to allow DNA to enter.

There are a number of ways in which DNA can be inserted into cells. One involves the use of physicochemical methods that essentially force DNA through the cell membrane into the cell. Once inside the cell, DNA structures initially reside "episomally," outside of the host genome. In this state DNA can reside and produce a gene product, but the DNA will not usually be replicated when the cell divides. Under appropriate conditions, such episomally located genes may, on occasion, become incorporated ("stably integrated" or simply "integrated") into the genome of the host cell when the host cell divides, by taking advantage of a normal cell process called homologous recombination. This occurs quite rarely in somatic cells. Although it is quite inefficient to rely on this as a method of gene insertion, it often turns out to occur frequently enough to be very useful.

The second category of DNA insertion techniques relies on viruses, which employ a number of different strategies to insert their genes into host cells. The best-known employ a class of viruses called retroviruses, which contain specialized mechanisms for efficiently inserting their genes into the genome of host cells when the host cells divide. These mechanisms can be used to produce retroviral vectors, which can very reliably, and permanently, introduce experimental genes into the genome of host cells (figure 20.4).

Some viral and physicochemical methods of inserting genes into cells are listed in table 20.1.

---

line). Thus, the genetic material associated with the packaging signal does not include genes for the essential viral proteins GAG, POL, and ENV. This results in packaging of the transgene using viral proteins produced by the helper cell; thus there is a viral particle that has no ability to produce any of its own proteins. This disabled virus can infect a target cell, but cannot reproduce. Instead of inserting viral proteins into the host cell when the host cell divides, it inserts the transgene. The viral proteins are then degraded, leaving no trace of the virus other than short DNA sequences that do not code for protein (i.e., the packaging signal and other small stretches of viral DNA that are involved in packaging, integration of the virus into the host cell genome, and initiation of DNA synthesis).

Table 20.1
Methods of inserting genes into cells

Technique	Are Dividing Cells Required?	Does It Work for Neurons?	Stable Integration
Retroviruses	Works only with dividing cells	Yes	Always
Herpes simplex virus	Nondividing cells	Yes	Not usually
Adeno-associated virus	No	Yes	Under some conditions
Calcium phosphate	Only for stable integration	No	Occasional
Electroporation	Only for stable integration	No	Occasional
Lipofection	Only for stable integration	Sometimes	Occasional
Impact with glass beads	Only for stable integration	Unknown	Occasional
Direct injection into cells with fine glass pipettes	Only for stable integration (can be used only with small numbers of cells)	Yes, for any cell type	Occasional

Note: Stable integration means incorporation into the genome of the host cell. Foreign genes may also reside episomally, that is, outside of the host genome. Such episomal genes are not necessarily replicated when the host cell divides. Stable integration of episomal DNA into the host cell's genome may occur when the host cell divides.

Gene Therapy

The above discussion considers topics that fall under the general heading of gene therapy. Gene therapy, as a general topic, has several forms. The two overall categories are germ line therapy (which is probably not applicable to humans) and somatic gene therapy (which is applicable to humans). Germ line therapy targets the entire organism through manipulation of the genome of germ line cells. This approach seeks to alter the genome per se, and the genetic alterations thus produced will be passed on to subsequent generations. Germ line modifications are done commonly in mice and in various submammalian organisms. It is generally, although not unanimously, agreed that the consequences of manipulating the genome are too unpredictable for use in humans.

The second general approach, the area considered in the earlier discussions in this chapter, is, to use the more technical term, somatic gene therapy. Somatic gene therapy is targeted to particular cell types with abnormalities. In other words, somatic gene therapy targets somatic cells (cells that are part of the body structure) rather than germ line cells. Therefore, any changes produced will not be passed on to subsequent generations. Somatic gene therapy has two forms: ex vivo (out of the body) and in vivo (in the body). The ex vivo approach involves genetic manipulation of cells in tissue culture, followed by transplantation into the body (in our case, into the brain). The in vivo approach involves genetic manipulation of cells without their removal from the body—in other words, transfer of DNA directly into brain cells. Although in vivo gene therapy does not really involve transplantation, it will be discussed briefly in chapter 24.

Genetic Engineering and Neural Transplantation

The idea of employing genetic engineering in neural transplantation first made its way into the literature in 1985, when Finch suggested that modification of cellular DNA might be employed to customize cells for neural transplantation. In the first experiment on modification of cells for neural transplantation, reported by Shimohama and coworkers (1989; see also Gage et al. 1987), cells were modified to produce a so-called reporter gene, which directs the production of the enzyme β-galactosidase. Production of this enzyme can easily be detected by specialized staining techniques. Although the production of this enzyme is not useful in itself, this experiment demonstrated the principle that cells could produce a foreign gene product following neural transplantation.

A more or less independent line of research, the development of immortalized cell lines, has evolved rather gradually. Its start might be dated from the development of the first intentionally immortalized cell lines (Geller and Dubois-Dalcq 1988; Major et al. 1985), or even the first use of tumors (which are merely aggregations of immortal cells produced by nature) for intracerebral transplantation in 1923 (Murphy and Sturm

1923). The first use of intentionally immortalized cell lines for intracere-bral transplantation was reported by Bredesen in 1990, and the first ex-ample of the use of intentionally immortalized cell lines to produce a functional effect in animals was reported by Anton et al. in 1994. This latter report, however, depended on additional manipulation of the cell line to produce a functional effect, so that the immortalized cell line in this case was actually employed as a vehicle for subsequent genetic manip-ulation. There are few studies in which unmodified immortalized cell lines have been found to be capable of repairing deficits in host brain function by transplantation. The development of cell lines for use in neural trans-plantation will be discussed in chapter 22.

For Further Reading

Kaplitt, M. G., and Loewy, A. D. (1995). *Viral Vectors: Gene Therapy and Neu-roscience Applications.* Academic Press, San Diego.

21

Growing Cells in Culture: Stem and Progenitor Cells

Neural transplantation as discussed thus far involves removing cells or tissue from one brain and transplanting this material directly into another brain. In recent years, however, it has become apparent that the future of neural transplantation will involve growing cells in culture before transplantation. There are many experiments on growing brain cells in culture, and most of these have involved isolating cells from the brains of fetal or embryonic animals, then manipulating the cells in some manner to stimulate growth. There are two fundamentally different goals of such studies. One is to obtain single cells—often called stem cells—that have the capacity to generate multiple cell types. Such cells might, perhaps, be used directly to repair relatively diffuse, generalized defects in brain function, or they might be induced to differentiate into specific types of cells before transplanting. An alternative goal is to employ cells that are more completely developed, and thus committed to a single, specific phenotype. Such cells might be employed to replace a specific population of degenerating neurons—for example, to replace dopamine neurons in Parkinson's disease or to substitute for chromaffin cells in the treatment of pain (chapter 14).

How, exactly, do we grow cells from the brain in culture? Once cells have differentiated into their mature neuronal form and adopted true neuronal phenotypes, they rarely divide. Nonetheless, when neurons are removed from the fetal brain, they can be kept alive in culture for extended periods. Occasionally, when cells are removed from a very immature brain, grown under standard cell culture conditions, and supplemented with appropriate growth factors, neuronal precursors will divide a few times before differentiating (e.g., Bouvier and Mytilineou

1995). In fact, coaxing cells to divide a few times before they are transplanted could greatly expand the available population of cells, so that many more cells are available for transplantation. For example, if the precursors of dopamine neurons are used and they can be induced to divide only three times, the number of fetuses required to be used in transplantation in Parkinson's disease would be reduced from about seven to only one for each human patient. Bouvier and Mytilineou employed very immature rat fetal cultures, and obtained growth of dopamine neuronal precursors by treatment with the growth factor basic fibroblast growth factor (FGF). Subsequently Studer and coworkers (1998) used a related method to increase the number of dopaminergic neurons prior to transplantation into rat brains. In their experiment, they first grew dopamine neuronal precursor cells in suspension with basic FGF; after basic FGF was removed, a considerable number of cells developed the dopaminergic neuronal phenotype. Clusters of these cells were found to affect amphetamine-induced rotation when transplanted into rat brains.

Although a few cell divisions may be useful, ultimately we would really like to be able to maintain the growth of cultured neurons for long periods of time. Rather than expanding a population of cells slightly, perhaps cultures could be maintained as a continuous source of cells. This is possible. When the culture conditions are changed slightly, it is possible to obtain extensive proliferation of neuronal stem cells or precursors in vitro. In 1992, Reynolds and Weiss discovered a technique for removing cells from the fetal or adult brain, growing them in culture, and subsequently inducing these cells to differentiate into neurons and glia. The technique was fairly simple: cells were removed from the brain and grown in suspension in the presence of a growth factor (either epidermal growth factor or basic FGF), without serum. Serum is often added to tissue cultures because it contains a number of proteins that enhance the survival, growth, and/or differentiation of many cell types and the attachment of cells to the substrate. Generally, culture media without serum favor the growth of immature, undifferentiated cells. After the cells had been grown for varying periods of time with epidermal growth factor and without serum, they were moved to a medium without epidermal growth factor, but with serum, and placed in culture dishes that had been coated (with poly L-lysine) to promote cell attachment. The cells then attached to the substrate and differentiated into astrocytes, oligodendrocytes, and neurons. This is the basic technique for growing neural stem cells in culture.

It was later found that cells from almost any part of the fetal brain could be grown using this technique (or variations of it using different growth factors or media supplements), but growing cells from the adult brain could work only if special populations of cells, located adjacent to the ventricles, were used (Weiss et al. 1996). Regions adjacent to the ventricles, termed the "subventricular zone," contain cells that continue to proliferate in the adult animals throughout life (Craig et al. 1996; Morshead and van der Kooy 1992). Normally, one purpose of these cells is to populate the olfactory bulbs (Craig et al. 1996; Lois and Alvarez-Buylla 1993). In many studies, cells have been grown from the fetal brain under similar conditions (Stemple and Mahanthappa 1997; Svendsen and Rosser 1995; Svendsen et al. 1995). Proliferating neuronal progenitor cells also can be obtained from the adult hippocampus (Gage et al. 1995) and the subventricular zone.

Neurons generated using the method of Reynolds and Weiss (1992) contained the neurotransmitters GABA and substance P. These neurons, as well as astrocytes or oligodendrocytes produced in culture, might be used in neuronal transplantation. Although cells can be grown from various fetal brain regions, these cells do not readily differentiate to form specific populations of neurons with defined phenotypes. For example, cells can be expanded from cultures taken from the fetal mesencephalon, but when they are grown in this manner for more than a few cell divisions, these cultures rarely if ever produce dopaminergic neurons.

Terminology and Orientation

This complex and rapidly evolving field is difficult to organize in a systematic manner so that it can be considered clearly and comprehensively. At the time of this writing, the topic of stem cell biology is evolving rapidly, and there are many unresolved issues.

First of all, what are the possible subdivisions of the general topic "growing cells in culture prior to transplantation"? One that we might consider is the limited goal of getting cells to divide a few times prior to transplanting them versus maintaining cells in culture indefinitely. Second, we might consider attempts to grow cells by manipulating their chemical environment versus altering the cells genetically so that they grow more readily in any appropriate environment. Third, we might grow immature neuronal precursors rather than cells that have already differentiated to form neurons or specific types of neurons. I have already touched upon some of these topics.

Often, the second choices in the three pairs go together; that is, normal undifferentiated neuronal precursors can divide a few times—perhaps quite a few—in culture. Usually, indefinite growth requires genetic modification, and often, more completely differentiated cells are the targets of genetic modification to make them grow better (since, otherwise, more mature cells often will not grow in culture). Techniques are, however, rapidly evolving to permit long-term growth of normal undifferentiated neuronal precursors. Also, there are genetically modified immature neuronal precursors. Furthermore, cells that have been genetically modified to stimulate their growth usually seem to stop growing when they are transplanted into the brain. Therefore, the subdivision of the topic implied by the titles of this chapter and chapter 22 does not quite make sense: immortal cell lines and stem cells are not necessarily two different things. Thus, to be more precise, this chapter considers the growth in culture of normal, unmodified cells. Chapter 22 considers the use of cultured cells that have been modified (either intentionally or through accidents of nature, i.e., tumor cells) for transplantation. However, genetically modified cells may behave like neural stem cells. Nevertheless, the discussion of genetically modified cells that behave as neural stem cells is reserved for chapter 22.

Therefore, there are two major categories of techniques used for growing cells from the brain in culture: (1) variations on the method of Reynolds and Weiss can be used to culture immature, undifferentiated cells from the brain and spinal cord, and (2) many studies have employed genetic modification of cells, transferring oncogenes into cells to stimulate growth. For purposes of discussion of the topic, this chapter is devoted to normal, unmodified cells, while chapter 22 is devoted to cells that have been subjected to genetic modifications or mutations in some form.

Some somatic cells, such as fibroblasts, can be removed and grown in culture for considerable periods; however, after about 45–50 cell divisions (sometimes as many as 100), normal cells stop dividing. Cells that have reached the 45–50 division limit begin to deteriorate, and are said to have undergone cellular senescence, a phenomenon first described by Hayflick (1965). This number of cell divisions is sometimes called the Hayflick limit. Cells that do not undergo cellular senescence are termed "immortal." Although cells generated using the technique of Reynolds and Weiss are not necessarily immortal, large numbers of cells can be generated in this way. The generation of immortal cells, which can be grown indefinitely in culture, will be discussed in chapter 22. This distinction is somewhat questionable, however, since normal stem cells of certain kinds, usually those obtained from very early developmental stages, may be immortal as well.

What Are Stem Cells, and What Cells Are Immortal?

Stem cells function in a number of organ systems to replace a population of mature cells that cannot divide to replenish themselves; examples of this situation occur for the epidermis (skin) and the hematopoietic (blood cell) system.

Stem cells are defined as follows (Alberts et al. 1994):

1. Stem cells are not terminally differentiated.
2. Stem cells are immortal, or at least can divide indefinitely over the lifetime of the animal.
3. When a stem cell divides, each daughter cell may either remain as a stem cell or undergo a pathway leading to terminal differentiation.

The brain is generated during fetal development. Although there may be some ongoing cellular replenishment, cell replacement in the mature brain is restricted to a very few cell types. Thus, with the exception of a few small regions (e.g., the dentate gyrus of the hippocampus), the brain generally is not being replenished on an ongoing basis by stem cells. Nonetheless, perhaps there are stem cells present in the brain, remaining there in a quiescent state, leftovers from development. Or perhaps stem cells could be c'>tained from the fetal brain, and by transplanting them into more mature brains, some degree of neural restoration could be produced.

Not all stem cells are alike; there are different stem cells for the hematopoietic system, epidermis, other tissues, and the brain. Neural stem cells are defined somewhat differently compared with stem cells in general: (1) neural stem cells are committed to a neural lineage, but retain the capacity to generate each of the major CNS cell types—neurons, oligodendrocytes, and astrocytes; (2) neural stem cells are self-renewing; and (3) neural stem cells can populate or repopulate developing or degenerating regions in the CNS (Flax et al. 1998).

In contrast, the alternative terms "progenitor cell," and "precursor cell" imply a cell type that is undifferentiated but has already moved along a differentiation pathway, and is destined to generate a particular cell type. Although cells that were generated in culture from the subventricular zone in the original study by Reynolds and Weiss (1992) can produce both neurons and glia, they appear to be restricted in the neuronal phenotypes that they can form. Thus, whether we should call these cells "neural stem cells" or "progenitor cells" is somewhat debatable. Generally, if a single cell can give rise to neurons (of any type), astrocytes, and oligodendroglia, it is called a stem cell.

Germ cells are immortal. This must be the case; all of the cells within your body, and all of the cells that are to form the bodies of all of your descendants, as well as all future germ cells, are to be derived from a single pair of germ cells. Thus, germ cells must be immortal. As the embryo begins to form, the earliest embryonic cells, termed embryonic stem cells, also are immortal. We would expect embryonic stem cells to be immortal, since they can differentiate into germ cells. And we know this to be the case empirically, since normal embryonic stem cells can form tumors, known as teratomas or teratocarcinomas, that can grow without limit and can be passaged from animal to animal, killing their hosts. Actually, a neural cell line, NTera2, has been derived from such a tumor and is being used for transplantation in rodents and human subjects (chapter 25).

Embryonic stem cells are totipotent, that is, any embryonic stem cell retains the capacity to regenerate an entire embryo. In other words, embryonic stem cells are completely undifferentiated: they can form all other cell types, including germ cells. During fetal development, the first specialization event is the differentiation of trophectoderm from the inner cell mass. The trophectoderm goes on to form the placenta and supporting structures, while the rest of the animal is formed from the inner cell mass. After this initial differentiation, none of the cells in the embryo remain totipotent; neither are they immortal. At each stage of development, cells become more and more specialized. At some stage of development, cells are present that give rise to neural stem cells. These cells have already undergone considerable differentiation; although they are immature, their range of possible fates is (presumably; however, see below) limited to the formation of various nervous system cell types. Neural stem cells, in contrast to embryonic stem cells, are not necessarily immortal. We do not know of tumors that consist of normal neural stem cells. Medulloblastomas, a type of CNS tumor, resemble neural stem cell tumors, but are generated by mutations.

Recently, however, it has been found that neural stem cells can be transformed into blood cells after transplantation into irradiated animals (Bjarnson et al. 1999). Conversely, blood cells (bone marrow cells) can be transplanted into the brain, although they do not necessarily develop neuronal or glial phenotypes (Schwarz et al. 1999). Thus, the differentiation capacity of neural stem cells is potentially very wide. One challenge is to direct the differentiation of stem cells into specific, defined phenotypes. A second is to develop methods by which such cells can be used to restructure the brain in a controlled, and limited, manner.

Therefore, we perhaps can have immortal cells through two routes. We can employ undifferentiated cells (stem cells), which are immortal, and later coax them into performing whatever function we need by application of various growth and differentiation factors and growth substrates. Or we can employ cells that are more completely differentiated, and have lost their immortality, by producing in these cells some alteration (generally a genetic alteration) to restore immortality. This latter approach is discussed in chapter 22. In this chapter, we will discuss two experiments that illustrate how normal, unmodified neural stem cells or neural progenitors might be used.

Dopamine Neurons from Progenitor Cell Cultures

As has been mentioned, neural stem cells can be cultured from the ventral mesencephalon, which is the normal source of dopaminergic neurons. These cultures, which have been studied by several groups, rarely, or never, become dopaminergic neurons (Ptak et al. 1995; Santa-Olalla and Covarrubias 1995; Mayer et al. 1993; Svendsen et al. 1995). A method by which ventral mesencephalic progenitor cells can be induced to form dopaminergic neurons has recently been discovered. Ling and coworkers at Rush-St. Lukes-Presbyterian Medical Center in Chicago (1998) started by growing cells from the ventral mesencephalon in suspension in serum-free medium containing EGF, very similar to the original method described by Reynolds and Weiss in 1992. Ling and coworkers tested a large number of molecules for their ability to induce a dopaminergic neuronal phenotype in mesencephalic progenitor cell cultures. Molecules tested included cytokines, which are known to be involved in the differentiation of stem cells of the hematopoietic system. One particular molecule, interleukin-1 (IL-1), caused a substantial number of these cells to begin to stain for tyrosine hydroxylase, a marker of dopaminergic neurons.

This treatment did not, however, cause the cells to have the physical form of dopaminergic neurons; they were rounded or irregular in shape, but did not have processes (figure 21.1, A). The number of tyrosine hydroxylase-containing cells was further increased by culturing the progenitor cells with normal striatal cells, but these cells still did not form processes. Addition of another cytokine, interleukin-11 (IL-11), to the mix induced some of the cells to have short processes (figure 21.1, B). Further addition of leukemia inhibitory factor (LIF), and GDNF caused the cells to become larger and more completely developed, with some processes, although they still did not look quite like dopaminergic neurons (figure 21.1, C). Finally, when the cells were grown in a mixture containing, in addition to serum, IL-1, IL-11, LIF, GDNF (figure 21.2), the medium from striatal cultures, and membrane fragments of cells from the mesencephalon, the progenitor cells became very well developed, appearing much like normal dopaminergic neurons (figure 21.1, D). Interestingly, these cells were obtained from embryonic mesencephalon of rat fetuses at 13.5 days of gestation, a time at which dopamine neuronal

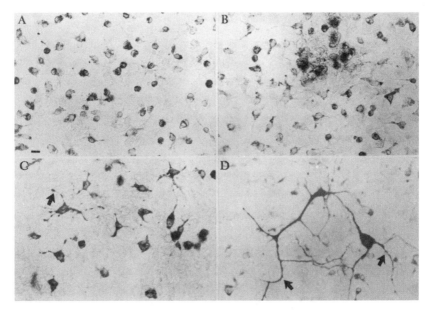

Figure 21.1
Cultured mesencephalic progenitor cells, showing effects of treatment with cytokines and growth factors to induce differentiation of these cells to form tyrosine hydroxylase-positive neurons according to the scheme illustrated in figure 21.2. When treated with interleukin-1, many of the cells expressed tyrosine hydroxylase (A). When treated with interleukin-11 as well, the cells were somewhat larger and resembled neurons (B). When leukemia inhibitory factor and GDNF were added, many of the cells developed multiple short processes and had larger cell bodies (C). Finally, with the addition of membrane fragments from the mesencephalon and conditioned culture medium from striatal cells, the cells began to resemble large, complex dopaminergic neurons (D). (From Ling et al. 1998; provided by Paul Carvey, Rush-Presbyterian-St. Luke's Medical Center, Chicago. Reproduced with permission.)

precursors normally are no longer dividing. Therefore, cells that are capable of becoming dopamine neurons are present in the mesencephalon *after* all of the dopaminergic neurons have already been born . . . apparently. Carvey has speculated that, just perhaps, dopaminergic neurons continue to differentiate from these cells at a very low rate even in adults.

This is a potentially very significant study for a number of reasons. First, it suggests a method by which dopaminergic neurons might be produced for neural transplantation. In fact, Carvey and coworkers

Cells from fetal brain adult subependymal zone or spinal cord

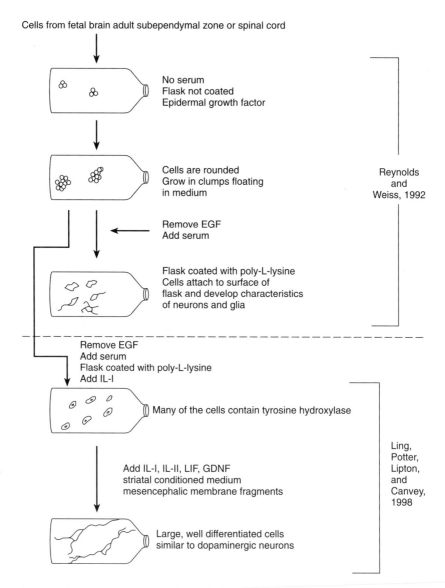

No serum
Flask not coated
Epidermal growth factor

Cells are rounded
Grow in clumps floating
in medium

Reynolds
and
Weiss, 1992

Remove EGF
Add serum

Flask coated with poly-L-lysine
Cells attach to surface of
flask and develop characteristics
of neurons and glia

Remove EGF
Add serum
Flask coated with poly-L-lysine
Add IL-I

Many of the cells contain tyrosine hydroxylase

Add IL-I, IL-II, LIF, GDNF
striatal conditioned medium
mesencephalic membrane fragments

Ling,
Potter,
Lipton,
and
Canvey,
1998

Large, well differentiated cells
similar to dopaminergic neurons

Figure 21.2
The scheme employed to culture progenitor cells from the brain and induce differentiation of these cells. First, cells are isolated and grown under conditions that
favor the survival of immature cells (no serum in the culture medium) and their
division (usually, epidermal growth factor or fibroblast growth factor in the medium), and that do not allow the cells to attach to the surface (flask not coated).
. The cells grow in floating clumps called neurospheres. The EGF is then removed,

(1999) have recently shown that these precursor cells, transformed into dopamine neurons, can be successfully transplanted into lesioned rats. More generally, both studies provide some indication of what may be required to provoke undifferentiated precursors of dopaminergic neurons into adopting a mature neuronal phenotype—information that may be needed, especially, for producing dopaminergic neurons from immortal cell lines. Even more generally, these data show that the factors required to induce immature neuronal precursors to adopt various mature neuronal phenotypes may be very complex.

Human Neural Stem Cells

Flax and coworkers (1998) recently obtained stem cells from the forebrain, adjacent to the ventricle, of a human fetus at 15 weeks' gestation, using methods akin to those described by Reynolds and Weiss in 1992 (see above). These cells were passaged weekly for more than one year, and thus did not exhibit cellular senescence. These cells were found to have several interesting properties. After the cells were placed in serum-containing medium, they were able to differentiate into neurons and oligodendrocytes, and when they were cocultured with tissue from mouse CNS, astrocytes also were formed. When cultured adjacent to cells with a genetic enzyme deficiency found in Tay-Sachs disease, these human neural stem cells were able to correct the enzyme deficiency, via diffusion of the enzyme from cell to cell. When transplanted into the brains of newborn mice, these human neural stem cells became integrated into several regions of the host brains, and exhibited properties characteristic of neu-

---

serum is added, and the flasks are coated with poly-L-lysine. This allows the cells to attach and differentiate into neurons and glia. This part of the technique was described by Reynolds and Weiss (1992).

The second facet of this method was described by Ling et al. (1998). When cells from the ventral mesencephalon are used, and interleukin-1 is added to the medium, many of the cells express tyrosine hydroxylase. When the cytokines interleukin-11 and leukemia inhibitory factor, as well as GDNF, fragments of membranes from the mesencephalon, and striatal conditioned medium, are added, the cells become large and well-differentiated, express tyrosine hydroxylase, and resemble dopaminergic neurons.

rons, astrocytes, and oligodendrocytes. Therefore, it seems to be possible to generate neural stem cells from human fetal brain tissue, and these neural stem cells can become extensively integrated into the brains of immature mice. Additional uses of similar cells are described in chapter 22.

Conclusions

The use of undifferentiated neural stem cells in culture may provide a means of generating cells that can be employed in neural transplantation without the need for genetically altering the cells. This topic is currently evolving very rapidly, and over the next several years, major advances in the ways normal neural stem cells can be employed in neural transplantation can be expected. In fact, human embryonic stem cells have recently been isolated. These cells are immortal, and when they are grown in mice as teratomas, they can differentiate to form neuronal precursor cells, among other cell types (F. J. Thompson et al. 1988). Nonetheless, for certain applications, this approach may have limitations. We may find that it is necessary to produce immortal cells with specific, predetermined phenotypic properties by intentionally producing genetic alterations in neural progenitor cells. The use of modified cells for neural transplantation, therefore, is the subject of chapter 22.

Further Reading

Snyder, E. Y., and Wolfe, J. H. (1996). Central nervous system cell transplantation: A novel therapy for storage diseases? *Curr. Opin. Neurol.* 9: 126–136.

22

Growing Cells in Culture: Immortal Cell Lines

What Is an "Immortal Cell Line"?

Cells may be obtained directly from an animal or a human donor: such cells are termed primary cells. In appropriate circumstances, some types of primary cells can be provoked to divide in tissue culture, but a limited number of divisions are possible, the maximum usually being about 45–50. Although this sounds like a lot, in practice this limit is reached fairly rapidly. Generally, it takes some effort to study the properties of a particular cell type, and by the time it has been determined that some particular cells are the ones you want to use, the limit is nearly reached. Cells that have reached this 45–50 division limit begin to deteriorate, and are said to have undergone cellular senescence, a phenomenon first described in 1965 (Hayflick 1965). Thus, even for types of cells like fibroblasts, which readily divide in culture, the generation of cells by culturing alone is limited. Most neurons, furthermore, do not divide at all, once they have reached their final stage of differentiation. The use of normal cultured cells for transplantation, such as the progenitor cells described in chapter 21, is a possibility, but has some limitations. A second possibility is the experimental modification of normal cells to produce immortal cell lines. Intentional modification of cells can also be used to generate cells with the properties of neural stem cells, which is discussed in this chapter (see "Type II Experiments," below).

The concept of immortal cell lines arises from studies of cells isolated from tumors. Tumors are typically generated from a single aberrant somatic cell that loses some of the normal controls of cell division and consequently gives rise to an essentially unlimited number of progeny. The

Table 22.1
Concepts and terms used in describing cell lines

Concept	Meaning
Clonal	All cells genetically identical
Immortal	Cells will grow indefinitely
Transformed	Cells will grow without attachment; cells are not contact-inhibited

exceptions are teratomas, which are derived from normal embryonic stem cells, as discussed in chapter 21. Cell lines can thus be isolated from tumors. Tumor cells are not subject to a limited number of divisions, and are said to be "immortal," since they can be grown in culture indefinitely. The use of such clonal and immortal cell lines similar to those obtained from tumors presents possibilities for obtaining essentially unlimited numbers of cells for transplantation, without the direct involvement of tissue donors. One cannot, however, make the unqualified statement that immortal cells are desirable for transplantation, unless cell growth can be absolutely controlled. We do not want to transplant cells into the brain that can develop into tumors.

In addition to immortality, tumor cells frequently have other properties that are definitely not desirable for transplantation. For example, when most kinds of normal cells are grown in culture, they stop growing when the culture dish is filled (at this point, the cells are described as being "confluent"). This property is called "contact inhibition." Some tumor cells will keep growing after confluence is reached, and will pile up in the culture dish—they are not contact inhibited. Cells that have this property are said to be "transformed," a property that is related to the ability of tumors to metastasize. Immortalized cells may or may not also be transformed. For transplantation, we have to be able to produce cells that are immortalized but *not* transformed (table 22.1). Cancer cells may have further abnormalities, such as the ability to attract the growth of new blood vessels and to pass through blood vessel walls.

Furthermore, for transplantation, although we want cells that can be grown indefinitely, we do not want these cells to grow constantly and uncontrollably all of the time. To produce cells that will grow indefinitely, but only when we want them to, in addition to having all of the other properties that we need, is a complex and major challenge. It will require reengineering the processes that have evolved to control cell growth, and therefore altering very basic biological processes of cells.

Why Do We Want to Use Immortal Cell Lines?

In my opinion, the future of neural transplantation is likely to involve the use of immortal cell lines. Or perhaps the near future will involve stem and progenitor cells, as discussed in chapter 21, while the more distant future will involve immortal cell lines. The use of immortal cell lines allows, in theory, for the possibility that a controllable, identical source of material could be ready and available for transplantation at all times. Thus, for humans, every transplant would be homogeneous, consisting of one kind of cell only, or perhaps two or three, rather than the mixture that is present in the brain. Every transplant would be identical, and sources of variation related to donor tissue and dissection techniques would be eliminated. No fetuses would be required, and there would be a greatly reduced problem of testing to rule out microbiological contamination. If routine clinical use of neural transplantation is to become a reality, immortal cell lines or some similarly controllable source of cells is, eventually, likely to be necessary.

An additional factor is that the use of immortal cell lines allows for the possibility of making further genetic modifications in cells prior to transplantation. In virtually every case, when we transplant cells into the brain as a treatment for some disease or disorder, we are using cells for some purpose that is slightly different from the purpose for which the cells were "designed." In some cases, it has been possible to employ cells that serve one purpose in the body, but happen to be fairly well suited for some particular use in brain repair, as in the use of chromaffin cells (normally part of the adrenal gland) for transplantation to alleviate pain, discussed in chapter 14, or the use of Sertoli cells from the testes because of their trophic and immunoprotective effects, as discussed in chapter 25. Although these cells work fairly well, they most probably are not *perfectly* suited for that purpose, and undoubtedly could work better if we were able to make slight modifications.

Even in the case of using fetal dopaminergic neurons for Parkinson's disease, there is room for improvement. Although these cells are being used for a purpose very similar to their normal function, there are some real differences. When we transplant them into the brain, we are asking these cells to survive in an unusual location and circumstance (the adult striatum, not the fetal ventral mesencephalon). We also hope that they will form functional connections in an adult brain, whereas they normally form connections in the developing brain. The immature brain provides a much more favorable set of circumstances for the development of neural connections. Perhaps for these reasons, we find that transplanted dopaminergic neurons often survive poorly and develop limited connections with the host brain. Thus, there is room for improvement even in this case. Perhaps the performance of these cells could be improved by genetic alteration.

It is conceivable that genetic alterations could be made in dopaminergic neurons or other kinds of cells without immortalizing them; however, this would mean that these alterations would have to be made separately for each individual case. It is also relatively difficult (although possible) to genetically alter cells that are not dividing. If we think about what we might like to be able to accomplish in the future, however, we might imagine that we would first make an immortal line of human dopaminergic neurons (for example). These cells could then be genetically modified so that we could destroy them with one hormone/drug, just in case it was necessary to remove them after transplantation (poor outcome, side effects, or whatever). We could have a second hormone that would be used to boost their production of dopamine. Other genetic modifications could increase these cells' resistance to suboptimal conditions for survival, so that few of them die after transplantation, and increase their ability to form new connections with the host brain. They perhaps could also be modified to be less antigenic, so that immunosuppression would not be needed. These cells could be grown in culture, and a batch would be removed whenever they were needed for transplantation into a human patient. Controls could be present to regulate their growth as well, but they would also have to be monitored to ensure that unwanted tumor-promoting mutations did not develop. Since these cells would all be identical, the total number transplanted into the brain would be far smaller than the total number implanted with fetal tissue grafts, thus decreasing the reaction of the host brain to the presence of foreign tissue. All of this is, actually, fairly realistic, and a goal that might well be reached (or a part of it, at any rate) over the next 20 years.

How Can We Intentionally Produce Immortal Cell Lines?

Immortal cells can be obtained from tumors, a situation that presents considerable difficulties, since tumor cells may form tumors after transplantation, and also because obtaining cells from tumors is a haphazard process. In addition, tumors do not really produce neurons, although they may produce some neuronlike cells or cells that can be induced to differentiate into neurons in culture. There are also a number of potential techniques for intentionally altering cells so that they can be grown in culture and used for transplantation. These techniques exploit several different avenues, described below.

There have been many experimental studies of these approaches, and they will not be discussed exhaustively here. A few of the most interesting and promising methods will be discussed, while others that are obsolete, have not yet led to interesting experimental studies of transplantation, or are not likely to be greatly explored in the near future will be omitted. For example, many cell lines have been generated as products of fusion between primary cells and tumor cells. Such "hybrid" cells—for example, cells that resemble catecholaminergic neurons—are useful for various purposes (Choi et al. 1991; Crawford et al. 1992); however, they are not likely to be useful for transplantation, since they have chromosomal abnormalities and many of the disadvantages of tumor cells. Thus, hybrid cells will not be discussed here.

Tumor Cells

Immortality is not an especially desirable property if it results in continuing cell division after transplantation into the brain; one would not want to harbor a group of cells continually and uncontrollably dividing inside the brain, since this would constitute a tumor. Transformation is even less desirable, because it can lead to the formation of metastatic tumors.

Tumor cells are often both transformed and immortalized. Certainly, nearly foolproof means of controlling unwanted cell division would have to be assured prior to employment of a tumor cell line for transplantation into human patients.

Several lines of cells that produce catecholamines or acetylcholine have been isolated from tumors and employed for transplantation. Despite the difficulties in using tumor cells for transplantation, some interesting observations have been made. One approach, by Gash and coworkers (1986), was to employ antimitotic agents, including mitomycin C, to render tumor cells amitotic. This led to an apparent persistence of the transplanted cells for extended periods following transplantation into primates.

A second, and perhaps more promising, approach to controlling the growth of tumor cells for intracerebral transplantation has been through encapsulation (Aebischer et al. 1991). The cell line most often used for this purpose is the PC12 catecholaminergic cell line derived from a rat pheochromocytoma, a tumor of the adrenal medulla (Greene and Tischler 1976). These cells are capable of producing dopamine and norepinephrine in large quantities, but form lethal tumors when transplanted into compatible hosts; for example, rats of the same strain from which the tumor arose. When transplanted into species other than rats, however, the tumors are rejected. Thus, PC12 cell grafts, or tumors, will not grow in humans, nor even in species closely related to rats, such as mice and guinea pigs.

There have been several reports of an interesting approach for using these cells in intracerebral transplantation. PC12 cells are grown in semipermeable capsules, then the capsules are transplanted into the brain (Aebischer et al. 1991; Tresco et al. 1992). This and similar methods are being developed by a private company in Rhode Island, Cytotherapeutics. The capsules confine the cells, preventing tumor formation. In addition, the capsules prevent cells and molecules that could cause graft rejection, specifically T cells and antibodies, from entering the capsule and rejecting the PC12 cell graft. This latter fact alone is not sufficient to allow for use of this method; however, there is a built-in fail-safe mechanism: if the capsules fail, the grafts will rapidly be rejected. Because the PC12 cells are from a species (the rat) that is so widely separated from the proposed host species (humans), the tumor would be easily and rapidly rejected in any but the most severely immunocompromised host. Simply by avoiding subjects with impaired immune function (patients with other kinds of grafts or with HIV, for example) the procedure could be made quite safe, in the sense that there would be little possibility of tumor formation. That is, if it works perfectly, the method could be quite safe.

This is not to say that capsule failure would be tolerable. The rejection of a graft would cause local tissue damage, so the possibility of capsule failure plus rejection should be avoided. Whether this method can be employed clinically, for transplantation into human subjects, is a serious question. It is not yet clear that sustained survival of significant numbers of PC12 cells can be maintained in such capsules for long periods of time, or whether they are capable of producing sufficient functional effects to be useful. Moreover, there are biomechanical problems related to the use of artificial capsules in the brain for extended periods, as well as possible capsule failure and other issues.

Immortalized Cell Lines Produced By Genetic Transfer of Oncogenes

The most recent, and probably the most interesting, method for developing immortal cell lines is through the use of oncogenes. A considerable number of cell lines have been developed using this method (H. Geller et al. 1991; H. Geller and Dubois-Dalcq 1988; Giordano et al. 1993, 1996; Jat et al. 1991; Renfranz et al. 1991; Ryder et al. 1990; Snyder et al. 1992; Whittemore and White 1993; Whittemore et al. 1994; Whittemore and Snyder 1996). Mammalian cells employ a complex series of biochemical events to regulate their division; for example, cells will grow only as needed during brain development, but remain under control at other times so that tumors do not form. Tumors develop when these growth controls become abnormal, such as through mutations. Certain viruses code for proteins that disrupt the normal cellular mechanisms of growth control, resulting in increased cell division and, sometimes, immortality. Normal cells also contain genes coding for proteins that can promote cell growth. These growth-promoting genes are called "oncogenes," because of their ability to promote tumor formation. Viruses contain oncogenes to promote their own reproduction, because their reproduction depends on reproduction of the host cell. It is clear that it is not sufficient simply to provoke cells to divide using oncogenes, since uncontrolled cell division is certainly not desirable. A number of additional strategies to obtain control over the production or function of the oncogenes are possible, and ultimately some such strategy would presumably be needed.

One of the most frequently used techniques involves the use of the gene coding for SV40 large T antigen, an oncogene derived from a monkey virus (Jat et al. 1986). SV40 large T antigen, also called SV40 large T protein, has numerous effects, including acting on proteins normally involved in limiting cell division. One of the proteins that SV40 large T antigen interacts with is called retinoblastoma protein or pRb in the scientific literature. This retinoblastoma protein controls the final step in a complex cascade of events controlling cell growth. When retinoblastoma protein is abnormal, the cell cycle can, under certain circumstances, continue when it would otherwise cease. In certain individuals with abnormalities in retinoblastoma protein, the frequency of tumor formation of certain kinds (retinoblastoma) is increased.

SV40 large T antigen binds to, and thereby blocks the function of, retinoblastoma protein. This property seems to be an important component of the cell growth–promoting properties of SV40 large T antigen, although the antigen does other things as well. Recently, a small fragment of the SV40 large T oncogene that effectively immortalizes neural cells but lacks some of the objectionable effects of the intact molecule has been identified (Truckenmiller et al. 1998). This may allow for production of neural cell lines with more complete neuronal properties.

In general, immortalization has the potential to become a unique and in some ways ideal genetic engineering strategy for transplantation of cells into the brain, because of the following considerations. Immortalization may require two genetic alterations, one to stimulate cell growth and a second to permit cellular immortality (that is, to circumvent cellular senescence). Cellular immortality may not impair the ability of neurons to differentiate. The genetic modification that is used to stimulate cell growth (e.g., transferring SV40 large T antigen into the cells), on the other hand, is needed only while the cells are in culture. If it were possible to turn this growth-stimulating genetic modification on and off whenever desired, one could produce cells that would behave like immortal cells in culture, growing indefinitely. When the immortalized cells were transplanted, the ideal strategy would be to reverse or remove whatever was done to achieve cell growth in culture, so that the cells would revert to being entirely normal cells. This is not as far-fetched as it might sound, since it is normal for genes to be turned on and off under many circumstances. There have been several studies along these lines (Hoshimaru et al. 1996; Westerman and Leboulch 1996). Moreover, continued growth of immortalized cell lines after transplantation into the brain is not generally observed, even without additional precautions. Therefore, although it cannot quite be done yet, the possibilities for use of this approach make it very attractive.

The first approach to "turning off" an immortalizing agent was through the use of a temperature-sensitive oncogene. There is a mutant form of the SV40 large T antigen that is thought to be effective only at relatively low temperatures (Jat and Sharp 1989). At body temperature, or perhaps slightly above body temperature, cells immortalized with this form (or allele) of the SV40 large T antigen, also called tsA58, may not divide. However, the expected inhibition of growth at body temperature seems to be incomplete, or at least somewhat unreliable. Thus, a temperature slightly above body temperature may be necessary for complete growth cessation, or additional supplementary means of inhibiting cell division may be needed. It also appears likely that the temperature-sensitive form may retain some of its effects (such as blocking of retinoblastoma protein) even at the higher temperatures. Thus, reversal of immortality produced by this mutant form of the SV40 large T protein at higher temperatures seems to be incomplete or perhaps entirely ineffective.

There are many possibilities for accomplishing reversal of immortalizing events. To give some idea of how this might be accomplished, one possibility will be described here. A potential method is through manipulating the promoter region of the oncogene that is used for immortalization. Promoters are sequences of DNA that determine whether genes will be used or not. There now are several methods through which expression (i.e., production) of a transferred gene can be controlled by chemical modulators that can be added to a tissue culture medium.

Understanding this approach requires some additional explanation. When cells are immortalized by genetic transfer of oncogenes, this involves insertion of DNA into cells. These DNA sequences contain two principal components: (1) a coding sequence, which specifies the actual amino acids in the final protein product, and (2) a promoter region, which (by interacting with cellular proteins) determines whether the DNA coding sequence will be transcribed (made into RNA) or will just sit there, unused.

There are many kinds of promoters (there are actually both promoters and enhancers; here we will use just the term "promoters" to describe the DNA sequences that influence whether genes are used), and they and related elements are the principal means used to determine what proteins will be manufactured by the cell. For example, muscle cells make myoglobin, and dopamine neurons make tyrosine hydroxylase. All cells contain the DNA for making both myoglobin and tyrosine hydroxylase, but most other cells do not need these particular proteins and do not manufacture them. Transcription factors are proteins that bind to promoter and enhancer regions of DNA and determine whether the coding part of the DNA will be transcribed. A complex pattern of transcription factor production determines the pattern of protein production by each cell, and hence the nature of the cell.

Some promoters are for "housekeeping genes," which serve very basic structural or metabolic purposes. Others are more specialized, used for functions of particular cell types, or during particular stages in the development and differentiation of certain cells. There are also viral promoters, which are employed by viruses to force cells to make viral proteins. Often, viral promoters are used in gene transfer experiments. Some viral promoter sequences that are frequently used are the Rous sarcoma virus promoter, the simian virus 40 promoter, and the cytomegalovirus promoter. These promoters are potent and relatively indiscriminate, which is why they are used here, and are useful in many circumstances. However, this is not necessarily the best situation for a promoter that is used to drive expression of an immortalizing gene.

What do we really want an immortalized cell, which is to be employed for transplantation into the brain, to do? In fact, we would like this cell to behave like an immortalized cell only when it is in tissue culture. When it is removed from culture and transplanted to the brain, we would prefer that it cease being immortal, and instead behave like an ordinary cell. This could be accomplished, most probably, by judicious use of promoters. Several promoters that can be turned on and off by externally added drugs or hormones exist; one such promoter is the ecdysone promoter, which is activated by the insect hormone ecdysone (No et al. 1996). Thus it is conceivable that an oncogene could be "turned on" while cells are in culture, but "turned off" after the cells have been transplanted into the brain. Since this hormone is not produced in the brain, or in mammals at all, it would not be present after the cells are transplanted and, therefore, the cells would presumably revert to normal behavior. Such potential refinements of the technology for immortalizing cells are likely to result in major improvements in this field.

For accuracy, it should be mentioned that immortalization of cells, especially human cells, is not simply a matter of controlling cell division. Producing immortal cell lines by simply forcing cells to divide can promote the development of chromosomal abnormalities, as a result of shortening of structures at the end of chromosomes that are called "telomeres." Obtaining immortal cell lines without chromosomal abnormalities may be best accomplished by gaining control over the enzyme "telomerase," which can add to telomere length (Bodnar et al. 1998; Jiang et al. 1999). The relative roles of telomerase and cell growth control in the immortalization of cells is, however, a complex topic which is beyond the scope of this book.

Creating Immortal Cell Lines: Two Strategies

There are two differing strategies or, in a sense, philosophies for developing immortal cell lines, whether through the use of the temperature-sensitive allele of SV40 large T antigen, v-myc, or other methods. One idea is to develop neuronal or glial cell lines with specific phenotypic properties, in order to replace specific types of brain cells that are lost. That is, cells which are always dopaminergic (cells that act like dopamine neurons in all circumstances, including in culture) might be made.

An alternative strategy for the development of immortalized cell lines for transplantation is the idea that cells can be made which will have different properties depending on the circumstances. These cells are genetically engineered counterparts of the neural stem cells described in chapter 21. Such cells are called multipotent. This means that they have the ability to differentiate into different kinds of cells, depending on their environment. This approach involves immortalizing progenitor cells or stem cells, as described in chapter 21. If one wants to replace dopamine neurons (according to this second strategy), one might develop cells that do not actually behave like dopamine neurons in culture. When transplanted into the brain, however, such cells might encounter signals that instruct them to behave like dopaminergic neurons. The example given, however, is rather extreme. Most probably, cells can have some ability to differentiate into more than one final type, but a cell that will "become a dopaminergic neuron" simply by virtue of being placed into the appropriate location in the brain is probably not realistic. Thus, the dopaminergic phenotype might have to be induced, at least in part, by exposure to various cytokines or other factors before being transplanted, as has been discussed in chapter 21.

The difference between these two strategies is rather complex, and there is neither a single "correct" approach nor an absolute difference between the two methods. Cells of the brain go through a series of steps in attaining their final, differentiated form. At an early stage of development, a single cell is capable of becoming a number of different types of cell; cells that are unrestricted in their potential for differentiation are called stem cells or neural stem cells. With each cell division, cells are gradually committed, or restricted, to becoming a smaller number of different kinds of cells. At the extreme, the entire organism begins with a single cell. Differentiation of neural stem cells, and further differentiation of these cells into neurons and glia with various phenotypic properties, is one phase of the overall process of cellular differentiation. Thus the difference between the approaches is not absolute. For example, one might imagine a cell that in culture is only partially a dopaminergic neuron, becoming a fully differentiated dopaminergic neuron only when it is in the brain, making contacts with other neurons. This sort of guidance toward a specific cellular fate occurs even for normal primary neurons. In fact, we can safely make a generalization: the earlier and less differenti-

Table 22.2
Contrasting approaches to the immortalization of cells

Type I: Phenotype Established in Brain after Transplantation	Type II: Phenotype Established in Culture
Multipotent Cells (Neural Stem Cells)	Unipotent Cells
Immortalized at an early stage of differentiation	Immortalized at a late stage of differentiation
May express multiple phenotypes	Express a single phenotype
Depend on environment for expression of phenotypes	Express phenotype independent of conditions, even in tissue culture
For replacement of cells in the injured brain, signals from the brain are required for expression of phenotype	Can be used to replace cells in the brain even if signals to specify cell phenotype are not present

ated the cells that are used, the easier they are to grow and immortalize, but the harder it is to make them differentiate into mature cells.

In practical terms, employing a multipotent immortalized precursor cell for transplantation presumes that if a cell is used which is near the final phases of differentiation, with one or two cell divisions remaining, the remaining aspects of differentiation can be achieved after transplantation into the brain, because of enhanced differentiation signals that are present there. In culture, despite our best efforts, signals for cellular differentiation might not be ideal, so that the cells would remain undifferentiated or incompletely differentiated. The contrasting strategy attempts to immortalize cells following, or during, their final division, so that commitment to a particular phenotype is assured or more nearly assured. This places less dependence on the host brain to specify phenotype, so that the cell line produced will always express only a single phenotype (behave like a single, particular type of cell). Depending on the purpose for which the cells are to be used, one or the other approach might be more useful (table 22.2). Thus, for some purposes it may be advantageous to employ very undifferentiated, immature cells as a starting material (type I experiments). Other goals might require cells that are at as late a developmental stage as possible as starting material for immortalization (type II experiments). Although I believe that the methods for producing immortal cell lines will gradually be improved over the next 10 years or so, a few examples of what has already been done with immortal cell lines and neural transplantation will be given for both approaches.

Type I Experiments

The Type I approach works better than anyone could have expected. Certain immortalized cell lines appear to be able to integrate into the host brain to a remarkable degree. It is not likely that the injured or mature brain contains all of the signals required to induce differentiation of cells into particular missing phenotypes following transplantation. Thus, there are bound to be some limitations of this approach. Nevertheless, it has been observed that the brain has a remarkable ability to induce transplanted immortalized cells to adopt various phenotypes, depending on the area of the brain into which they are transplanted. In some cases, the injured brain even seems able to guide transplanted cells to adopt phenotypes of missing cells.

One of the most remarkable and extensive studies of transplantation of immortalized cells is the study by Evan Snyder and coworkers reported in 1992. These experiments employed cells immortalized from fetal rat cerebellum using the v-myc oncogene. A number of cell lines were isolated, and found to have variable properties despite being derived from single clones. One cell line, clone C27–3, was chosen for transplantation studies. When these cells were transplanted into the newborn rat brain, they were found to express different morphologies, depending upon exactly where in the brain they were transplanted. In some locations, the cells behaved like neurons, while in slightly different locations, the same cells behaved more like glial cells. The transplanted cells assumed properties that very closely resembled those of normal host neurons and glial cells, and even formed contacts with host cells.

The nearly complete integration of these cells into the host brain structure suggests that such cells might be used for transplantation and delivery of factors into the brain in a therapeutic manner. Evan Snyder and coworkers are extensively exploring such possibilities (e.g., E. Snyder et al. 1995; E. Snyder and Wolfe 1996), including the development of human stem cells for delivery of genes to the brain (Flax et al. 1998). For example, Snyder and coworkers (1995) employed a mouse with a genetic deficiency in the enzyme β-glucuronidase, an animal model of Sly disease, or mucopolysaccharidosis VII. This kind of disorder is called a lysosomal storage disease, because of the accumulation of molecules comprised of protein and/or carbohydrate in subcellular organelles called lysosomes, and progressive enlargement of these structures. The cell line C17.2, which has normal activity of the enzyme β-glucuronidase, was transplanted into the brains of these animals. These animals normally show accumulation of glycosaminoglycans (molecules comprised of protein and carbohydrate), which eventually causes degeneration of both neurons and glia. Transplanted cells distributed diffusely through the brain and greatly decreased the lysosomal enlargement usually seen in these animals (figure 22.1).

Additional experiments showing variable differentiation of a single cell line were reported by Shihabuddin and coworkers (1995, 1996) and by Onifer and coworkers (1993). Some of these experiments involved the use of adult host animals rather than the newborns used by Snyder and coworkers. These investigators earlier developed a line of cells derived from the fetal rat raphe nucleus, called RN33B, which in many respects behave like neurons in culture (Whittemore and White 1993). These cells were transplanted into several places in the brain; depending on the location into which they were transplanted, they assumed properties that differed quite markedly. When transplanted into the spinal cord, corpus callosum, or most parts of the hippocampus, they exhibited an elongated, bipolar shape. In contrast, when transplanted into the cerebral cortex, the same cells developed multipolar morphologies (Shihabuddin et al. 1995, 1996; see figure 22.2). Some transplanted cells in the cerebral cortex were, in fact, very similar to normal cortical neurons. It is interesting that the cell line used in these experiments had a particular defined phenotype, yet was capable of considerable variation following transplantation.

The development of multipotent cell lines is an interesting area that could follow a number of different courses in the future. The observation that some immortal cell lines can adopt variable phenotypes after transplantation in different locations is interesting: Is it possible that there are local signals in the brain, especially in the injured brain, which can simply direct cells to adopt certain "useful" phenotypes, and that these cells will

I.

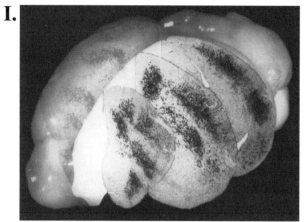

II.

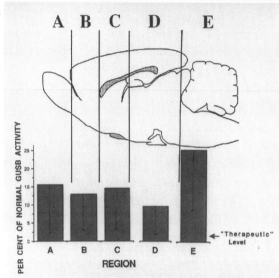

III.

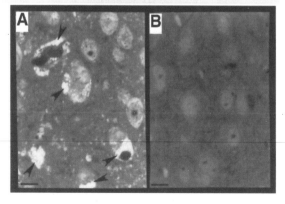

then go on to do whatever is needed to repair local damage? Surprisingly, sometimes this does seem to be the case in animal studies. Nonetheless, we cannot assume that this will be a general feature of transplanted immortal multipotent cells.

In a demyelinating disease, for example, multipotent cells (cells with a variety of potential phenotypes) transplanted into the brain may be able to detect local signals indicating that oligodendrocytes are missing. These cells may then differentiate into oligodendrocytes, and remyelinate local areas of demyelination. Perhaps, especially in immature animals, this

Figure 22.1
Illustration of the use of a cell line to partially correct a genetic degenerative disorder. A cell line, C17.2, which has normal activity of the enzyme β-glucuronidase, was transplanted into the brains of animals with a genetic deficiency in the activity of this enzyme. These enzyme-deficient animals are direct analogues of the human disorder mucopolysaccharidosis type VII. These animals normally show accumulation of glycosaminoglycans (molecules comprised of protein and carbohydrate) in subcellular organelles called lysosomes, which eventually cause degeneration of both neurons and glia. This kind of disorder is called a lysosomal storage disease, because of the accumulation of material in lysosomes that cannot be degraded. Transplanted cells distributed diffusely through the brain and greatly decreased the lysosomal enlargement usually seen in these animals.

I. A computer reconstruction of the brain of a mature animal that received transplanted C17.2 cells. These cells have been modified with the lacZ gene, so that they can be labeled with a blue reaction product. A newborn animal received a transplant of C17.2 cells, which were found to have migrated and distributed throughout the brain.

II. Distribution of the activity of the enzyme β-glucuronidase throughout the brains of animals with mucopolysaccharidosis type VII. The animals normally do not have this enzyme, but C17.2 cells have substantial enzyme activity. The data shown are enzyme activity levels as a percentage of normal enzyme activity. In liver and spleen, restoration of enzyme activity to between 2 and 5 percent of normal is sufficient to correct the degenerative disease.

III. Illustration of lysosomal storage in animals with β-glucuronidase deficiency, that is, mucopolysaccharidosis type VII. In (A), an untreated animal is shown. The lysosomes are distended, and appear as vacuoles (holes, or bubble-like structures) in the cortex of an eight-month-old animal that did not receive a transplant. (B) In a similar region from the brain of an animal with transplanted C17.2 cells, these vacuoles are greatly decreased, and the brain is nearly normal. Scale bar: 0.02 mm. (Photograph from E. Snyder et al. 1995. Reprinted courtesy of Evan Snyder, Harvard University, with permission.)

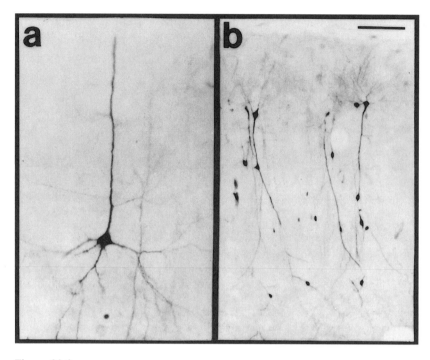

Figure 22.2
A single clonal cell line can adopt different phenotypes after transplantation, depending on where in the brain it is transplanted, even in adult host animals. This figure depicts cells from the RN33B cell line after transplantation into the cerebral cortex (a) or the hippocampus (b), showing that a single cell line can adopt different characteristic morphologies in different locations. In a scanning electron microscope picutre of the RN33B cell line being grown in culture, attached to plastic dishes (c), the extensive formation of processes by these cells is apparent. (Photograph courtesy of Scott Whittemore, University of Kentucky. Pictures (a) and (b) reproduced from Shihabuddin et al. 1996, with permission.)

might work sometimes—this would have to be determined empirically. But more probably, the adult brain does not contain all of the necessary differentiation-inducing signals, and cell-cell signaling processes may be abnormal in the diseased brain, so that signals for differentiation may not be available. Therefore, in many circumstances it may be more advantageous to employ cells that are already irrevocably committed to the appropriate and desired phenotype (in our case, cells that already are committed in culture to being oligodendrocytes). Such committed cells

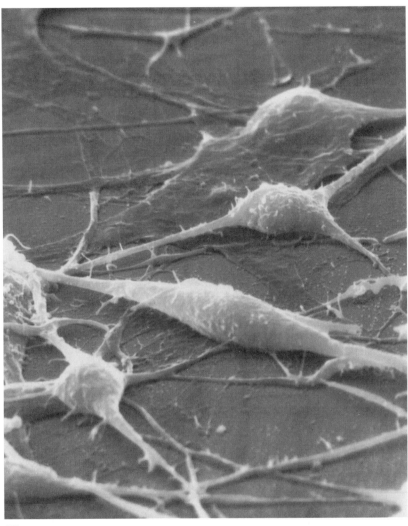

(C)

Table 22.3
Two related concepts involving cellular differentiation

Phenotypic commitment	The stage of development of a cell following which it is committed to developing only a single phenotype, that is, a single set of properties. After commitment to a single phenotype (for example, a dopaminergic neuron), a cell must either become that phenotype or remain undifferentiated.
Terminal differentiation	Development of a cell's final form, following which reversion to an earlier undifferentiated, and multipotent, phenotype is no longer possible.

would express the oligodendrocyte phenotype following transplantation, without any instructions from the host brain.

There is a third possibility: cells with multipotent properties might be used for transplantation into the brain after a phenotypic commitment is induced in culture prior to transplantation (table 22.3). The molecular signals that induce cells to become committed to particular phenotypes are rapidly being identified. These signals may be applied to multipotent cells in vitro, so that they are committed to a particular phenotype before they are transplanted. An excellent example of this strategy is the studies on mesencephalic cell differentiation by Ling and coworkers (1998), discussed in chapter 21. In this study, using normal cells, a dopaminergic neuronal phenotype could be induced by a combination of growth factors, cytokines, and tissue extracts. Thus, cells may be provoked to undergo terminal differentiation either before or after transplantation by exposing them to appropriate factors. In this way, multipotent cells may be useful for transplantation even when the brain does not express the signals needed to induce differentiation in the desired direction.

Another possibility, emphasized by E. Snyder and coworkers (1992, 1995; Snyder and Wolfe 1996), is to use multipotent immortalized cell lines as "vehicles" for subsequent modification to deliver specific factors or exogenous genes into the CNS. At least some of these cell lines show an extraordinary ability to become very completely integrated into the host brain and quite widely distributed, with virtually no evidence of host immune or glial reaction. Such cells could be ideal candidates for additional modifications to permit delivery of growth factors or other substances into the brain for therapeutic purposes.

Type II Experiments

A large number of immortalized cell lines with specific properties have already been created from CNS cell cultures. These include cells with serotonergic properties, dopaminergic properties, GABAergic properties, and undifferentiated cells that have the capacity to adopt various forms after transplantation. Eaton and coworkers (1997) found that immortalized serotonergic cells can be used to alleviate pain in animal models. In our laboratory, for example, we have developed a series of cell lines from the rat striatum that make GABA (Giordano et al. 1993, 1994, 1996). One of the clearest and most immediate goals of making an immortalized neuronal cell line is the production of dopaminergic neurons. This goal has not been achieved entirely, although there are several cell lines with partial dopaminergic properties. Some of the most extensive experiments along these lines were reported by Anton and coworkers (1994). These studies employed a cell line from the rat mesencephalon, immortalized with the temperature-sensitive SV40 large T antigen. Although the cell line was not really dopaminergic, slight tyrosine hydroxylase (TH) immunoreactivity was detected in the cells. The approach used by Anton and coworkers, however, was to make a further genetic modification in the cells, by introducing the TH cDNA into the cells by retroviral infection techniques. Thus, the cell line used had two successive genetic modifications. First, they were immortalized by the introduction of SV40 large T antigen, and then induced to make more TH by introduction of the TH cDNA. This resulted in a cell line that did, in fact make lots of TH, but differed from dopaminergic neurons in two important respects: (1) the cells made L-DOPA, but not dopamine, and (2) when transplanted into the brains of animals, these cells did not form connections with the host brain. Nevertheless, the cells were capable of ameliorating some of the manifestations of substantia nigra lesions in both rats and monkeys. This is the most effective of the attempts to produce an immortal cell line that can be used for transplantation in Parkinson's disease. There is also a second study in which a human immortal glial cell line was used to express tyrosine hydroxylase, and these cells were also effective in a rodent model (Tornatore et al. 1996).

Nonetheless, these experiments do not come close to fulfilling the ultimate goal of producing an immortalized dopaminergic neuron. Ideally, methods would be developed that would allow cells to be grown in culture, but to become more or less normal dopaminergic neurons when transplanted into the brain. Such methods would, almost necessarily, depend on the normal physiological processes that cause cells to become dopaminergic neurons, experimentally changing only their propensity to divide in tissue culture.

The events that prompt cells to adopt a mature, differentiated form include both external signals, some from neighboring cells, and internal events. Recently, some of the events that normally induce cells to become dopaminergic neurons have been discovered. Dopaminergic cells develop in the embryonic brain in proximity to "floor plate" cells, a cell type that is present in an embryonic structure called the floor plate. When cells from the embryonic brain that would not ordinarily become dopaminergic neurons were cultured with floor plate cells from the embryo, the floor plate cells were able to induce some of the cells to behave very much like dopaminergic neurons, due to contact with a cell surface protein (Hynes, Porter, et al. 1995; Hynes, Poulsen, et al. 1995). Another recent study has identified a transcription factor called Nurr1, which is necessary for cells to become dopaminergic neurons (Zetterstrom et al. 1997).

In summary, what I have called the type II approach seeks to obtain cells with a differentiated phenotype in culture before they are transplanted into the brain. This might be accomplished by immortalizing cells after they have become committed to a particular phenotype, or by influencing them to become committed to a particular phenotype in culture, after they have been immortalized. In contrast, the type I approach described above seeks only to immortalize cells that have the *potential* to become cells of the desired phenotype. Then cells are transplanted into the brain, and the host brain is depended upon to influence the cells to develop a particular desired phenotype.

Genetically Altered Mice

One of the most versatile methods of producing immortal cell lines involves the use of genetically altered mice. There are two different methods for producing genetic alterations in mice. Transgenic mice have additional genes inserted more or less randomly into the genome. Gene targeted mice have genes that are either deleted (knockout mice), modified, or altered by the insertion of genes into specific targeted locations in the genome. The methods for producing such animals will not be described here in detail. For the interested reader, the book *Gene Targeting* by Sedivy and Joyner (see list for "Further Reading") provides a description of the technology that is comprehensible to the nonscientist. It should be emphasized that these methods *cannot,* under any circumstances, be employed to produce human cell lines, since that would entail interference with the human genome and the production of genetically altered fetuses, clearly an unacceptable proposition. Still, the technique is very useful in animal models, and there may even be human applications of another kind, which we can speculate about at the end of this section.

The initial idea was to randomly insert the SV40 large T gene into mice (Jat et al. 1991). This method leads to indiscriminate expression of SV40 large T antigen. More sophisticated versions of this idea use transgenic mice that express the oncogene driven by a selective promoter (Suri et al. 1993). As has been mentioned, various proteins are selectively produced by certain cell types. Control of the expression of proteins is mainly exercised by a region of the gene that precedes the coding region, and is called the promoter. Thus, the enzyme tyrosine hydroxylase is produced in catecholaminergic neurons mainly because these neurons produce the appropriate transcription factors to activate the tyrosine hydroxylase promoter.

It is possible to insert oncogenes into specific locations in the genome, or to link oncogenes with specific promoter sequences, so that the appropriate sequences become joined with oncogene coding sequences. This results in a foreign gene (a transgene) being produced only in selected cell types. In our case, the transgene is an oncogene, usually SV40 large T antigen. If SV40 large T antigen (for example) is coupled to the tyrosine hydroxylase promoter, it will be produced only in cells that express tyrosine hydroxylase—that is, in cells that make the tyrosine hydroxylase protein (i.e., catecholaminergic neurons). Using this and similar strategies, selective cell types can be targeted for immortalization and cultured directly from the brains of mice. This procedure has been used to produce a number of cell lines, including catecholamine-producing cell lines (e.g., Suri et al. 1993).

As has been mentioned, human cell lines cannot be made in this way: we certainly cannot produce transgenic humans with viral oncogenes! Before leaving this topic, however, let's consider whether transgenic animal cells that could be useful for human therapy might be produced.

First, let's not limit this to mice. A larger animal, somewhat closer to humans phylogenetically and in physical size, would be better. Chimpanzees or any larger primate would probably not be practical—for a variety of reasons—but what about pigs? The first step would be to alter the pigs so that their cells are not very likely to produce immunological reactions in humans. This might not be an insurmountable problem, since CNS cells and especially neurons are not strongly immunogenic anyway, and neurons can be transplanted across species with the aid of only modest immunosuppression. Through the use of selective breeding and/or gene targeting to modify immunogenic proteins expressed by pig neurons, it might be possible to breed a strain of pigs that could be used as a source of cells for brain transplantation in human subjects. There is at least one biotechnology company engaged in this kind of enterprise. Although this project might take a while, it seems within the realm of possibility. Whether this strategy would have any advantage compared with producing human cell lines in culture is questionable. Which leads us to the next topic.

Human Cell Lines

Although it is conceivable that animal cell lines could be used for transplantation in humans, cell lines derived from human tissue are likely to be ultimately more useful. It is possible to develop human glial, and probably eventually neuronal, cell lines from human fetal brain tissue using cell cultures. The first human CNS cell line produced was the glial cell line developed by Major and coworkers in 1985. More recently, Whittemore and coworkers (1994) developed two astrocyte cell lines from human spinal cord, using retroviral transfer of the temperature-sensitive SV40 large T antigen. Further developments in techniques for cell immortalization are likely to result in cell lines that are ultimately more useful. In all likelihood, we are now at the beginning of the development of techniques for the production of neural and glial cell lines. After hundreds or thousands of human cell lines, with ever-improving properties, have been produced over perhaps 10 years, we will begin to see lines that are realistically suitable for transplantation into the brains of human patients.

Further Reading

Cepko, C. L. (1989). Immortalization of neural cells via retrovirus-mediated oncogene transduction. *Ann. Rev. Neurosci.* 12: 47–65.

Gage, F. H., Wolff, J. A., Rosenberg, M. B., Xu, L., Yee, J.-K., Schults, C., and Friedmann, T. (1987). Grafting genetically modified cells to the brain: Possibilities for the future. *Neuroscience* 23: 795–807.

Geller, H. M., Quinones-Jenab, V., Poltorak, M., and Freed, W. J. (1991). Applications of immortalized cells in basic and clinical neurology. *J. Cell. Biochem.* 45: 279–283.

Sedivy, J. M., and Joyner, A. J. (1992). *Gene Targeting.* W. H. Freeman, New York.

Snyder, E. Y. (1995). Immortalized neural stem cells: Insights into development; prospects for gene therapy and repair. *Proc. Assn. Am. Physicians* 107: 195–204.

Snyder, E. Y., Park, K. I., Flax, J. D., Liu, S., Rosario, C.M., Yandava, B. D., and Aurora, S. (1997). Potential of neural "stem-like" cells for gene therapy and repair of the degenerating central nervous system. *Adv. Neurol.* 72: 121–132.

Whittemore, S. R., Eaton, M. J., and Onifer, S. M. (1997). Gene therapy and the use of stem cells for central nervous system regeneration. *Adv. Neurol.* 72: 113–119.

Whittemore, S. R., and Snyder, E. Y. (1996). Physiological relevance and functional potential of central nervous system-derived cell lines. *Mol. Neurobiol.* 12: 13–38.

23
Genetically Modified Cells for Producing Neurotrophic Factors and Neurotransmitters

One approach to genetic engineering of cells for use in neural transplantation is to start with a more or less neutral cell type, and to modify these cells so that they produce a therapeutically useful biochemical. This involves inserting genes into cells prior to transplantation, to coax cells into producing substances that they otherwise would not. Although this feat can be accomplished quite routinely, considerable improvements in the methodology need to be made, especially if this technology is to be used in human therapy. Particular improvements that are needed involve improved control and predictability of the amounts of protein produced. Genetic alteration of cells can be done more successfully using current technology if the target cells are only maintained in culture, rather than transplanting them into an animal. As improvements appear, we are likely to see an increasing emphasis on this technology in neural transplantation.

Most studies using this approach fall into two broad categories: (1) experiments on delivery of growth factors and (2) experiments in which cells are made to produce neurotransmitters or neurotransmitter precursors. This approach has been used experimentally to produce a wide variety of substances, including neurotransmitters and their precursors, such as L-DOPA and GABA, and growth factors, including NGF, GDNF, bFGF, and BDNF. In these experiments, cells are modified to act as biological manufacturers of individual chemical substances, but otherwise do not necessarily perform all of the functions of neurons or glial cells. Therefore, altering cells to make foreign proteins will always have some limitations. Neurons do not, of course, simply make neurotransmitters: they release neurotransmitter in a controlled manner at synapses that have been formed with other cells. This occurs in response to appropriate inputs from other neurons. Simple manufacture of neurotransmitter and its delivery to localized regions of the brain is likely to be effective only in a few very special circumstances. Treatment of pain, for example (see chapter 14), is a distinctly possible circumstance in which effects might be produced by simple production of neurotransmitters or neuromodulators. If we can find therapeutic reasons for delivering growth factors into the brain, delivery by genetically modified cells is a promising approach. For this kind of application, it seems likely that engineering cells to produce a single chemical substance may turn out to work quite well, since growth factors may be effective when administered diffusely.

What Kinds of Cells Can Be Used for Starting Material?

Virtually any cell type is a potential candidate for genetic modification. Cell lines can be used; often, a cell line that already has some of the desired properties can be enhanced by genetic manipulation. When cell lines are used, the modification need be made only once, and an unlimited supply of cells can then be produced for transplantation. Alternatively, it is possible, at least in theory, to remove cells from the host by biopsy, modify them in culture, and then transplant them into the brain. In humans, this would mean modifying a patient's *own* cells in culture. (The possibility of modifying cells *without* removing them is discussed in chapter 24.) This approach is limited to cell types that can be removed by biopsy and subsequently be propagated in culture. In practice, this is a severe limitation, and only a relatively few cell types can be profitably used in this manner.

Primary cell types that are good candidates for biopsy, genetic manipulation, and subsequent transplantation include endothelial cells, muscle cells, olfactory epithelial cells (or ensheathing cells), macrophages, and fibroblasts. Although it would be inconvenient (e.g., requiring brain biopsy), primary glial cells might be used in this way. Despite the technical obstacles, there are obvious advantages to the use of glial cells as a starting material: they belong in the brain. Since no cell is entirely neutral (all cells produce biologically active molecules), there may be substantial advantages in using glial cells as a starting material, since they are perhaps less likely to cause unexpected adverse effects by producing unwanted substances. The use of primary cells is also limited by the fact that this approach requires custom modification of cells for each individual. In most cases, the unpredictability of genetic modification with current technology may make this approach impractical.

The problem of what kind of cell to start with is quite complex. If we employ, for genetic modification, a cell type that is easily obtained (e.g., fibroblasts, muscle cells), we may ultimately find that these cells produce unwanted effects after we transplant them into the brain. Using glial cells as a starting material would largely overcome this potential problem. If we are going to contemplate using glial cells, however, there are the problems of obtaining the cells (requiring a significant surgical procedure) and of growing and genetically modifying them in culture (which is especially difficult with glial cells from mature donors). This is probably impractical. Thus, in order to use glial cells as a platform for genetic modification, it may first be necessary to develop improved methods for making immortalized glial cell lines (see chapter 22). This would allow immortal cell lines, rather than glial cells obtained directly from patients, to be used for genetic modification.

Another restriction on the kinds of cells that can be used is that cells are not always biochemically equipped to process foreign proteins efficiently. Thus, it is not always a simple matter of inducing any cell to make a protein. Depending on the particular protein, foreign proteins may be unstable in cells that do not normally make that protein (Wu and Cepko 1994). In addition, mechanisms to employ proteins efficiently may be fairly specialized. Thus, genetically modifying cells so that they produce neurotransmitter may not be very useful; neurotransmitter processing and release by cells is a very complex process. On the other hand, employing cells to produce growth factors is, in many ways, less complex, since growth factors might be effective if they are produced slowly and steadily. Using genetically modified cells to manufacture growth factors could, therefore, turn out to be quite useful.

Growth factors are protein molecules that promote the growth, differentiation, and survival of other cells. The more specific term "neurotrophic factor" is used to describe molecules that have trophic effects (i.e., promote growth, differentiation, and survival) for neurons. The first such factor to be discovered was nerve growth factor (NGF), discovered and isolated by R. Levi-Montalcini and coworkers more than 40 years ago (Levi-Montalcini 1987; Levi-Montalcini et al. 1995, 1996). NGF was initially observed to have trophic effects on peripheral sympathetic (noradrenergic) neurons and immature peripheral sensory neurons only. Although it was long suspected that there would be other neurotrophic factors, few were known until the 1980s. This field received a tremendous boost when it was found, by Hefti and coworkers (1984, 1986), that NGF has trophic effects on acetylcholine-containing neurons in the brain. Many additional neurotrophic factors are now known, among them factors that affect specific types of CNS neurons. Some of the neurotrophic factors that have been most extensively studied are basic fibroblast growth factor (bFGF), ciliary neurotrophic factor (CNTF), glial-derived neurotrophic factor (GDNF; see chapters 10 and 24), neurotrophin–3 (NT–3), and brain-derived neurotrophic factor (BDNF). Each is effective for certain types of neurons. The factor that is most effective for promoting differentiation of dopaminergic neurons is GDNF.

Growth Factor Delivery by Genetically Modified Cells

The first experiment in this area was published in 1988 by Rosenberg and coworkers. These investigators studied the ability of cells that produce nerve growth factor (NGF) to prevent degeneration of acetylcholine-containing neurons (cholinergic cells) in the septum following severing of their axons. The fimbria-fornix connects acetylcholine neurons to their targets in the hippocampus. These cholinergic neurons require NGF for survival; normally, this is obtained from their target cells by transport from the hippocampus. Therefore, when the fimbria-fornix pathway is cut, severing the axons of these neurons, many of them die. Earlier, Hefti (1986) and Kromer (1987) had shown that NGF injections could prevent degeneration of these cholinergic cell bodies when their axons were severed. In the experiment by Rosenberg and coworkers, fibroblasts were modified to produce NGF, then transplanted into the site of the fimbria-fornix injury. About half of the cholinergic neurons died when the fimbria-fornix was cut. In animals with the NGF-producing fibroblast transplants, the death of cholinergic neurons was found to have been largely prevented when the animals were examined after two weeks. Presumably, this occurred because the transplanted cells supplied NGF that substituted for the NGF the cells would normally have obtained from their own brain, by transport via their axons. This study in 1988 was the first example of using genetically modified cells to deliver a growth factor to the CNS. Additional experiments published within a few years improved substantially on this basic idea (Ernfors et al. 1989; Kawaja et al. 1992).

There has recently been a considerable effort to employ a variety of growth factors as pharmacological agents in the treatment of human disease, a subject that in general is beyond the scope of this book. There have been no dramatic success stories, although there are some promising possibilities (see Yuen and Mobley 1996). There have been several problems with delivering growth factors systemically, as drugs. These include a high frequency of side effects, perhaps related to effects of growth factors on systems other than the intended target.

There is at least one paradigm in which growth factors have been used in animals, where the possibility of human use seems quite reasonable. This involves an animal model of Huntington's disease. (These studies are discussed in more detail in chapter 17.) Frim, Short, and coworkers (1993) employed a Huntington's disease model in which striatal neurons were destroyed by the excitatory toxin quinolinic acid. For this study, a line of immortal rat fibroblasts (Rat1 cells) that had been modified to produce NGF was used. These cells were transplanted into the corpus callosum of rats, just above the striatum; cells that had not been modified were used as a control. Seven days after the cells had been implanted, quinolinic acid was infused in order to lesion the striatum. When the animals were examined after 18 days, it was found that the NGF-producing cell grafts had decreased the size of the lesions markedly, and resulted in a large increase in the number of acetylcholine-producing neurons that survived the lesioning. In comparison with animals that had not received grafts, or that had received grafts of the original Rat1 cells, the size of the lesions had been reduced by about 80 percent. The NGF-producing grafts did not decrease the size of the lesions on the opposite side of the brain. Thus, it appeared that the distance over which the secretion of NGF was effective was limited to a few millimeters. Several additional studies have shown that delivery of neurotrophic factors, including CNTF and NGF, into the brain can decrease brain injury produced by excitotoxic molecules in Huntington's disease models (see chapter 17).

A major limitation of such studies is the duration of growth factor production. In both of the studies described above (Rosenberg et al. 1988; Frim, Short, et al. 1993), NGF production by the transplanted cells diminished quite rapidly over the course of a few days or weeks. In the Frim, Short, et al. (1993) experiment, the NGF-producing cells were for the most part found to have stopped producing NGF by between 7 and 18 days after transplantation, even though the cells had survived and remained healthy. Only a few NGF-positive cells were found, generally at the edge of the grafts. The procedure was effective because the trauma occurred all at once, a few days after transplantation, when the effect of NGF produced by the cells shortly after implantation was still being exerted. Presumably this procedure would not be effective in a chronic illness, where the loss of cells occurs gradually, over an extended period of time. Thus, it will ultimately be necessary to obtain continuous protein production not for days or weeks, but for years or even decades. The cessation of expression of transferred genes therefore continues to be a major problem for this area of study. Several studies have more recently obtained continuous growth factor production from transplanted cells for relatively long periods, a couple of months. Nonetheless, continuous and reliable production of growth factor presumably would be needed for a period of years, and levels of protein production by cells after transplantation in human subjects could be subject to unacceptable variations.

Also, excessive production of growth factors could be undesirable; for instance, peculiar effects such as growth of neurites from other regions into the proximity of growth factor delivery could occur. It may be necessary, therefore, to have some means of controlling the amounts of growth factor that are produced. Current thinking is that the striatal damage in Huntington's disease is related to the formation of insoluble protein clumps (chapter 17). This may be quite different from the animal models that are currently used, and whether neurotrophic factor delivery can prevent the consequences of this kind of damage is not clear.

Thus, cells can be engineered to produce a number of growth factors, including NGF, BDNF, bFGF, GDNF, and CNTF. As information on possible uses of these growth factors in disease states becomes available, new uses are likely to be found. The major technical problem at present is the gradual loss of expression of transferred genes. This difficulty is likely to be solved by use of alternative promoters and cell types as vehicles for gene delivery. Technical problems for the future may include the development of methods for regulating levels of growth factor production and eliminating the production of unwanted substances by transplantable cells.

Genetic Engineering of Cells to Make Neurotransmitters: L-DOPA in Parkinson's Disease Models

There also has been considerable work in the area of modifying cells to make neurotransmitters; much of this has been devoted to the enzyme tyrosine hydroxylase, which catalyzes the synthesis of L-DOPA from tyrosine. Since L-DOPA is effective as a treatment for Parkinson's disease when administered systemically, it has often been presumed that cells which produce L-DOPA would, in themselves, be useful for transplantation. Other studies have investigated the possibility of making cell lines that produce acetylcholine or GABA (e.g., Eaton, Plunkett, et al. 1999; Ruppert et al. 1993; Giordano et al. 1993). Cells that produce opiate peptides for use in pain syndromes (chapter 14) would seem to be another (perhaps more likely) possibility (Eaton, Lopez et al. 1999). At the present time, however, most of the effort on this topic has involved cells that produce L-DOPA and/or dopamine.

With regard to the issue of genetically altering cells to produce neurotransmitters, it must be noted that whereas growth factors can be effective if secreted diffusely, neurotransmitters are normally produced by neurons and released into synapses, in response to neuronal activity. Parkinson's disease is probably (or perhaps partially) a specialized and unique example. Normal dopaminergic neurons work by releasing dopamine into synapses, and possibly by releasing it more diffusely as well. L-DOPA, the precursor of dopamine, has therapeutic effects when administered systemically, probably related to conversion to dopamine in residual nerve terminals. In the late stages of Parkinson's disease, L-DOPA loses its effectiveness, however, probably because the ability of the injured striatum to store dopamine and buffer L-DOPA conversion and dopamine release is impaired. It is not entirely clear whether, especially in late stages of the disease, the release of L-DOPA alone would be sufficient to produce a therapeutic benefit.

It is possible, for example, that residual dopaminergic neuron terminals are required for the beneficial effect of L-DOPA. In that case, it might be the case not only that delivery of dopamine (rather than L-DOPA) is required, but also that it is necessary to deliver dopamine at synapses. Probably, at least for most transplantation purposes other than Parkinson's disease, it will ultimately be necessary to re-form functional synapses, not simply deliver a neurotransmitter or neurotransmitter substitute. At the present time, we cannot rule out the possibility that even Parkinson's disease requires regulated release of dopamine at synapses for a therapeutic effect, especially in late stages of the disease.

Thus, in producing cell lines that are capable of being employed in Parkinson's disease, a major issue is What is a sufficient level of function? Is neurotransmitter, or L-DOPA, release enough? Will it be possible to convert a more or less "neutral" cell into a substitute neuron? If it is the case that neurotransmission and synaptic connections are needed, rather than just production of neurotransmitter, substitute cells probably will not be adequate. There may be a few cases where production of neurotransmitter alone will be sufficient. Possibly Parkinson's disease is a unique or rare case in that regard, although evidence that it can be treated by transplantation of cells that make L-DOPA is quite weak.

There are several additional issues related to the use of cell lines that produce the enzyme tyrosine hydroxylase, which catalyzes the conversion of tyrosine to L-DOPA. One is that many cell types do not contain a cofactor which is required for catalytic activity of the tyrosine hydroxylase (TH) enzyme. This cofactor can be provided to culture media, but is not so easily delivered to the brain. There have been many studies in which this issue has been ignored. Recent experiments show that delivery of TH alone, without cofactor, is ineffective (Mandel et al. 1998).

The first studies on the use of genetically engineered cells that produce TH for neural transplantation were reported in 1989 and 1990. These experiments employed several cell types, such as rat and mouse fibroblast cell lines, modified to produce the tyrosine hydroxylase enzyme. The results presented in the earliest experiments were, to say the least, somewhat equivocal (e.g., Freed, Geller et al. 1990; Wolff et al. 1989) and will not be detailed here.

Subsequent studies improved on the earliest results. Horellou et al. (1989), Horellou, Brundin, et al. (1990), and Horellou, Marlier, et al. (1990) obtained behavioral effects and release of dopamine from genetically engineered cells transplanted into the rat striatum. Fisher and co-workers reported in 1991 on the effects of primary fibroblasts modified to produce L-DOPA. In their experiment, primary fibroblasts from inbred rats were used, so that a single line of fibroblasts could be developed and used in multiple animals. The use of primary cells, derived directly from an animal (as opposed to immortalized cell lines) avoided the potential problem of continued growth of the transplanted cells and tumor formation. A single clone of cells that expressed high tyrosine hydroxylase activity was isolated. These cells, when transplanted into the brains of animals with substantia nigra lesions, reduced rotational behavior substantially after two weeks. In control animals, which received grafts consisting of fibroblasts transduced with a reporter gene (β-galactosidase), the transplants had no effect. The reductions in rotational behavior were maximal after two weeks and declined gradually thereafter; about half of the effect had been lost by two months after transplantation. The cells continued to express TH two months after transplantation, although weakly. There also was a considerable accumulation of debris and fibrous material associated with the grafts. Although there is certainly room for improvement—the gradual loss of TH activity being a major issue, as well as potential problems with the use of fibroblasts as a cell type, because of the production of extracellular matrix material by these cells—this study suggests that this approach may work in principle.

There are still major problems with the idea of using cells to produce tyrosine hydroxylase. These include (1) doubts concerning the ability of the cells to produce functional quantities of L-DOPA because of the requirement of tyrosine hydroxylase for a cofactor that is not produced by most cells; (2) the long-term stability of tyrosine hydroxylase production; and (3) the reliability and stability of behavioral improvement that is seen. It appears that the retroviral promoters used to regulate gene expression for neural transplantation generally lose their effectiveness following implantation into the brain, so that tyrosine hydroxylase activity becomes "turned off" shortly after transplantation. Expression of tyrosine hyroxylase has been observed for only a few weeks in most studies. Although there have been examples of expression for as long as several months, production of the exogenous gene products usually decreases over, at best, a several-month time frame.

There is a possibility that cell types more closely related to the original primary cells, in this case dopaminergic neurons, not only would function in a more complete manner but also would produce exogenous gene products for longer time intervals. Suppose we had a line of dopaminergic neurons that could be grown in culture; these would be the ideal vehicle for genetic modification for transplantation in Parkinson's disease. Although it has not yet been possible to produce entirely typical immortalized mesencephalic dopaminergic neurons, immortalized mesencephalic cells with partial dopaminergic properties have been produced. There has been one study of this type: Anton et al. (1994) studied transplants of an immortalized mesencephalic cell line. The immortalized mesencephalic cells were initially found to express very weak tyrosine hydroxylase— almost none, actually—but were modified to express high levels of tyrosine activity by further manipulation with retroviral vectors (this study is described in more detail in chapter 22). This latter approach has several distinct advantages. One is that such cells are less likely to deliver undesired bioactive molecules which could produce unexpected effects. Another is that enhancement of the production of normal cellular products may be more successful, in that it would be more consistent with their normal physiology. In other words, a cell that normally produces low levels of TH may be more likely to respond favorably to efforts to enhance TH production—for example, make the cofactor required for TH activity. Finally, the immortalized counterparts of dopaminergic neurons might have all of the relevant cellular machinery needed to deliver dopamine via synaptic release.

A somewhat less ambitious idea than using immortal dopaminergic neurons has been to employ other cells that have the capacity to produce dopamine rather than only L-DOPA (figure 23.1). One approach has been the use of cells that already have the ability to convert L-DOPA to dopamine, such as pituitary At20 cells (Horellou et al. 1989). These cells,

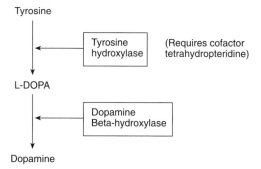

Tyrosine

Dopamine

Figure 23.1
Steps involved in the enzymatic production of dopamine, starting with the amino acid tyrosine. Tyrosine conversion to L-dihydroxyphenylalanine (L-DOPA) is catalyzed by the enzyme tyrosine hydroxylase (TH). This is the rate-limiting step in the process, that is, increases or decreases in TH activity translate into corresponding changes in dopamine synthesis. Tyrosine hydroxylase requires tetrahydropteridine (which is not present in all cells) as a cofactor. Dopamine β-hydroxylase then catalyzes the conversion of L-DOPA to dopamine.

unfortunately, are tumorigenic, but methods to employ this strategy might be developed using nontumorigenic cells. Another method, investigated by Kang and coworkers (Kang 1998; Kang et al. 1993; Wachtel et al. 1997), used two separate populations of cells: some of the cells were altered to produce L-DOPA, while others were engineered to produce the L-DOPA decarboxylating enzyme. Depending on the proportions of the two cell types used, different amounts of L-DOPA and dopamine could be produced in tissue culture. This is another interesting possibility that could be explored in the future.

γ-Aminobutyric Acid (GABA)

There have also been a number of attempts to develop cell lines that produce the neurotransmitter GABA (e.g., Ruppert et al. 1993). GABA, being an inhibitory neurotransmitter, is of particular interest for transplantation in epilepsy. In addition, cells that produce GABA might be used for transplantation in movement disorders, to decrease overactivity of various output nuclei. For example, removal of parts of the globus pallidus has therapeutic effects in Parkinson's disease (Baron et al. 1996;

Vitek et al. 1997). There certainly could be advantages to inhibiting over-activity in this nucleus by transplantation of GABA-producing cells rather than removing the tissue completely. As has been done for Parkinson's disease models, GABA-producing cells might be obtained by introducing the gene for glutamic acid decarboxylase (GAD) into "neutral" cells, such as fibroblasts or muscle cells, and transplanting these cells into the brain. Alternatively, immortalized cells that produce low levels of GABA might be used (Giordano et al. 1993, 1994, 1996). Enhancement of GABA production by such cells might be an especially effective and useful strategy, analogous to enhancement of tyrosine hydroxylase activity in cells from the mesencephalon as done by Anton et al. (1994) and described earlier. Recently, transplants of cells engineered to express the GAD enzyme, and produce GABA, have been shown to be effective as transplants in animal models of neuropathic pain (Eaton, Plunkett et al. 1999). Although thus far it has been explored only minimally, the development of GABA-producing cells for use in neural transplantation is a very interesting possibility.

Conclusion

The notion of genetically engineering cells to produce particular proteins and then transplanting these cells into the brain is, in essence, a sophisticated type of pharmacological approach. Polypeptides of various kinds—ranging from short five-amino acid neuromodulators to larger molecules—for example, growth factors that are comprised of hundreds of amino acids—are very important pharmacological mediators. A great deal of effort in pharmacology is directed at the development of small nonpeptide substances that can be administered systemically as drugs, and mimic or replace peptide molecules. There also have been a number of attempts to treat diseases by administering growth factors either systemically or directly into the brain.

Delivery of growth factors via transplantation of genetically engineered cells has considerable potential for use in disease treatment and prevention. Compared with systemic delivery, or even with diffuse and widespread delivery into the brain, delivery via transplanted cells has both advantages and disadvantages. Some of the disadvantages are that transplanted cells require surgery, that doses are not easily regulated or adjusted, and that the procedure would be either irreversible or reversible only with a second surgery. Nonetheless, the advantages are substantial. Genetically engineered cells can deliver a growth factor to a very localized region of the brain, so that other regions would be affected minimally or not at all. This is likely to greatly decrease the incidence of side effects. Moreover, delivery can ideally be continuous, at a constant level, and in amounts that are physiologically appropriate, and (at least potentially) can be continued for long periods without interruption or decrement. For these reasons, the use of cells to deliver peptides and especially growth factors for the treatment or prevention of brain disorders has a very high therapeutic potential.

Further Reading

Fisher, L. J., Chalmers, G. R., and Gage, F. H. (1994). Use of genetically modified cells to deliver neurotrophic factors and neurotransmitters to the brain. In *Providing Pharmacological Access to the Brain: Alternate Approaches*, T. R. Flanagan, D. F. Emerich, and S. R. Winn (eds.), pp. 329–333. Academic Press, San Diego. Methods in Neurosciences, vol. 21.

Gage, F. H., Kang, U. J., and Fisher, L. J. (1991). Intracerebral grafting in the dopaminergic system: Issues and controversy. *Curr. Opin. Neurobiol.* 1: 414–419.

Glass, D. J., and Yancopoulos, G. D. (1993). The neurotrophins and their receptors. *Trends Cell Biol.* 3: 149–155.

Levi-Montalcini, R. (1987). The nerve growth factor 35 years later. *Science* 237: 1154–1162.

Levi-Montalcini, R., Skaper, S. D., Dal Toso, R., Petrelli, L., and Leon, A. (1996). Nerve growth factor: From neurotrophin to neurokine. *Trends Neurosci.* 19: 514–520.

Loughlin, S. E., and Fallon, J. H. (eds.). (1993). *Neurotrophic Factors.* Academic Press, San Diego.

24
Direct Gene Transfer

The preceding chapters discussed the possibility of altering cells in culture, and then using these cells for transplantation into the brain. This is sometimes termed the ex vivo approach to somatic gene therapy. The contrasting approach, in vivo somatic gene therapy, involves genetic manipulation of cells in their normal environment. Although this does not involve transplantation, it is very much related to the technology of neural transplantation, and thus a brief discussion of this topic will be included.

The principle of this type of experiment is to introduce genetic material into existing cells within the brain. There are many techniques for inserting genes into cells, based on physicochemical methods of interfering with the ability of cell membranes to exclude outside DNA, that are used in vitro. These standard methods cannot, in most circumstances and at the current level of technical development, be employed in normal cells in vivo, because (1) they are generally too harsh and damage a significant number of cells, (2) they often require a degree of manipulation and control that can be used only in tissue culture, and (3) such methods usually are effective in transferring DNA into only a fraction of the target cell population. Nonetheless, there are some exceptions. Lipofection, transfer of DNA using detergent-like reagents to penetrate cell membranes, has been used in animals in vivo for the delivery of genes into the lung and can sometimes be used in the brain. As these methods are improved, delivery of genes into endogenous brain cells with lipid-based reagents may become feasible. Nonetheless, the technology of transferring genetic material into endogenous cells has become of great current interest mainly because of relatively new and rapidly emerging technologies for employing disabled viruses for DNA delivery.

Most effort so far has involved viruses of the Herpes simplex, adenovirus, or adeno-associated virus type (e.g., Bowers et al. 1997; Davidson et al. 1993; Dobson et al. 1990; Federoff et al. 1992, 1997; A. Geller et al. 1990; Horellou et al. 1997; Johnson et al. 1992; Le Gal La Salle et al. 1993; Mandel et al. 1997, 1998; Xiao et al. 1997). These viruses normally are effective in inserting their genetic material into nondividing cells. Usually genes delivered by these viruses do not become incorporated into the host cell's genome, but nonetheless can direct the production of proteins. Such episomal genes are not passed on to descendant cells effectively, but neither do they require that the cells which are infected be in a dividing state. Thus, there is the potential of using these viruses to deliver genes into existing brain cells.

The details of these techniques are somewhat complex, and at this time methods for their use are still evolving. The mechanisms by which viruses are employed to deliver genes into cells are beyond the scope of this book, but one interesting example, the adeno-associated virus, will be described here.

In general, viruses are subverted for use in gene delivery (or as vectors) by removing their ability to produce crucial structural proteins. These structural proteins, required for replication and/or encapsulation, are produced separately, usually by genes contained in a host cell. If the virus no longer can produce essential structural proteins, then it cannot be infectious, and thereby can be rendered safe for use in gene delivery.

The adeno-associated virus (AAV) has several quite interesting properties. First, it is not infectious by itself, requiring adenovirus (or certain other similar viruses, i.e., helper virus) for infection. In the presence of helper virus, AAV undergoes a "lytic" infection cycle, in which the virus replicates and destroys the host cell. In the absence of helper virus, however, AAV enters an alternative pathway termed latent infection. Under these conditions, AAV can become integrated into a host cell's genome and remain there indefinitely, over the course of many cell divisions, without any discernible adverse effects on host cell function. This tendency for latent infection is the property that makes AAV especially attractive

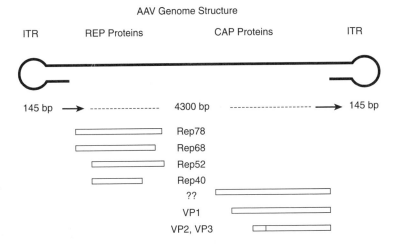

Figure 24.1
This and the following two figures explain how the adeno-associated virus (AAV) is employed to transfer genes into cells. The AAV genome consists of a single, linear DNA molecule. At the ends are the ITRs, inverted terminal repeats, which are important in the insertion of the AAV genome into the genome of target cells. The remainder of the DNA codes for several proteins that are important in viral replication (REP proteins) and capsule formation (CAP proteins), indicated by the rectangular bars. Use of AAV as a gene transfer vector is based on removal of the REP and CAP coding sequences, and replacement of them with the gene or genes that are to be transferred. A cell is used to produce the AAV vector; this cell produces the REP and CAP proteins in addition to the recombinant AAV genome. (Adapted from Bartlett and Samulski 1995.)

for use in gene therapy (see Mandel et al. 1997, 1998; McCown et al. 1996; Xiao et al. 1997).

The structure of AAV is exceedingly simple (figure 24.1): its genome is simply a linear stretch of single-stranded DNA, about 4,700 base pairs total. At each end is a 145 base-pair segment called the inverted terminal repeat (ITR). In between the ITRs are the sequences that code for the proteins used by the virus for replication and encapsulation.

If one creates an artificial structure by replacing all of the AAV except the ITRs with DNA that contains sequences coding for other proteins (such as a reporter molecule—in other words, a marker—β-galactosidase,

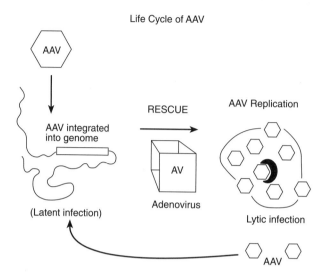

Figure 24.2
The normal AAV life cycle. After infection, AAV becomes integrated into the genome of the host cell. In human cells, integration occurs at a specific location in the genome. At this stage, the virus is "latent," or inactive, producing no viral proteins. When cells bearing integrated AAV are exposed to adenovirus, the AAV can be "rescued" from its latent state, replicate, and destroy the host cell. That is, rescued AAV causes a lytic infection. Recombinant AAV, modified for use as a gene delivery vector, cannot cause lytic infection because the genes required for replication of the virus, as well as the capsule proteins, have been removed. (For further information, see Bartlett and Samulski 1995.)

or whatever we are interested in), and by producing the replication and encapsulation proteins separately, the DNA flanked by the ITRs will be packaged to produce a virus. The replication and encapsulation functions will have been performed in a separate host cell, in the presence of helper virus. The AAV particles are then separated from the helper virus, resulting in AAV that does not have the capacity to produce any of its own proteins. In this form, the ITRs are employed as gene delivery vehicles (figures 24.2 and 24.3). In this way, virtually any gene can be delivered for use in gene therapy using the AAV vector.

These particles have the ability to enter host cells of a wide variety of types. Once they are inside, the capsule proteins are degraded, leaving only the DNA. Since the only part of the original AAV that remains at this point is the two ITRs, this would seem to be a perfect gene delivery vehicle. However, there remains the problem of the capsule proteins; although they are not capable of transferring any genetic information, either the intact capsule proteins or degraded fragments of them do have the potential capacity for inducing immune responses. Viral proteins also may be directly toxic to host cells.

When AAV is employed as a gene delivery vector, the product is a linear DNA segment in a protein capsule that allows the DNA to enter cells. Once inside a target cell, the altered AAV genomes can be useful in gene therapy in two ways. The ITRs and certain viral proteins appear to recognize specific sequences in the human genome on chromosome 19, where they mediate integration into the genome. However, since viral proteins are needed for site-specific integration to take place, the DNA alone, and thus the viral vector, may mediate the integration process (although not the integration to a specific site). Integrated structures can remain stably integrated into the genome over many cell generations in dividing cells. In most cases, it appears that integration requires cell division, although it is thought that integration may infrequently occur without it. The second mechanism is that, in nondividing cells, AAV may remain intact episomally, directing protein expression in the absence of integration. Protein expression from nonintegrated AAV may continue for extended periods in the brain.

Despite potential difficulties, the AAV system is one of the most promising for gene delivery directly into endogenous brain cells; remaining problems include possible immune responses to capsule proteins, and means of circumventing such reactions may eventually be found. Although it may be possible to deliver DNA into cells in the brain using nonviral vectors (for example, lipofection techniques), the most promising and probably the most efficient systems for delivering genes directly into cells within the brain are likely to be based on viral vectors. Each vector system has unique properties, with attendant advantages and disadvantages. Herpes simplex virus has received a great deal of attention because it has a natural affinity for the nervous system and can reside within neurons in a latent state, without apparent adverse effect, for extended periods of time. Herpes simplex can be cytotoxic, however, and much of the effort in developing this virus involves eliminating its ability

Old Method for Producing rAAV

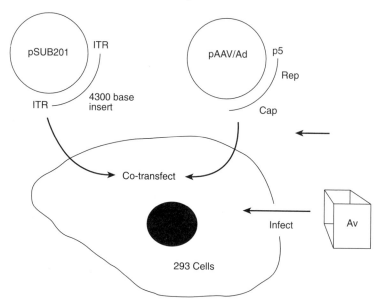

Lyse cells, liberating rAAV particles, AV, and debris

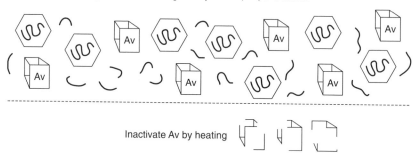

Inactivate Av by heating

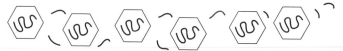

Purify rAAV particles by CsCl centrifugation

to produce toxicity. Strategies for employing Herpes simplex as a gene delivery vector are currently being developed, and will not be described in detail here.

Applications

The notion of using viral vector systems to deliver genes into endogenous brain neurons is in its infancy. Many experiments along these lines are on the order of demonstration, using well-described test systems to demonstrate the practicality of this approach. Several experiments have, for example, used viral vectors to show that when tyrosine hydroxylase is produced by endogenous neurons and/or glia, positive effects can be obtained in established animal models of Parkinson's disease. It is unclear what the net result of a situation in which glial cells, rather than neurons, were producing the neurotransmitter would be. One recent study by Mandel and coworkers (1998) employed an adeno-associated viral vector to deliver the genes for both TH and the cofactor-synthesizing enzyme into the striatum of rats. The combination of both genes, but not TH alone, was found to result in L-DOPA production and decreases in apomorphine-induced rotation. The adeno-associated viral vector was found to have transduced TH mainly into neurons. TH expression was also maintained for at least six months. This study suggests that it may eventu-

---

Figure 24.3

AAV vector production. The genes coding for viral REP and CAP proteins are contained in one plasmid (pAAV/Ad), and the viral ITR sequences and the gene of interest are contained in a second plasmid (pSUB201). Both plasmids are transfected into a host cell, in culture (293 cells). Subsequently, the host cells are infected with adenovirus, thereby rescuing the latent AAV. The recombinant AAV then replicates, using the viral genes from the pAAV/Ad plasmid. This results in the production of infectious recombinant AAV, assembled with CAP proteins coded for by the pAAV/Ad plasmid. The recombinant AAV does not, however, contain any of the genes necessary for viral reproduction or capsule formation, and thus can be separated from adenovirus, purified, and used for gene delivery. For further information, see Bartlett and Samulski 1995, and Ferrari et al. 1997.

Newer methods of AAV vector production, described by Xiao and coworkers (1998; not illustrated) employ a third plasmid (pXX6) in place of the adenovirus; this third plasmid performs the functions of adenovirus required for viral replication, and eliminates the problem of possible contamination of recombinant AAV with infectious adenovirus.

ally be possible to develop techniques for treating Parkinson's disease or other neurotransmitter-related abnormalities by direct gene transfer into the brain.

It is probable that the idea of delivering genes into endogenous neurons would allow for many possibilities that have not been thought of as yet, but are very novel and interesting. The notion that delivery of genes into endogenous neurons could protect neurons from degeneration is especially attractive. It also may be possible to induce rather minor alterations in the functioning of endogenous neurons or glia to improve brain function in certain diseases. In fact, the possibilities for the use of this approach are almost unlimited.

One recent study on the delivery of a trophic factor (glial-derived neurotrophic factor, or GDNF) to protect neurons from injury, by Choi-Lundberg and coworkers (1997), will be described here as an example. In this case, an adenovirus vector was used for gene delivery (adenovirus and adeno-associated virus are two different viruses). There has also been a successful study of this type using adeno-associated virus (Mandel et al. 1997).

The adenovirus vector was constructed to code for human GDNF, and as controls a mutant (inactive) form of GDNF, with a 12 amino acid deletion and a marker gene (β-galactosidase) were used (Choi-Lundberg et al. 1997). It was shown that infection of cultured cells (PC12 cells) with human GDNF led to the production of biologically active GDNF in significant quantities. To test for effects of this vector on degeneration of dopaminergic neurons in animals, the adenovirus-GDNF vector (or one of the controls) was injected just dorsal to the dopaminergic neurons in the substantia nigra. (Axons from these dopaminergic neurons project to the neostriatum.) To identify a subgroup of these neurons, a fluorescent tracer, fluorogold, which is transported back down the axons, was injected into the striatum. Seven days after injection of the vector and the fluorogold, the neurotoxin 6-hydroxydopamine was injected in the same place as the fluorogold. Since both were injected in the same location, the 6-hydroxydopamine kills more or less the same neurons that were labeled with fluorogold. The question, then, was whether the adenoviral vector was able to protect the fluorogold-labeled dopaminergic neurons from death induced by the 6-hydroxydopamine.

In fact, the degree of protection was remarkable, with more than half of the dopamine neurons being protected from injury. The lesions decreased the number of fluorogold-labeled neurons by 60 percent or more, indicating a 60 percent loss of neurons. The neuronal loss was between 60 and 75 percent in various control groups that were treated with inactive viral vectors. In the animals that received the virus encoding active GDNF, however, the loss of dopaminergic neurons was only 22 percent—in other words, about two thirds of the neurons were protected. The results are indeed remarkable, especially since 6-hydroxydopamine is an artificial toxin, and is not likely to be a normal cause of dopaminergic neuron death in Parkinson's disease. This is, therefore, a very promising finding regarding the use of growth factors to protect neurons against toxic injury.

In this study, as in the experiments on protection of neurons from injury in Huntington's disease models, it should be remembered that the toxic insult occurs over a very brief time period. In contrast, in the disease itself (both Parkinson's disease and Huntington's disease), the toxic process is very protracted. Whatever is killing the neurons is doing so slowly, over a very long time, probably many years. Presumably, this would mean that any treatment, such as CNTF or GDNF delivery, would have to be continued over many years as well. Achieving constant, long-term production of proteins in the brain from viral vectors, such as adenovirus, continues to be an obstacle. Nonetheless, it is a technical obstacle only, and presumably it can be overcome sooner or later. It is more important to emphasize that we have a principle to work from: we think that we may already know a means of preventing or arresting the progress of some degenerative brain disorders once a few technical problems are overcome.

Further Reading

Federoff, H. J., Brooks, A., Muhkerjee, B., and Corden, T. (1997). Somatic gene transfer approaches to manipulate neural networks. *J. Neurosci. Meth.* 71: 133–142.

Neve, R. L. (1993). Adenovirus vectors enter the brain. *Trends Neurosci.* 16: 251–253.

VII
Conclusions

25
Conclusions

In considering what might be possible in the future, and where we might be 20, 40, or 100 years from now in the realm of brain repair, we might first decide how far we *want* to be able to go, and then, how we might be able to get there.

Replacing the Brain—All at Once or a Little at a Time

If, for the moment, we forget about what is possible and what is not, first of all there are limits imposed by the nature of the brain. I think that most of us would agree that once replacement reaches a certain point, the individual is lost and the exercise of "brain repair" becomes meaningless. As in previous hypothetical cases, we can consider the extremes. Suppose it became possible, somehow, to implant an *entire* fetal brain or, since we are being fanciful, the entire brain and spinal cord, into a person with an advanced neurodegenerative disorder. Let's say that this new brain could even be induced to form appropriate connections with the optic nerve, cranial nerves, and spinal nerves, and function in an entirely normal manner.

I think it's fairly obvious that this procedure would be useless. Since the new brain would not possess *any* of the characteristics of the original person, it would (at best) produce a creature more or less akin to a large and awkward newborn human infant. It would be worse than cloning the original person because, in contrast to a clone, the brain and body would not mature together. This situation would almost certainly result in major—and perhaps monstrous—abnormalities. Imagine a brain maturing in the manner of an infant, or in fact a fetus, inside the body of a fully grown adult. It's pretty obvious that this would cause difficulties, so instead of dwelling on this, let's devote our thinking to something a little less extreme.

How about this possibility? We gain the ability to replace any part of the brain, but instead of replacing the entire structure at once, we do it in stages. We replace a few regions, wait a while, then replace a few more, until the entire brain and spinal cord have been restructured. What would happen? Perhaps the individual's characteristics would be retained by the parts of the brain not replaced, and the new parts could be "trained," or would somehow assume the properties of the host individual. It might be akin to a prolonged period of partial infancy. Perhaps this would not be possible in its extreme form (replacing the entire brain). There are likely to be structures that cannot be replaced, or can be replaced only with a substantial loss of fidelity.

We might also imagine that the more replacements we perform, the more the overall integrity of the brain and its coordination with the body become compromised. This might be something like the movie *Multiplicity,* in which the leading actor (Michael Keaton) has himself cloned. The first copy is quite helpful, working efficiently and making life easier (in some respects) for the original. When the cloned copy is used as a template to make another clone, however, peculiarities are seen: the clone-of-a-clone looks like the original, but behaves very strangely.

As a general issue, the use of multiple transplants is a possibility that we should consider. Of course, we won't be cloning adult humans to help with the housework . . . at least, not right away. Performing multiple surgical procedures to implant cells and otherwise alter neural circuits is, however, a distinct possibility. At some point, will the individual become unrecognizable? Can a substantial part of the brain be replaced? What would happen if it could?

I think that, in fact, the *Multiplicity* cloning example is rather the way that this would work. After a certain amount of mucking around with the brain, things would start to work not quite as well as before. I don't think it will ever be possible to replace—say—half or even a tenth of the brain without its being quite noticeable in a major way, even to a casual observer. Since the brain functions as an integrated whole in many respects, no replacement strategy will ever result in the replacement parts working together with the whole in quite the same way as in the original. Thus, with multiple transplantations or other kinds of surgical intervention in the brain, we would probably see a gradual erosion of the integrity of the brain and the individual as a large amount of intervention is cumulatively performed. So, what is okay and what is not?

Suppose we have a situation in which an individual has Parkinson's disease, receives a transplant for that, subsequently develops cancer, and receives a second transplant into the spinal cord to relieve pain. I think that most people would find this acceptable; two transplants for two serious but unrelated problems. In each case, the transplant in clearly intended to influence a defined, local circuit rather than to produce fundamental modifications in brain circuitry. This is an example of two transplantation procedures being used, neither of which is likely to disturb the overall integrity of the brain. The number of cells transplanted would probably amount to perhaps one-millionth of the total in the brain.

Let's look at another example. Suppose we develop a cell type that is capable of repairing the brain following stroke. This is not entirely farfetched. Let's say that these are undifferentiated cells with the capability of differentiating into both neurons and glia after being transplanted, and also produce trophic factors that promote recovery in nearby cortical tissue. The neurons that arise from these cells can replace lost cortical neurons and develop connections with host neurons to a considerable degree. Cells that perform some of these functions have already been developed, as discussed in chapters 21 and 22. In addition, Sertoli cells, obtained from the testes, have been found to promote recovery in the rat model of Parkinson's disease, apparently by secreting trophic factors that influence nearby cells (Sanberg et al. 1997; figure 25.1). These cells also can suppress rejection of nearby grafts (Sanberg et al. 1996). A human cell line derived from a teratocarcinoma, which can be stimulated to differentiate into neurons, has also been employed for transplantation. Based on rodent experiments in which these cells produced behavioral recovery following injury (Borlongan et al. 1998), these cells have recently been transplanted into the brains of human patients in an attempt to treat basal ganglia stroke (Kondziolka et al. 1999; cf. Fackelmann 1998). The first 12 patients to receive the procedure were transplanted with either 2 or 6 million cells. There were no serious adverse effects,

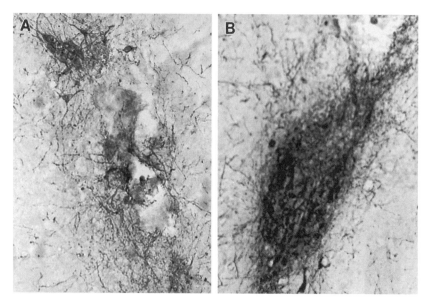

Figure 25.1
Promotion of the survival of transplanted rat dopamine neurons by co-transplanted rat sertoli cells. (A) Rat ventral mesencephalon clone, 7 days after transplantation to the rat striatum. (B) Transplants of rat ventral mesencephalon
combined with rat Sertoli cells. As can be seen by comparison of the two photographs, the co-transplanted Sertoli cells greatly increased the survival of dopamine
neurons. (Photograph courtesy of A. Willing and P. Sanderg, Dept. of Neurosurgery, University of South Florida, Tampa. Willing et al. 1999, with permission.)

and some signs of possible improvement (Kondziolka et al. 1999). It is
believed that these cells are likely to function mainly by producing trophic
effects on nearby cells, although the formation of connections with host
neurons is not inconceivable. Even if this procedure does not work especially well, improvements in the methods for obtaining cells to influence
nearby neuronal circuits in a beneficial manner following injury can be
expected over the next several years (chapter 22). This study may signal
the beginning of a new type of clinical application of neural transplantation, in which immature cells are permitted to develop and become integrated (in some manner) with the host brain structure.

Whatever type of cell is used, the connections with host neurons will
not be complete, and they will not be *exactly* like the connections of

the original neurons. Long-distance connections would, probably, not re-form as readily as local circuits. However, most stroke victims recover considerably without transplants or any sort of intervention. Let's imag-ine that these transplanted cells are capable of both accelerating the rate of recovery and increasing the extent of recovery following stroke, and that one type of cell can be used for transplantation into all parts of the cerebral cortex. None of those assumptions are unreasonable.

In an individual who has had one stroke, these cell transplants would be helpful. Two or three strokes would probably not change the favorable nature of the response to the transplants. But what would happen to someone who had 10, 100, or even 1,000 strokes, and received cell trans-plants for all of them? Well, from a practical standpoint, if someone had numerous strokes (probably more than 20 or 30) they would be occurring so frequently that surgery and recovery could not keep up with the injury, and the general trauma of repeated surgery and anesthesia would begin to counteract the benefits of the transplants. But let's forget about that for now, and instead think about this on a more theoretical level. Let's consider what might happen to cortical *function* in someone who received 100 or 1,000 cell transplants for stroke.

This is a much tougher question. I really don't know the answer with any degree of certainty. Even under the best of circumstances, it would at least require some time for the transplanted cells to become integrated with the host brain. The connections that the transplanted cells form would not be precisely like the original. For the new circuits to become fully integrated would certainly require months, if not years. Even after maximal recovery, there would probably be some degree of functional degradation. This degradation of brain function would probably not be noticeable after two or three procedures, but after (for example) 100 cell implantations, things probably would start to get murky.

Remember that we are talking about an injured brain. Even in an indi-vidual with an intact brain, implanting cells into 100 locations in the cerebral cortex would certainly be disruptive. And here we are con-sidering someone with brain injury and major functional impairment. Would the transplants cause improvement? Maybe. Would the im-provement come at the expense of the person's individual identity? Proba-bly—but since the person is already severely impaired and maybe even noncommunicative, we might not know the difference. We might not, for example, recognize a degradation of the personality. Once a patient has had 100 strokes, we might see a greater recovery than would otherwise occur, but this recovery would be at such a rudimentary level that we might not recognize whether the personality was altered or not. Let's say the patient becomes able to eat with assistance, gets out of bed, and recovers a vocabulary of 100 words or so. Would we know whether or not the personality had been altered?

There are lots of issues here, but the interesting one is What degree of intervention alters brain function so drastically that it is no longer worthwhile? I don't know exactly, but we can certainly assume that it would be somewhere between performing one or two grafts and attempting to restructure the entire brain. I can't define this issue in a way that would point to a discontinuity or a factor that could form the basis for a rule or guideline. I do, however, suspect that a large number of transplants forming connections with a host brain would begin to disturb the integrity of the brain even more than the injury itself.

Again, we are speaking hypothetically: in someone who had experienced 100 strokes, the situation would probably be hopeless. So let's consider something more limited. Let us imagine that we are able to measure the functional integrity of the brain as a parameter *independent* of the individual's functional impairment. Thus, our imaginary subject might be unable to speak, move, or respond in any manner. But perhaps the subject retains certain sensory inputs and is able to exercise cerebral capacity by reminiscing about past experiences, fantasizing, and imagining. We somehow can measure this ongoing integrated cerebral activity: let's say, with functional MRI (magnetic resonance imaging). We can also give it a number: normal cerebral function is 100 units or 100 percent. We find that our apparently unconscious, unresponsive person who has had 100 strokes retains 50 units of cerebral function!

Creating this scenario allows us to think about this in a more concrete manner. With each stroke, some cerebral function units are lost. Let's say that we lose 10 units with the first stroke, and a little bit more with each subsequent stroke. I would guess that after one stroke, the transplant could improve matters, and more cerebral function units would be recovered than without the transplant. The brain is resilient and redundant, and compensation for minor disturbances can occur. In addition to a collection of local circuits performing specialized functions, the brain functions as an integrated whole. When there is more and more damage, this integrated functioning will begin to be degraded. Perhaps after a certain number of strokes—5, 10, or 20? Of course, it would also depend on the severity of the strokes—the capacity of transplants to improve local functioning would begin to be counteracted by disturbances in the *overall* functioning of the brain. Thus, perhaps after one or two strokes, or maybe four or five, transplants might improve matters, but after a large number of strokes, the transplantation procedure would make matters worse.

Therefore, my guess is that we would have the following result. Our subject begins with 100 units of cerebral function. One stroke causes a loss of 10 units; 90 units remain. Spontaneously, the subject recovers to 95 units, and with a transplant, to 99 units or maybe even to 100 units. After experiencing 100 strokes, however, the subject deteriorates to 50 cerebral function units. We now make transplants into all 100 stroke sites (none of this, obviously, is practical). The transplants would promote local recovery at each individual stroke site, and in the process form and/or modify connections with neighboring neurons. With this many transplants, however, perhaps the positive effect on local recovery would begin to be compromised by disturbance of the overall integrity of brain function. Thus, I would guess (and really, this is no more than an educated guess) that the subject with 100 strokes would lose 50 units of cerebral function, but with 100 strokes plus 100 transplants, this subject might lose even more.

Brain Development and Integrity, and a Model

In order to appreciate my reasoning regarding this multiple transplants/stroke issue, I would like to talk a little about the development, integrity, and overall complexity of the brain. First of all, when a transplant is made into the mature, or even partially mature, brain, we have a situation which is quite different from that which is in effect while the brain is developing. Even though transplants often develop connections with the host brain, they do so under a very different set of conditions than those in the developing brain. In the developing brain, many factors promote the development of pathways, extension of neurites, and migration of neurons. It is not simply a matter of re-creating each of these to obtain new connections in the adult. The brain develops as a whole, as a single, integrated unit, so that a complex and highly orchestrated sequence of events takes place around the development of neuronal interconnectivity.

We might also think a little about the complexity of neuronal interconnectivity and overall organization of the CNS. For this exercise, we will not concern ourselves with the processing of information within cells, and we will mostly ignore the vast population of glial cells (these greatly outnumber neurons, and also contribute to information processing). We will consider only the physical connections between neurons.

Each neuron has both inputs, received mainly via dendrites and synapses on the cell body, and outputs, delivered via axons. Dendrites can extend for some distance, and axons can extend many centimeters. Both dendrites and axons can branch extensively. A single neuron may have many thousands of inputs and outputs; possibly 10,000 is an average number, but some neurons are thought to have nearly 1,000,000 connections with other neurons. It is thought that there are on the order of 10^{12} neurons in the brain. If each neuron makes connections with 10^4 other neurons, the complexity of the overall structure is vast (to say the least). There is probably a chain of connectivity that results in all neurons being connected to all other neurons. Thus, neural circuitry cannot be thought of as being comprised of an array of small circuits, each having a few thousand or a few million connections. Instead, the nervous system is one vast circuit with a "billion billion" connections that matures as a whole, and continues to evolve throughout life.

Forget about any analogy with a computer: The *internal* processing of information within a single cell is as complex as, or more complex than, the workings of any computer. The brain is more akin to a few billion (actually, a thousand billion) computers connected by a few thousand cables for each computer, plus billions of technicians (maintenance technicians) climbing throughout and constantly tinkering with the cables, and lots of other activity as well. The computers are not located in a nice, organized office building: they are piled up in a gigantic and apparently haphazard heap at least the size of a large office building. They are mixed up with cables, technicians, and various other gadgets (akin to glial cells) that influence the computers, supply power, work on internal mechanisms, and insulate the cables.

If one computer with its associated equipment occupies one cubic meter (not an unreasonable assumption, since neurons occupy only a small fraction of the volume of the brain), a structure with 10^{12} computers would be about the size of Mount Everest!

In our model, however, we must imagine a degree of plasticity and flexibility that is not present in any computer. First, the internal workings of the computer can modify themselves in response to inputs and interactions with the local environment. The connections are not wires making hard connections with other computers; they are relatively ethereal, making connections of various flavors and strengths. The connections are also plastic; although they do not grow over long distances, they are subject to local modifications. This machine has many wonderful properties, through being incredibly plastic and able to modify itself in response to the environment, and also has a unique "personality" and specialized skills and attributes.

The wonderful properties of this machine, however, come at a great cost: repairs are difficult. Minor, routine repairs take place automatically, within the machine, as a result of internal plasticity mechanisms. Once in awhile, however, a disease or catastrophic event occurs within the machine that overwhelms the internal plasticity mechanisms: some sort of internal corrosion, or perhaps a meteor strike. Then we have a problem. The cables are composed of an unusual material that is recycled when damaged. They require inputs and outputs to maintain their integrity. When a cable is cut, it simply evaporates, leaving no trace of its former presence. Even the gadgets that had been there to insulate the cables (the oligodendrocytes) move away, leaving no trace of their former locations. The structure is very delicate as well. Sometimes the cables evaporate if we just touch them.

When the cables were routed in the first place, specialized technicians (let's call these construction technicians) were around to help get the cables to the right places. But once the cables are finished, the construction technicians disappear, and only the maintenance technicians remain. So how do we repair this? If one, or one million, of the computers crash while the machine is being built (and the construction technicians are still around), the machine will fix itself, or perhaps we can throw more computers on top of the heap and everything will take care of itself. The cables will start to grow out from the computers, and the construction technicians will be there to make sure the cables go to the right places.

But how can we repair this structure in a mature, finished computer heap when a malfunction overwhelms the internal mechanisms for restructuring and repair? Well, there is no circuit diagram. There can't be one: the structure is too vast, every structure is unique, and we can't get inside to trace the wires, because every space is filled so there's no room to move around. There are general outlines, but the details cannot be mapped.

We might try throwing some new computers on top of the heap and waiting for cables to grow out from these computers. But since there are no construction technicians around to route the cables (there are only the maintenance technicians), they don't grow far and don't connect very well. We can throw in some construction technicians, but they wind up being lost, because the landmarks they need for wiring are gone. We can also try to stuff some computers inside the mass (this is what we are doing with transplants), to a place where we know some of the cables are supposed to connect. This might work somewhat, but since only the local cable connections re-form, we get only a partial restoration.

Thus, one problem will be the huge number of longer cable connections. Although we do not have a detailed circuit diagram, we do have a general idea of where the cables need to go. But there are no construction technicians to guide the cables, so they are lost. And if construction technicians are sent in to help, they get lost, because the signposts and pathways are gone. We can physically go inside and lay a pathway of guiding material, which does help somewhat, but everything we do causes a certain amount of damage in itself, so that the repair efforts are clumsy in comparison with the elegance of the initial construction. We must, in essence, repair the damage with tools such as huge cranes and drills. In order to replace a computer bank located far inside the structure (let's say a mile down), we must reach the location by drilling through the overlying structures!

If we take a look at the problem of repairing the brain in this way, it is obvious that there are going to be some limits on what we can do. We can't, and may never be able to, rewire the brain as though it were a large, complex version of a television or a computer. We can coax it into cooperating with minor repair efforts, but we may never be able to patch things up after major damage. To continue the analogy, if an explosion occurs deep inside the structure, destroying miles of cables and thousands of computers, efforts to repair the damage by pouring in new computers (in some manner) may help a little, or perhaps even quite a bit, but it is unlikely that we can ever fix things completely. Over the next 20 years, we will probably see many refinements (some of which will certainly be remarkable) in our ability to repair brain injury. But I think we will always find that our efforts to repair the damaged adult brain will have a minuscule impact in comparison with the structural adjustments that take place during brain development. Unrealistic expectations in this respect are probably counterproductive, in that aiming for the impossible may tend to discourage research from focusing on achievable goals, or to place less value on goals that are reached.

Building New Brains or Artificial Brains

What about the opposite possibility—the popular science fiction idea of removing, simulating, or copying the brain and inserting it into a new body, or into an artificial body. In my opinion, this is fundamentally impossible to accomplish in any useful manner. In contrast to the idea of replacing or restructuring the damaged brain, here we are considering the possibility of housing the brain (or in some sense the "essence" of the brain) in a new vehicle. This could be conceived of as either physically removing the brain and putting it into a new body (something that has, in fact, been considered more or less seriously), or as somehow copying the unique "consciousness" of a particular individual, whatever that means, and inserting that consciousness into a new body or some other appropriate housing.

Regarding the scenario of removing the brain and transplanting it into a new body (this appears occasionally in science fiction), I don't believe that it is possible to perform this manipulation in any productive or meaningful manner. Inducing a transplanted brain to reconnect with the rest of the body is not sensible, not useful, and probably not possible. The process of reprogramming the brain so that it can reconnect with the body would undoubtedly produce severe changes, probably altering functions beyond those primarily involved in sensory and motor control. Furthermore, I am sure that to most people, transplanting entire brains would be a reprehensible idea. Transplanting livers, hearts, skin, and corneas makes sense, but the whole body (or the whole brain; transplanting the brain is the same thing as transplanting the body), no.

There is an interesting notion that appeared in a series of popular science fiction books by Poul Anderson (1993, 1994). I found the premise of these books to be fascinating. The culture envisioned in this series develops a technology that makes it possible to read out the personality of important individuals (the primary tool being a sort of sophisticated, but vaguely described, electroencephalographic recording) and download these personalities into artificial brains. The artificial brains can be stored in containers about the size of a shoebox, or they can be placed in robotlike bodies of various kinds (e.g., a bipedal model or a kind with wheels). "Downloads"—only a few exist—are generally not completely happy about their condition. Not many people wish to become downloads, and most of those who do, eventually terminate themselves or become insane.

In these books, it becomes possible to download personalities from humans to machines long before it becomes possible to create artificial intelligence capable of substituting for the human brain (hundreds of years before!). When artificial intelligence is finally created, however, it immediately begins to work at improving itself, becomes more and more intelligent, has greater wisdom than the human mind, links up to form a unified intelligence complex, and quite rapidly takes over the planet. Humans become subservient to this grand artificial intelligence—and it is hard to object, since the artificial intelligence runs the planet more efficiently and sensibly than humans had been able to. No wars, no conflict, no waste, the ecology improves, and so on. The artificial intelligences have merged into a single, intercommunicating entity . . . of course!

What of the above is possible, and what is not? I think that some form of human brainlike artificial intelligence is possible (there already are some computer simulations of human thinking and various kinds of artificial intelligence). Maybe not likely, and not coming soon, but possible. I believe it may be possible to create artificial devices that are essentially indistinguishable from human intelligence. They might not have all of the properties of the human brain, they might be very large and unwieldy, and they probably could not exist without human assistance, but probably an artificial intelligence can be made with properties that, to an observer, are indistinguishable from human consciousness, free will, and decision making. Such devices would not, however, be simple extensions of present-day computers. A more plastic and complex machine would likely be required. Moreover, I don't think that artificial intelligence is likely to get out of hand and start running the planet, enslaving the human population in the process.

What about the "downloads"? In the book *Harvest of Stars* (Anderson 1993), downloads appear centuries prior to the advent of artificial intelligence. The concept made a pretty good story; however, I think that, in contrast to artificial intelligence, downloads are fundamentally impossible. The workings of a specific individual human brain are too complex, too subtle, and too dependent on experience to be copied in this manner . . . certainly not to a machine. I don't believe that it would even be possible to copy one individual to a clone of that individual, unless perhaps under very highly controlled conditions.

What do I mean? The experiences of normal maturation interact with the brain—and with the body—in a very complex fashion, even influencing the body and the brain physically. In a mature individual, it might be possible to copy the physical structure of the brain to a limited degree, but only insofar as the structure is determined genetically. Those aspects of brain structure and function which are molded by interactions with the environment could not be copied. It might be possible to create two clones (or identical twins, although twins are mirror images and are not actually identical), raise them in two separate but identical artificial environments, and wind up with two mature individuals who are essentially identical. Even this assumes that it would be possible to create artificial environments that could nurture a normal human being. But, obviously, we are getting very far away from copying the brain as originally imagined. None of this has much connection to the science of repairing the brain in a mature individual.

An alternative to the downloading idea, which might actually be possible, would be to observe a particular individual's decision-making process, deduce a set of rules and principles, and apply these to a model system to create a decision-making machine. In the book, the downloads are employed because of the perceived importance of certain individuals for their leadership and decision-making capacities. A duplicate decision-making machine might certainly be made in a black-box manner, by copying the behavior of the individual, not by mimicking the brain itself. Facetiously, we might suggest that the technological process envisioned in *Harvest of Stars* (Anderson 1993) was, in fact, an erroneous technology in which the characters in the book *believed* that they were downloading the workings of the brain, but in fact were simply producing a machine that copied the decision-making and other personality properties of the individual through some artifactual and erroneous (but realistic) process. How could they know that the decisions made by the machine were, in fact, the same as those the original would have made? The decisions were reasonable, and apparently consistent with the original person, but each decision was unique. Perhaps the download was simply listened to in the manner of an idol or a religious icon, obeyed with blind faith.

For the same reasons, replacing entire brains will not be either reasonable nor feasible. The notion that if one's brain deteriorates, it might be possible to duplicate the brain and replace it entirely, is a purely imaginative concept. And, for pretty much the same reasons, it won't be useful to transplant any large part of the brain. We can make minor adjustments, and we can try to tap into mechanisms that the brain itself uses to compensate for minor injury, but I don't think that major restructuring of the brain, in the sense of replacing all or large parts of it or putting it into a new housing, will be possible.

This might be a good place to mention a new, and rather remarkable, development in the realm of brain-computer interface technology. Philip R. Kennedy and Roy A. E. Bakay at the Department of Neurosurgery, Emory University, and Community Neurological Clinic, Duluth, Georgia, have developed a technique that allows for the development of a direct connection between the brain and a computer. This can permit, in a limited form, neural output from paralyzed patients to be used for communication with a computer interface. This was accomplished by using fragments of peripheral nerve that were incorporated into the tip of recording electrodes. The peripheral nerve fragments induced ingrowth of myelinated neural fibers from the patients' cerebral cortex. After a period of time had elapsed to allow for axonal ingrowth, this permitted stable recordings of action potentials to be made from endogenous neurons, and the output signals could be decoded and used as computer commands. In two paralyzed patients tested so far, one patient was able to send on-off signals to a computer (Kennedy and Bakay 1998) The second patient, also paralyzed, was able to send more complex signals to a computer, to manipulate a cursor, and operate icons by "thinking" of particular muscles. After several months of effort, the patient was able to perform more complex tasks, i.e., typing short messages when presented with a keyboard on the computer screen (Bakay and Kennedy 1999). These signals can be employed for communication purposes, or perhaps to control muscle stimulators; at least, this kind of system has the potential to enrich the quality of life for certain select patients that are completely paralyzed.

Limitations of Brain Repair

At this point, I would like to take a step back and talk about the structure of the brain in a slightly different way. If we consider the communication between neurons only (glial cells communicate with neurons as well, adding further complexity), there are on the order of 10^{12} neurons. As was discussed in the previous section, each neuron communicates with many other neurons, often with many thousands of them. Each neuron contributes its own information-processing capacity to the complexity of the circuit. Because of the extensive connectivity between neurons, in all probability every neuron is in indirect communication with every other neuron, forming one immense circuit.

If the brain were to operate in the manner of a computer—for example, as a fixed circuit—the loss of any connection (or group of like connections) might be expected to cause a catastrophic failure, as in a computer function. Again, obviously, the brain could not operate in this way. The brain has a degree of plasticity and adaptability that allows it to substitute for lost components and remodel itself in response to environmental inputs and to minor injury. Although neurons themselves are not replaced—or, to be more correct, are replaced only in certain select locations and circumstances—their connections show a great degree of adaptability. Connections between neurons may be physically modified, and the functions of connections may be altered in response to injury of adjacent or interacting elements. Thus, the brain does not function as a circuit, but more like a processor that responds to external conditions, using a set of instructions contained in the genome. Redundancy and plasticity allow the brain to function quite normally in the face of considerable injury.

In cases where injury or disease mechanisms overwhelm the various fail-safe redundancy and compensatory mechanisms that are inherent to brain function, functional losses are experienced. This is the case in many sorts of brain damage and disease, where noticeable and permanent functional deficits are seen only after brain damage becomes considerable. A great deal of functional recovery is seen in most cases of stroke, for example. Parkinson's disease is a carefully studied example of this phenomenon: functional deficits are not noticeable until about 80 percent of the dopaminergic neurons are lost.

I believe that, in general, we are successful in repairing the brain when we can tap into its restructuring capacity, in one sense or another, to assist the recovery process when it becomes overwhelmed. I think it is probable that virtually all successful brain repair strategies, knowingly or unknowingly, will exploit this capacity of the brain to compensate for minor damage. In some cases, severe damage results in obstacles that compensatory mechanisms cannot overcome, and we may be able to artificially provide more appropriate conditions for recovery. For example, in cases where the capacity for growth of interneuronal connections is a limitation, we may be able to provide more appropriate growth substrates. It may also be possible to deprogram the brain a bit so that it reverts to a slightly earlier developmental state in localized regions, thereby facilitating recovery. In other cases, however, recovery will be inconsistent with continued normal functioning of the brain, or may produce crippling alterations of other brain functions. In certain cases, recovery would require adaptations that are not part of normal brain function, and in such cases, repair may be impossible. The presence of such limitations is probably not a bad thing; in fact, it is likely that such limitations prevent us from doing things that would go beyond what we would want, or should want, to do. This conclusion is, however, somewhat speculative.

It is quite popular to think that technology will eventually be able to "do anything." I don't believe that this is true, and there probably are conceivable types of brain repair/reconstruction goals that simply cannot be accomplished. Blind faith in the invincibility of technology is usually associated with a degree of fuzziness about the basic principles involved. A reasonable example, again drawn from science fiction, is the idea of human travel to other star systems. When the physical limitations are not well understood, travel to other star systems can be entertained as a more realistic possibility. Since we now know, however, that a spacecraft would require about 40,000 years to reach the nearest stars if traveling at a rate of 60,000 miles per hour, we probably won't be going to neighboring stars anytime soon! In reality, the speed of light limitation is not the most fundamental problem: the difficulty is more one of carrying sufficient fuel and materials to reach great enough velocities. If the speed of light were 186 million, rather than 186 thousand, miles per second, this would help in some ways, but it would still be hard to get there in the extreme. Well, maybe there are "wormholes" that interconnect stars (a popular science fiction way of circumventing the speed of light), but probably not (at least, not that humans can pass through!). Still, I think that we will be traveling to other star systems before we can transplant personalities or download individuals from one body to another!

We have already established (to my satisfaction, at least) that we can't replace entire brains, or most of the brain. We also cannot download the brain and personality of particular individuals to computers, nor can we construct some kind of artificial brain program to replace our brains. Let's take a look at some "ultimate" brain reconstruction scenarios from another, more realistic angle.

Recall the earlier example of repairing stroke injury with multiple transplants. Since we are being fanciful, let's consider an even more ultimate possibility. We will try to make a self-renewing brain. For this exercise, let us imagine that we are dealing with an individual who has a global degenerative disease that results in a gradual and progressive degeneration of neurons throughout the brain. Suppose we can create a stem cell that is committed to becoming a neuron, and that is engineered so that a differentiation program is triggered by signals received from nearby degenerating cells. We will transplant these engineered cells into areas of the brain where degenerating cells are likely to occur. Or we might endow them with the ability to migrate throughout the brain and distribute themselves. All of this is probably feasible. We will call these "sentinel cells" for now.

When, subsequent to cell death or degeneration, appropriate signals are received, a nearby sentinel cell, or two or three, will divide once. At each division, one of the two daughter cells remains a sentinel, and the other differentiates into a neuron or glial cell of a type appropriate to its surroundings. Let's call the neurons derived from sentinel cells "sentinel neurons." Once differentiated, the sentinel neurons extend processes and form connections with nearby neurons. All of this might be possible; however, there still are limits. Note that I (carefully) specified *nearby* neurons; long-distance connections would still be a problem. So these sentinel cells might greatly aid in promoting local recovery following brain injury, and in this manner perhaps would slow the process of degeneration. There still are limits, however, and complete restructuring still will not be possible.

Why should we not expect to be able to program cells to re-form long-distance connections? If we can do all of these things with cells, why can't we completely restructure the brain? We can replace cells to any degree we wish, and we probably can induce long-distance growth of fiber tracts, but individual axons cannot retrace the paths of lost predecessors and find the appropriate targets on their own. There are several related questions about this issue: (1) Why can't axons find their way in the mature brain? (2) How do axons find their way during development? (3) Can we alter the mature brain so that it acts like a fetal brain in terms of providing axonal guidance? To answer the last question, we can, but only for localized regions that can be targeted and manipulated. We cannot alter the fundamental physiology of the brain so that it acts like an immature brain, for this would also alter very basic properties of the brain that are essential to its nature. In contrast to the (possibly) unlimited potential for manipulating isolated cells, there are limits on the degree to which we can restructure and manipulate the brain; they cannot be circumvented except at the cost of losing fundamental properties of the human brain and mind. The brain matures as a whole, as one integrated unit. The scaffolding for development and mechanisms for maturation unfold together, in an intricately orchestrated process. We will not be able to reprogram isolated circuits, cells, or sections of the brain to dedifferentiate and reintegrate themselves into the whole, because we would find it necessary to recapitulate the entire process of brain development to do so, thus losing the individual whose brain we are trying to repair.

To explore the possibilities and biological limitations of brain repair, we will make one last attempt to dream up a technological marvel. We will explore the limits of what we can do and, if we take this step, whether we would get a result that is desirable. We will look at two possibilities. The end result of the first is essentially the same as the "sentinel cell" example. The second possibility is a little different. This time, we will start with cells normally residing in the brain rather than transplants.

Our goal is to reprogram a resident cell type—perhaps microglia—to function differently, in a manner that is conducive to brain repair and regeneration. This can be done by introducing genes into cells that are present in the brain. Perhaps for this purpose we will use microglia, altering them by injecting or otherwise delivering a gene-delivery vector of some type. Let's say we can introduce into these cells genes that allow them to become multipotent, differentiating into cells which can mature into neurons or glia of various types. Becoming neurons, these cells will occupy locations formerly occupied by degenerating neurons and reestablish connections with nearby neurons. This will produce essentially the same result, with the same limitations and possibilities, as the "sentinel neuron" example described above. So now let's go on to the final possible ultrafantastic approach. (This is not going to be practical either, which will lead us to the conclusion that our ultimate goals should be relatively modest.)

Starting with the germ line instead of selected somatic cells, we will introduce modifications into the human genome that permit brain cells, both neurons and glia, to become self-renewing. When brain injury occurs, they will divide and adopt an immature state with unlimited growth potential, to replace cells that are lost. In this manner, the brain will develop an unlimited ability to repair itself. This is akin to the workings of the brains of animals such as salamanders.

What is wrong with this goal? We probably would wind up having brains with about the degree of adaptability and flexibility as those of the salamander. The evolutionary cost of having a brain with this kind of morphological plasticity (or regenerative potential) is that most of the behavioral repertoire must be written into the genome. In order to have a brain that learns from experience and adapts to the environment, one must also have stability and retention of learned skills and information. Thus, I believe that if we were to gain the ability to replace components of the brain without limit, no matter what tactic we use, eventually we would come to the point that replacement results in the loss of experience and personality, and results in fundamental changes in the functioning of the human brain. So here we have come up against a second kind of limit: if we make the brain completely plastic, we will erase fundamental aspects of the way in which the human brain works. Admittedly, this scenario is quite unrealistic, since hardly anyone would seriously entertain the possibility of invasively altering the human genome.

I am not, however, claiming that if we introduce any sort of added plasticity in the adult brain, we will necessarily erode fundamental properties of the human mind. But such an alteration would have to be selective and carefully targeted to specific diseases. Adverse consequences could result from restructuring the brain *in advance* so that it responds to injury in a fundamentally different way, and becomes able to adjust to major debilitating injury. We may very well be able to assist in functional recovery by promoting neural plasticity in restricted brain regions without such obstacles. Hardly anyone would claim that aiding the spinal cord in recovering after injury would erode human consciousness.

Perhaps, to look at this issue in another way, it would be useful to view the nervous system as having a kind of hierarchical organization. Recognize, however, that this is a great oversimplification, of a kind that scientists universally despise, and the nervous system is not really organized in this manner. But I still think it is useful. At one end of the hierarchy is peripheral nerve, where long-distance connections regenerate quite readily (although usually not accurately, depending on the kind of injury). Peripheral nerve responds to injury by simple regrowth. At the other end of the hierarchy is the cerebral cortex, which is quite plastic and shows evidence of recovery from fairly substantial injury. Apparently, however, it does so not mainly by regrowth and regeneration, but by reorganization of adjacent brain regions, allowing for functional substitution and adaptation. The physiology of the response to injury is pretty much the same throughout the brain. In some subcortical regions, there is a degree of physical restructuring, but the response to injury in most regions of the brain appears to involve mainly reorganization of uninjured circuits rather than structural regrowth.

What might be the evolutionary reason for this difference between peripheral nerve and CNS—which, physiologically, largely boils down to a structural difference between peripheral nerve and CNS myelinated tracts (discussed in chapter 2, under "Cellular Components," and in chapter 18, under "Studies by Richard Bunge and Mary Bunge")? Again we are guessing, but it seems probable that if there were a degree of plasticity in the adult mammalian CNS akin to that in peripheral nerve or the invertebrate brain, it would be inconsistent with the fundamental nature of the mammalian brain. In the formation of the mammalian brain, a certain amount of detail is encoded in the genome, but most of the behavioral repertoire, and thus most of the detail of brain organization, depends on experience. If the cortex were to be completely restructurable in the adult, much of the experience-dependent behavioral repertoire would be erased in the process. This hypothetical erasure process would go beyond even knowledge (e.g., typing skills), and would include fundamental parts of the behavioral repertoire that are acquired in infancy.

In lower organisms, where much of the information required for normal functioning is encoded in the genome, unlimited plasticity is possible. Structural reorganization would not result in either behavioral incapacitation or reversion to an infantile behavioral repertoire.

Therefore, we may have a sort of multilevel nervous system in which there are several kinds of structures. For each structure, the kind of manipulation that is possible is dependent on the contribution of that structure to human "nature"—personality, consciousness, and so on. For

Table 25.1
Four general divisions of the nervous system

Structure	Response to Injury	Contribution to consciousness	Physiological Structure
Cerebral cortex	Reorganization only	Large	Oligodendrocytes (CNS)
Subcortical brain	Reorganization, some structural adjustments	Some	Oligodendrocytes (CNS)
Spinal cord	No regeneration	Negligible	Oligodendrocytes (CNS)
Peripheral nerve	Regenerates	Essentially none	Schwann cells (PNS)

Note: CNS—central nervous system structural organization includes myelination by oligodendrocytes, no separate pathways for individual neurites. PNS—peripheral nervous system structural organization includes Schwann cells that are dedicated to individual axons and basal lamina that encircle individual fibers.

convenience, let's call this "consciousness." The unaided response to injury and our ability to manipulate various structures are roughly related (table 25. 1).

Thus, for the entire CNS, we are "stuck" with a CNS cellular physiology, even though there are some places (e.g., the spinal cord) that (it seems!) could be more plastic with little risk to human consciousness. Thus, in the spinal cord we can probably intervene to any degree we desire, restructuring it surgically or reengineering it so it can respond to injury in a more favorable manner, without risk to human nature, individuality, or consciousness. For other reasons, however, reengineering the spinal cord ahead of time, in uninjured individuals in anticipation of injury, is probably not a good idea. In peripheral nerve, too, we probably can intervene freely. In the cerebral cortex, most probably there is ultimately less that can be done. As was discussed earlier in this chapter, we probably can implant cells two or three or four times following a stroke or other injury without producing a noticeable erosion of consciousness or personality. Interventions that aid or accelerate reorganization of areas adjacent to injured parts of the cortex can likely be undertaken more freely. We probably cannot aim (even as an "ultimate" dream) to promote actual regeneration in damaged cortical areas. Beyond that, however, our efforts are probably best directed at preventing stroke, degeneration, or injury and its sequelae.

Conclusion

The question, then, is would any of these radical strategies, or any other strategy that I haven't thought of, make any sense even if it were possible and even if it did not change the way in which the brain processes information? The problem is that replacing all or much of the brain, even if it were possible to do so accurately, would change the individual. The end result would not be a "repaired" version of the original person, but a different person.

This engenders considerations not unlike those related to human cloning. Cloning oneself would produce an individual physically similar (in some ways) to the original. Of course, it would produce an infant, and the mature person could be quite different. The nature of the individual is only partly encoded in the physical structure of the brain, and in the aspects of this physical structure that are genetically determined. The individual is shaped largely by experience, with experiences as an infant and child being especially important.

So there is no sense in which our ultimate goal is to completely restructure the brain. Then what is our ultimate goal? I would say that it is to be able to repair localized damage of the brain and spinal cord, induced by trauma or disease, accurately and reliably. A goal with still higher priority will be to prevent such damage from occurring in the first place. Our limitation will be that major parts of the brain cannot be replaced. We can prevent degeneration without limit, but once brain circuits are lost, we will find that we can replace only specific circuits with specific functions. Regardless of how skilled we become in repairing the brain, limitations on the degree to which we can practice this repair will remain.

This leads us to the conclusion that our ultimate goals in brain repair strategies are not radically different from the kinds of things that we are trying to perfect now. Thus, we may be able to aid the restructuring of the cerebral cortex following injury, but we probably can't physically replace much (or any significant part) of the cerebral cortex. In certain subcortical nuclei, we can certainly replace some cell populations, but it is not likely that entire nuclei can be replaced. We can, perhaps, modify endogenous brain cells by introducing into them genes that allow them to respond to injury more favorably. Similarly, however, we can't go so far as to endow neurons with the ability to entirely regenerate their connections following axotomy. The cells that we employ for transplantation probably can be modified as well. Perhaps in culture we can generate cells that exceed the efficiency of the original cells; possibly our modified cells could grow axons more vigorously in the mileau of the mature brain, or perhaps they would have augmented levels of metabolic activity.

For spinal cord injury, in those cases where spinal cord function is completely lost, any sort of recovery is better than none. There is not much danger of producing major personality changes by manipulating the spinal cord, nor is producing additional damage a major concern. Thus, we are likely to see attempts to produce functional recovery in the spinal cord that involve relatively heroic measures; for example, combined surgical manipulation, transplants, growth factors, implantation of growth substrates, and interventions to prevent further degenerative changes. Such advances, which involve major restructuring and multiple interventions, are more likely in the spinal cord than most parts of the brain.

Fundamental improvements in the ways we approach preventing or delaying degenerative changes are quite likely. We may be able to better identify causes of degeneration, whether these have a basis in genetic defects, exposure to toxins, or acquired disease. Blocking degeneration with strategies related to growth factor treatment is also likely to see a great emphasis in the future. And we may be able to make great strides in identifying the causes of degenerative disorders, so that they can be predicted. This may result in an increased emphasis on brain repair strategies, proactive steps to prevent neurodegeneration. Implantation of cells that secrete growth factors or other substances which bolster cells against neurodegenerative changes, for example, may become increasingly emphasized, as opposed to replacing cells after they have been lost.

Moreover, when neurons are damaged, they may cease to function long before they actually die. During this period, recovery remains possible, and might be promoted either by removing the cause of stress or injury, or by strategies such as administration of growth factors. Any such strategy aimed at preventing degenerative changes does not face the innumerable and sometimes insurmountable obstacles that impede restructuring of the damaged brain.

Overall, in the future, we are likely to see vast improvements in the management and treatment of brain disease when the overall picture is considered. If an armamentarium of treatments that can be used to produce minor brain repair and restructuring becomes available, these treatments may come to have an impact which is far more than minor. The possibility of employing brain repair strategies in early stages of disease, before major structural damage occurs, in combination with strategies to prevent further degeneration as well as pharmacological treatment and retraining techniques, may have an enormous overall impact on the outcome of neurodegenerative disorders.

Glossary

acetylcholine   A neurotransmitter employed by certain neurons in the brain and at the neuromuscular junctions of mammals. It is thought that neurons which employ acetylcholine as a neurotransmitter are particularly susceptible to degeneration in patients with Alzheimer's disease.

activated microglia   Microglia, a glial cell type that serve a number of immune system functions in the CNS, are activated by chemical mediators, and gain the ability to migrate and phagocytize debris.

adipose tissue   Fatty tissue. Contains primarily fat cells, which consist mostly of fats stored in triglyceride form. Fat cells also contain other normal cellular components, including cell membranes, cell nuclei, and other structural proteins.

adjuvant   A material that aids or enhances. Adjuvants are employed in immunology to enhance local immune responses. Substances such as mineral oil and the cell walls of certain bacteria produce an increased immune response when locally administered into or under the skin. Adjuvants are commonly used to assist in the production of antibodies and to provoke autoimmune responses.

adrenal chromaffin cell   An epinephrine- or norepinephrine-producing endocrine cell that is found in the adrenal medulla, the central part of the adrenal gland.

adrenal cortex   The outer region of the adrenal gland, which contains primarily the cells that secrete adrenal steroid hormones.

adrenalectomize   To remove the adrenal gland; adrenalectomy is removal of the adrenal gland.

adrenal gland   A gland located at the superior part of the kidney that contains the adrenal cortex (the outer part) and the adrenal medulla (the core region).

adrenaline   See epinephrine.

adrenal medulla   The core region of the adrenal gland, the most prominent cellular feature of which is the adrenal chromaffin cell.

afferent   A neuronal input, toward a particular target.

agnosia   Loss of comprehension.

allele   A particular form of a gene. For example, if I have gray eyes, and you have brown eyes, you have a different allele of the gene that controls eye color than I do.

allograft   A graft from one individual to another of the same species.

Alzheimer's disease   A progressive disease typically beginning in the fifth decade of life, and resulting in general dementia and brain atrophy.

anterior   The front. In humans, anterior is toward the abdomen. In four-legged animals, anterior is toward the head.

anterograde   Along an axon in the direction away from the cell body, toward the distal part.

anterograde tracing   The process of tracing the path of axons from the cell body toward their terminals. This was formerly accomplished by severing the axons, or damaging the cell bodies, and searching for the degenerating fibers that were produced. Modern methods employ chemical substances, often wheat germ agglutinin coupled to horseradish peroxidase, a fluorescent substance called DiI, or a lectin called PHAL, which is injected near the cell bodies. There are very sensitive methods to detect these substances after they have been transported along the course of the axons of the injected cells. In the case of DiI, the chemical is not transported, but simply diffuses along the axonal membrane.

antibody   A protein molecule, produced by B lymphocytes, that interacts with (binds to) an antigen. Most antibodies are of the IgG type, which contain two regions that bind to target proteins.

antidiuretic hormone   ADH, or vasopressin, a hormone produced in the supraoptic and paraventricular nuclei of the hypothalamus. It is secreted from the pituitary gland, and has the effect of concentrating the urine and thereby decreasing water loss.

antigen   A material, usually a protein, carbohydrate, or (sometimes) nucleic acid or synthetic molecule, that elicits an antibody response.

aphasia   An impairment of speech.

apoptosis   The process through which cells undergo programmed death. It also can be triggered by events such as serious DNA damage.

aspiration   For this book, this term is used to describe the pulling of tissue into a small opening in a metal or glass tube by application of a vacuum.

astrocyte   A type of glial cell that has starlike processes radiating from the cell body, and serves a number of functions related to support of and communication with neurons.

autograft   A graft within an individual animal, from one part of the animal to another.

autonomic ganglia   Small clusters of neurons, outside the central nervous system, that are part of the autonomic nervous system.

axon   The process, or extension, of a neuron that sends impulses to other cells. Axons conduct action potentials, sometimes for long distances, by a process that involves exchange of ions with the surrounding medium.

axotomy The process of severing an axon from a nerve cell.

basal lamina A sheathlike covering, composed of protein with carbohydrate components, that surrounds various tissues, especially peripheral nerve fibers.

base In molecular biology, it indicates a single DNA segment. A string of three bases comprises a codon, which codes for one amino acid.

BDNF Brain-derived neurotrophic factor, a member of the NGF family.

blind In reference to experiments, to test effects of procedures such as administration of drugs or transplantation. "Blind" means that steps are taken to ensure that the evaluators, patients, and those administering treatment are unaware of whether the animal or human is receiving active treatment or a control procedure. Expectations about outcomes of procedures often play a large role in the results: for example, testers may unwittingly convey their expectations to the subjects, which in turn may have a large effect on the outcome of a trial. For this reason, clinical trials are almost always conducted "blindly."

blood-brain barrier A structure whose basis is tight junctions between the cells that line blood vessels (endothelial cells). It prevents substances in the blood from reaching the brain. Compounds that are soluble in lipids (such as alcohol, abused drugs, and many drugs used for treating CNS disorders) are not excluded by the blood-brain barrier because they pass directly through cell membranes. Other compounds, such as certain amino acids, are actively transported into the brain by endothelial cells.

bradykinesia Slowness or retardation of movement seen in Parkinson's disease.

brain stem The lower part of the brain, between the cerebral hemispheres and the spinal cord.

catalepsy A trancelike state in which animals or humans do not respond to their environment. Used to test effects of drugs that block dopamine receptors in the striatum.

catecholamine A series of compounds, chemically characterized by having a catechol ring and an amine group, that serve as chemical messengers. The primary catecholamines that are active in vertebrates are dopamine, norepinephrine (noradrenaline), and epinephrine (adrenaline).

caudal Toward the tail (see rostral).

caudate nucleus A subcortical region of the brain that is important in the control of movement and mood.

caudate putamen In rats and other rodents, the caudate nucleus and putamen are not separated by a band of white matter and thus are collectively known as the caudate putamen

cavitation The formation of empty (that is, fluid-filled) cavities, sometimes observed in the spinal cord long after severe spinal cord injury. Spinal cord cavitation also occurs in the degnerative disease known as syringomyelia.

cDNA Complementary DNA, the DNA corresponding to a sequence of messenger RNA (mRNA). Some of the cell's DNA (introns) is omitted when it is transcribed to messenger RNA. Thus, the sequence of the messenger RNA corresponds to the structure of the cell's proteins, while the cell's DNA does not. In order to construct DNA that is of the same structure as the proteins, a copy must be made from the RNA. These DNAs, which are complementary in structure to the mRNAs, are called cDNAs. The original DNA, as present in the genome, is called genomic DNA.

cell adhesion molecules   Molecules responsible for adhesion of adjacent cells to one another.

cell body   The body of a cell, as distinct from its processes. The cell body of a neuron is often called the perikaryon (region around the nucleus).

cell cycle   The series of events that comprise cell division through mitosis, complete cell division, and preparation for a subsequent division. When a cell—for example, a neuron—has stopped dividing, it is said to have withdrawn from the cell cycle, or to have exited from the cell cycle by entering a G0 phase.

cell line   A clonal (identical) population of cells derived from a single cell that can be propagated indefinitely (i.e., is immortal). Such cells can be isolated from tumors or produced in culture by various methods, as described in chapter 22.

cell recognition molecules   This term is used to indicate the fact that cell adhesion molecules may serve purposes other than simple adhesion, such as signaling and interacting with interior components of the cell.

cellular senescence   The process of cellular aging, through which somatic cells lose the capacity to divide. In most cells, this occurs after about 50 cell divisions.

cerebrovascular accident   Neurological impairment resulting from an interruption in local blood supply. Also called "stroke."

cholinergic   Refers to neurons that employ acetylcholine as a neurotransmitter.

choreiform   Describes involuntary twisting, twitching, or dancelike movements characteristic of Huntington's disease.

chromaffin   Used to describe the catecholamine-containing cells of the adrenal medulla. The term was originally derived from the chromaffin granules, structures within the cells that store catecholamines and have a particular staining property.

chromaffin cell   The catecholamine-producing cells of the adrenal medulla. These were classically recognized by their chromaffin granules, which can be distinguished with a staining procedure using potassium bichromate.

chromosome   A large DNA molecule that contains a number of genes.

clonal cell line   A genetically identical collection of cells derived from a single cell.

clone   The genetically identical progeny of a single cell.

CNTF   Ciliary neurotrophic factor, a protein molecule that has trophic effects on certain types of neurons.

cogwheel rigidity   A type of rigidity characteristic of Parkinson's disease, in which the limbs have a ratcheting, irregular stiffness or rigidity when moved.

constitutive   Expresses a particular property regardless of environmental conditions. Thus, if a cell type produces L-DOPA only when stimulated by the growth factor GDNF, or only after it is transplanted into the brain, L-DOPA production is not constitutive. If L-DOPA is produced in tissue culture without additional growth factor stimulation, and after transplantation into any part of the brain, L-DOPA production is constitutive.

contact inhibition   Inhibition of growth by contact with other cells, observed for most normal cells in culture. Cancer cells do not show contact inhibition.

contralateral   On the opposite side of the body.

control group   A group of animals or humans subjected to a treatment as similar to an experimental treatment as possible, with the active component omitted; employed for comparison. See chapter 5.

contusion   A bruise or impact injury that does not produce an open wound.

corpus striatum   A term for the caudate nucleus, putamen, and globus pallidus. Same as striatum.

cortex   Outer layer, from the Latin *cortex* (shell or outer covering). The cerebral cortex is also called the "neocortex," in reference to its development late in phylogeny. In addition to the cerebral cortex, the cerebellum has a cortex, as do the adrenal gland and other structures.

corticosteroids   Several hormones released by the adrenal cortex that play a role in the regulation of a number of metabolic functions, including mineral and electrolyte metabolism and immune function.

corticotropin-releasing hormone   A hormone produced in the hypothalamus that promotes the release of adrenocorticotropic hormone (ACTH), which in turn promotes corticosteroid release from the adrenal cortex.

cyclosporine   An immunosuppressive drug, used in transplantation to inhibit graft rejection.

cytokines   Peptide messenger molecules that are involved in the regulation of immune system cells. Some cytokines influence cells of the nervous system.

cytoplasmic extension   A process extending from the cytoplasm of a cell, the nature of which is not known. If one observes a cell extending a process, but this process is not known to be a neurite, and the cell may or may not be a neuron, it is safer to call the process by the more general term "cytoplasmic extension."

degenerate   To die or deteriorate.

dementia   Impairment of cognition and intellectual function.

dendrite   A process of a neuron that is specialized to receive messages.

diencephalon   A general term for the subcortical region of the brain that includes the hypothalamus and thalamus.

differentiation   Cell differentiation refers to the process of cellular maturation, during which a cell acquires properties that are unique to its particular type and that are required for the cell to perform its functional role. As a cell passes through various steps of differentiation, it acquires (or "expresses") more and more unique properties. At early stages of development, there are relatively fewer cell types present in the body. During maturation, cells differentiate, so that a greater and greater diversity of cell types is present.

distal   Away from, or along an axon in the direction away from, the cell body; opposite of proximal.

DNA   Deoxyribonucleic acid, the genetic material.

dopamine   A neurotransmitter that is important in the transmission of messages from substantia nigra to the neostriatum, and in several other pathways. Neurons that use dopamine as their neurotransmitter are lost in Parkinson's disease. Dopamine is a member of the catecholamine family.

dopaminergic   Utilizing the neurotransmitter dopamine.

dorsal   Toward the back. In humans, dorsal is usually the same as posterior. In four-legged animals, dorsal is usually upward, or the same as superior. Opposite of ventral.

dorsal root   The spinal nerve root that conveys sensory input to the spinal cord.

double blind   Similar to the term "blind," and originally used in reference to clinical trials, double blind means that neither the patient nor the evaluator knows the nature of the treatment (i.e., active drug or placebo). In the context of the relatively complex nature of clinical studies of transplantation, in theory a double-blind experiment would require that the patients be evaluated by someone other than the surgeon, and that the person performing the transplantation surgery would have no direct contact with the patient subsequent to the surgery. This is because it is not possible for the surgeon to be blind to the nature of the transplantation surgery, and because if the surgeon were to assist in evaluation of the patient subsequent to the transplantation, even just by interviewing or visiting the patient, the expectations of the surgeon regarding the outcome of the procedure could be unintentionally transmitted to the subject. In addition, this ensures that the individuals rating the outcome evaluate the subjects in an unbiased manner.

dystonia   Abnormal muscle contractions that may cause twisting or spasms.

ectopic   Refers to misplacement, or placement of an organ or tissue in other than its normal location.

efferent   An output; that is, a neuronal pathway traveling away from a designated location.

electrolyte   A charged substance, or ion derived from a salt (such as sodium, potassium, or chloride) that maintains the composition and concentration of dissolved substances, and the balance of electrical charges in blood and body fluids.

embryonic stem cell   A cell type present in the immature embryo prior to differentiation of any specific cell types. Embryonic stem cells are immortal, and any individual embryonic stem cell is totipotent, that is, able to regenerate an entire embryo.

encapsulation   Placement of tissue inside a capsule.

endothelial cell   A type of flat cell that lines blood vessels.

enhancer   A segment of DNA that binds protein molecules which enhance transcription, but not by participating directly in the process of transcription. Enhancers often can work in either direction, and often at some distance from the transcription start site.

enzyme   A protein that promotes, or catalyzes, biochemical reactions.

epinephrine   A catecholamine hormone secreted by the adrenal gland, in response to activation of the sympathetic nervous system. A relatively few neurons in the brain utilize epinephrine as a neurotransmitter. Epinephrine is derived from norepinephrine by the action of the enzyme phenylethanolamine N-methyltranferase (PNMT), and norepinephrine is derived from dopamine by the action of the enzyme dopamine β-hydroxylase (DBH). Epinephrine is also called adrenaline.

episomal   Genetic material, or DNA structures within a cell, not associated with the chromosomes; that is, nonchromosomal DNA.

epitope   The region of an antigen that binds to an antibody.

excitotoxic   Refers to the process of death or damage of neurons produced by prolonged excitation, via activation of excitatory amino acid receptors. Excitotoxic compounds include kainic acid, ibotenic acid, and quinolinic acid. (Also excitoxicity, excitotoxin.)

exon   A stretch of DNA that codes for protein.

experimental autoimmune encephalomyelitis (EAE)   An autoimmune inflammatory disease of central nervous system myelin, induced by immunization of animals with CNS tissue. In susceptible animals, this provokes an autoimmune reaction directed against their own CNS myelin, especially in the spinal cord. This disorder resembles multiple sclerosis and is often used as a model for that disorder.

experimental design   The scheme for the conduct of an experiment. It may include the number of subjects or animals, the type of controls, the duration of testing, the order of testing, and the comparisons from which conclusions will be made.

express   This term is used to convey the fact that cells are actively producing a certain substance.

extracellular matrix   The material, composed primarily of proteins, carbohydrate, and associated water molecules, that fills the space between cells.

ex vivo   Out of the body. In genetic engineering, refers to procedures that are performed on cells in culture, that are then to be returned to the body by transplantation.

fiber   A term often used to refer to the processes of neurons. It may refer to the entire assembly of process plus sheath. The term "neurite" refers to the neuronal process only.

fibroblast   An undifferentiated cell type, normally present in many tissues, that produces extracellular matrix and from which specialized connective tissue cells can develop. Fibroblasts can differentiate into cells of several types, including chondrocytes (cartilage cells), osteocytes (bone cells), adipocytes (fat cells), and smooth muscle cells. Fibroblasts are capable of migrating into the sites of tissue injury and proliferating to form scar tissue, and are easily grown in tissue culture. Many immortalized lines of rodent fibroblasts have been developed by extended growth in tissue culture—for example, the NIH 3T3 mouse fibroblast cell line.

fluorodopa   A compound used to detect the presence of the terminals of dopaminergic neurons in PET scanning. It is taken up by the terminals of dopaminergic neurons.

forebrain   The anterior part of the brain during embryonic developement. As the brain matures, some rearrangement takes place so that not all forebrain structures remain in the anterior part of the brain in the adult.

FY506   An immunosuppressive drug, used in transplantation to inhibit graft rejection.

Gelfoam   A gelatin-based sponge material that is frequently used for neurosurgical procedures in animals to help stop bleeding and to fill the space created by removal of tissue.

gene   A sequence of DNA that codes for a protein product, or that directs the production of a species of mRNA.

gene targeting   The process of modifying the DNA in a cell or an intact organism by selective modification of a known gene.

gene therapy   Replacement or alteration of DNA for therapeutic purposes. See chapter 20.

genetic engineering   The science of altering DNA for some defined purpose. See chapter 20.

germ line cells   Cells that participate in the reproductive process, and carry genetic material on to succeeding generations through the natural reproductive process (i.e., sperm or ova). Also called germ cells. All other cells of the body are somatic cells.

germ line therapy   Genetic engineering applied to germ line cells. See chapter 20.

gestational   Refers to the day of fetal/embryonic growth in utero. A 17-day gestational fetus is 17 days post conception.

globus pallidus   A subcortical nucleus that participates in control of motor functions, and is part of the striatum.

glyoxylic acid   A compound that can be used to induce histochemical fluorescence of catecholamines.

growth cone   The leading segment of a growing axon, which contains components specialized for axonal growth, such as the protein GAP–43. The growth cone is somewhat larger than the trailing parts of the axon, and from it very fine processes, known as filopodia, are extended to explore and select the terrain over which the growth cone will proceed.

growth factor   A protein molecule that promotes the growth, differentiation, and survival of other cells.

gyrus   One of the convolutions, or raised portions, of the cerebral cortex. The plural form is gyri.

Hayflick limit   The number of divisions, usually 45–50, that can occur in normal somatic cells prior to the onset of cellular senescence.

hematopoietic system   The system from which all blood cells are generated.

histochemical fluorescence   This term is used to refer to a method of chemically reacting catecholamines in tissues with formaldehyde vapor or glyoxylic acid (on microscope slides) to induce the formation of fluorescent molecules that can be examined using a fluorescence microscope.

histochemistry   A general term describing the use of chemical reactions to identify particular biochemicals in thin sections of tissue taken from the brain or other organs.

histology   Microscopic examination of tissue using thin slices (sections), or occasionally flattened structures such as the iris.

homeostatic/homeostasis   Describes the process of controlling functions that regulate internal body states at an optimal level. Such processes as control of body temperature, blood pressure, hydrational state, and blood glucose level are often described as homestatic functions.

homograft   An obsolete term for a graft from one animal (or human) to another of the same species.

horseradish peroxidase   An enzyme that is used as a marker molecule for tracing neuronal pathways, among other purposes. It is used mainly because it is convenient to stain, using one of several chemical reactions.

huntingtin   The protein molecule that is abnormal, containing an excess number of glutamines, in patients with Huntington's disease.

Huntington's disease   A degenerative disorder that usually has its onset in the thirties or forties and primarily involves the neostriatum. The most notable symptom is choreiform movements.

hybrid cells   Cells created by fusion of two cell types, usually tumor cells and normal cells. These cells contain DNA from both cell types, and usually behave like tumor cells while retaining some of the properties from the nontumor fusion partner.

hybridoma   A cell produced by fusion of a tumor cell with an antibody-producing cell. Used to produce antibodies.

hyperactivity   A greater amount of behavioral activity than is normally seen. In the present context, hyperactivity is used to refer to animals that show greater locomotor activity than normal animals in enclosed testing chambers.

hypogonadism   Dysfunction of the gonads (ovaries or testes).

hypophysectomy   Removal of the hypophysis (pituitary gland).

hypophysis   The pituitary gland.

hypothalamus   An area at the base of the brain, near the pituitary gland, that is important for the control of homeostatic and endocrine functions.

ibotenic acid   An excitatory compound that acts as a glutamate agonist, and can be used to kill neurons when injected directly into the CNS. It is classified as excitotoxic because it kills neurons through inducing excessive activation.

immortal   A term employed to describe cell lines that are not subject to a limited number of divisions prior to cellular senescence. Normal cells from the body can divide only a limited number of times in culture before they become senescent and lose the capacity for further division. Some cell types, such as most neurons, normally do not divide at all, either in tissue culture or in their normal environment. Immortal, or immortalized, cells also are not limited by certain other requirements that limit the growth of nonimmortal cells.

immunohistochemistry   A technique used to identify particular molecules in cells (such as cells in the brain) by their reaction to antibodies. For example, cells that react with an antibody to the enzyme tyrosine hydroxylase are said to be tyrosine hydroxylase positive, or TH+.

immunoreactive   Reacts with antibodies directed to a particular substance. For example, neurons that contain the enzyme tyrosine hydroxylase are often referred to as "tyrosine hydroxylase immunoreactive neurons" because the neurons are stained using an antibody that binds to tyrosine hydroxylase. Thus, if the cells are stained, they appear to contain tyrosine hydroxylase. Because the tyrosine hydroxylase is not measured directly, but only inferred to be present because it binds to the antibody (the antibody might bind to other substances—although steps are generally taken to ensure against such problems), the cells are described as being tyrosine hydroxylase immunoreactive, sometimes abbreviated TH+. In almost all (but not necessarily all) cases, tyrosine hydroxylase immunoreactive cells do contain that enzyme.

immunosuppress/immunusuppressant   Having the property of suppressing immune function. Immunosuppressant drugs are used to inhibit the rejection of brain and other types of grafts.

inferior   An anatomical term that indicates below or beneath.

inner cell mass   The inner layer of cells that forms at the time of the first specialization of the developing embryo; it goes on to form all of the cells of the body, including germ cells.

in situ   In its position; without being disturbed.

interneurons   Neurons that connect only to other neurons in their immediate vicinity. In contrast, the term "projection neurons" is sometimes used to refer to neurons that project to distant regions of the brain.

intron   A segment of DNA that interrupts the coding sequences (exons) and does not code for protein. Much of intron DNA appears to be "noise," although introns may have functions that are not presently known.

in vitro   A process or event that is studied in a biological culture system. Translates as "in glass," although modern culture systems almost always employ plastic, rather than glass, culture vessels.

in vivo   In the body, or within a living organism. Translates as "in life."

ion channel   Structure in cell membrane, consisting of protein, that allows charged ions to pass into or out of the cell, through the cell membrane. Ion channels open or close in response to signals, especially changes in charge differential between the interior and exterior of the cell, or in response to attachment of neurotransmitters to the ion channel protein.

ischemia   Impairment of blood supply. Usually causes CNS damage due to insufficient supply of oxygen and glucose.

isograft   A graft from one animal to another genetically identical animal. In humans, a graft from one homozygous twin to another would be called an isograft. Same as syngraft.

kainic acid   A substance derived from a form of seaweed, structurally analogous to the excitatory amino acid glutamic acid; it interacts with brain receptors for excitatory amino acids. Most CNS neurons are excited by kainic acid. When exposure of neurons to kainic acid or to other excitatory amino acids is excessive or prolonged, they may be killed. This is termed excitotoxicity. Excitatory amino acids such as kainic acid are often injected into local regions of the brain to produce loss of neurons and mimic various forms of brain injury.

kindling   A procedure used to induce an experimental model form of epilepsy in animals that involves repeated, spaced stimulation (usually electrical stimulation of the brain) leading to generalized seizures.

L1   A cell adhesion molecule that is present on axons and Schwann cells, and promotes the growth of axons.

laminin   A molecule composed of protein and carbohydrate (i.e., a glycoprotein) that is sometimes present in extracellular matrix, and is a prominent component of basal lamina. In many situations, the presence of laminin promotes the growth of neurites.

lesion   An area of injury. In the brain, a lesion or lesioned area usually is a location in which the neurons have been destroyed.

Lewy bodies   Rounded, pigmented structures found within neurons in the substantia nigra, the locus ceruleus, and other locations that are characteristic of Parkinson's disease.

lipophilic   Having an affinity for lipids (fatty substances). Since cell membranes are constituted of lipids, lipophilic chemicals can penetrate through cell membranes.

LTR   An area of retroviral DNA that inserts the viral DNA into the DNA of the host when the host cell is dividing, and induces the host cell to express the downstream DNA sequence.

macula   The center of the retina, where the highest density of photoreceptor cells occurs.

magnocellular neurons   Large neurons, located in the hypothalamus, that produce vasopressin.

medium spiny neurons   Large neurons in the neostriatum that receive inputs from the substantia nigra and cortex, and give rise to the major output pathways from the neostriatum.

melanin   A biological pigment found in neurons in the substantia nigra; it is also produced in the skin and other pigmented structures (e.g., eyes) through a different process.

mesencephalic flexure   A characteristic feature of the midbrain, just rostral to the pons, that is where the dopamine neurons of the substantia nigra are located.

mesencephalon   The midbrain. The substantia nigra is located in the mesencephalon.

messenger RNA (mRNA)   Nucleic acid that is the template for production of protein. It is formed from DNA by the process called transcription.

microglia   A type of glial cell present in the CNS that is derived from the mesoderm (i.e., connective/lymphatic/muscle tissue layer of the embryo), and thus is not part of the neuronal/astroglial/oligodendroglial lineage. These cells serve neuronal support functions and functions related to immune surveillance.

mitosis   Cell division by somatic cells in which each daughter cell contains a replica of the genetic material in the original cell. Mitosis is distinguished from meiosis, which is the process of cell division employed by germ cells. Meiosis involves two successive cell divisions, chromosomal rearrangement, and daughter cells containing half of the DNA of the parent cell.

monoclonal antibody   An antibody made by hybridoma cells that has the property of being a single, identical antibody molecule. In contrast, antibodies produced in a living animal consist of a collection of slightly different molecules.

mucosal cells   Cells that line the small intestine and possess microvilli, called the brush border. These cells produce digestive enzymes.

multipotent   A term used to describe a cell having the (potential) ability to differentiate into more than one final cell type.

neocortex   The cerebral cortex, that is, the outer, convoluted part of the brain, not including the cerebellar cortex.

neonatal   The period of development shortly after birth.

neostriatum   The caudate nucleus and putamen. In rodents, the caudate nucleus and putamen are combined, whereas in primates the two structures are separate.

nerve growth factor   (NGF) The first neurotrophic factor discovered, it promotes the growth and differentiation of certain types of neurons. Cells that were first known to be affected include peripheral sympathetic neurons and peripheral embryonic sensory neurons. More recently, it has been found that cholinergic neurons (which use the neurotransmitter acetylcholine) are also affected by nerve growth factor.

neural stem cell An undifferentiated precursor cell having the capacity for self-renewal; it can differentiate to form neurons, astrocytes, and oligodendrocytes. (This definition is provisional; a precise definition has not been agreed upon by the scientific community.)

neurite A general term used for a process or extension of a neuron. These may be either dendrites or axons, or they may be processes that have not entirely differentiated into axons or dendrites.

neurofilaments Filamentous proteins found in axons that are important for axonal structure and function.

neuroleptic A term used to describe dopamine antagonist drugs, such as chlorpromazine (Thorazine) and haloperidol (Haldol), used in the treatment of psychosis.

neuromodulator A soluble chemical that acts as a messenger to influence neuronal function.

neuronal fibers A general term used to describe the processes of neurons, including dendrites and axons; it also may be applied to axons with associated structures (e.g., myelin).

neurotrophic Refers to something that promotes the growth, differentiation, and survival of neurons.

neurotropic Refers to something that attracts the growth of neurites.

neurotrophic factor Protein molecule that has trophic effects (i.e., promotes growth, differentiation, and survival) for neurons.

node of Ranvier The gap between myelinated sections of a peripheral nerve, corresponding to the interface between two Schwann cells.

nonspecific In the context of neural transplants, "nonspecific" indicates an effect caused by tissue injury, or by the surgery itself, rather than a physiological function of the transplanted tissue.

norepinephrine A small molecule, classified biochemically as a catecholamine, that serves as a biological messenger. Norepinephrine functions as a neurotransmitter for certain neurons in the CNS and as a hormone when secreted by chromaffin cells of the adrenal medulla. Also called noradrenaline.

NT–3 Neurotrophin–3, a neurotrophic molecule of the NGF family.

nucleus This term refers to (a) the nucleus of a cell, which is the central part of the cell that contains the DNA or genetic material, or (b) a subcortical brain region that contains a collection of neuronal cell bodies.

nucleus accumbens A subcortical region of the brain that receives a high density of dopaminergic terminals from dopamine neurons located in the ventral tegmentum.

nucleus basalis of Meynert (NBM)   A nucleus located in the forebrain that contains a large number of acetylcholine-containing neurons which project to the cerebral cortex. Also called nucleus basalis.

olfactory tubercule   A subcortical region that receives dopaminergic inputs from neurons located in the ventral tegmentum.

oligodendrocyte   One of the types of CNS glia. Oligodendrocytes are the CNS myelin-producing cells.

oncogene   A gene that promotes the formation of tumors. Some oncogenes are derived from viruses, while others are present in the mammalian genome but do not result in tumor formation most of the time. Most oncogenes simply promote cell division.

opiate   A chemical compound with analgesic properties that is derived from the opium poppy and is related to opium.

opioid   A drug or compound with actions similar to those of opiates. "Opioid" is a more general term, and includes compounds that are not chemically related to opiates.

osmolarity   A measure of the total concentration of soluble materials (mainly salts) in a fluid, such as serum or urine.

paraplegia   Paralysis of the lower part of the body, including the legs.

parenchyma   The main part, or the central region.

parkinsonism   The state of having symptoms of Parkinson's disease.

Parkinson's disease   A disorder primarily of motor function, caused by degeneration of the dopamine-containing neurons in the striatum.

peptide   A molecule consisting of a string of two or more amino acids.

perikaryon   The part of a neuron close to, or around, the nucleus.

peripheral ganglia   Small collections of neurons located outside the central nervous system.

PET   Abbreviation for positron emission tomography. An X-ray-like technique similar to CAT scanning, it produces a three-dimensional image of the brain. Rather than showing the brain substance, however, PET scanning measures the relative amounts of particular chemicals in particular brain regions. In neural transplantation, PET scanning is often used to measure the concentrations of fluorodopa in particular brain regions, which indicates the presence of, and relative amounts of, terminals of dopamine neurons.

p53   A protein produced by normal mammalian cells that can promote DNA repair, inhibit cell division, and, under extreme circumstances, trigger programmed cell death.

phenotype   The physical properties of a cell, or animal, that comprise the sum of influences of the cells' genetic material and its interaction with the environment during maturation.

phenotypic   Refers to the properties of a mature differentiated cell or an entire organism. They are not simply part of the genetic properties of the cell, but depend on the interaction between the environment and the genome.

phylogeny   A term used to describe the hierarchy of organisms from the simple to the more complex. In a rough way, phylogeny is derived from the evolutionary development of organisms, with the more complex or phylogenetically higher animals having appeared later in evolution.

pia mater   A thin membrane that covers the brain; it is the innermost of three such membranes collectively called the meninges. Also called the pia. The three meninges are the pia mater, the arachnoid, and the dura mater.

placebo   An inactive substance given to patients in place of an active drug, sometimes to satisfy the wish of a patient to receive a medicine when none is needed. In drug trials, an inactive medicine is often administered in order to simulate effects of a drug other than the active pharmacological properties. This allows actual therapeutic effects to be distinguished. Often, the expectation of improvement will in itself cause improvement, so that in order to distinguish real effects, changes induced by medicines are compared with effects produced by a placebo.

plasticity   This term is used to describe a variety of changes that may occur in the brain. In its most general form, "plasticity" refers to any change in the brain that is enduring. Thus, if the efficiency of transmission between two synapses is enhanced by repetitive use, and this enhancement persists after the repetitive use has ceased, it is a form of plasticity—that is, an adjustment in the way the brain is functioning. Other forms of plasticity consist of formation and loss of synapses, growth of axons and dendrites, and development of barriers that prevent contacts between adjacent neurons.

polypeptide   A polypeptide is a string of more than 10 amino acids. Short strings (10 amino acids or fewer) are generally referred to as peptides.

posterior   Toward the rear. In two-legged animals posterior is the same as dorsal, while in four-legged animals, posterior is the same as caudal.

postsynaptic   The receiving side of a synapse. A neuron that is on the receiving end of a synapse is often referred to as a postsynaptic neuron.

precursor cell   A cell that is destined to become a particular cell type but has not yet differentiated into that cell type.

prefrontal cortex   The most anterior part of the frontal cortex.

presynaptic   The sending side of a synapse. A neuron on the sending end of a synapse is often referred to as a presynaptic neuron.

primary cells   Cells obtained directly from a donor animal or human subject. Cells that have been modified or propagated in culture are not primary cells.

process   An elongated extension of the cytoplasm of a cell. Many cells have processes; for example, oligodendrocytes have processes that terminate in myelin sheaths. The processes of neurons are longer and more complex than those of any other cell type.

progenitor   A cell line that gives rise to more fully differentiated cell types, but has a restricted potential for differentiation. The distinction between neural stem cells and neural progenitor cells has not been strictly defined.

promoter   A DNA sequence that initiates transcription of a downstream DNA sequence by binding to proteins that in turn bind to RNA polymerase. Promoters must be used in gene therapy for initiation of transcription of a cDNA that is part of a retroviral vector inserted into another cell.

pronation-supination   A test used to assess motor function in patients with Parkinson's disease. Subjects are asked to place their hand on a flat surface and alternately place palm up, palm down, palm up, and so on, as rapidly as they can.

proximal   Close to, or in the direction of, the cell body.

putamen   A nucleus that is part of the striaum; it usually shows the largest loss of dopamine in Parkinson's disease.

pyramidal   Refers to the shape of a population of neurons in the neocortex. These neurons have a triangular shape and usually have long axons that project to other regions of the brain or other parts of the cortex. (In contrast, interneurons have short axons connecting to the same region of the cortex.)

quadriplegia   Paralysis that involves all four limbs.

quinolinic acid   An acid that causes neuronal excitation and can be used to damage the CNS, as an animal model of Huntington's disease.

reafferent   Describes the restoration of an afferent, or neural input.

receptor   Protein molecule embedded in cellular membranes that detects extracellular messenger molecules, especially neurotransmitters. Synaptic transmission involves release of neurotransmitter at synapses. Following release, neurotransmitter diffuses across the synaptic cleft and is sensed by receptor molecules in the postsynaptic neuron.

reporter gene   A gene that is introduced into cells for detection purposes. Often, reporter genes are used to test procedures for gene introduction, that is, to determine whether a method for transferring genes into cells is working effectively. Commonly used reporter genes are firefly luciferase, β-galactosidase, chloramphenicol acetyltransferase, and human placental alkaline phosphatase.

restriction enzyme   An enzyme derived from bacteria that is able to cut DNA in specific locations. The name is derived from the fact that these enzymes restrict the infection of bacteria by viruses.

retinitis pigmentosa   A progressive degenerative disease of the retinal photoreceptor cells.

retinoblastoma (Rb) protein   A protein normally produced by mammalian cells that inhibits cell division by binding proteins that drive cell division. Proteins bound to Rb protein are released when the Rb is phosphorylated.

retrograde   In an axon, refers to the direction toward the cell body, or the proximal part. The opposite term is anterograde.

retrograde tracing   An anatomical technique that exploits the tendency of neurons to transport chemical substances from axon terminals back to the cell body. Thus, the source of cells that send axons to a particular location can be determined by injecting these chemical substances.

retroviral vector   A disabled retrovirus that is used for transferring foreign DNA into cells.

retrovirus   A virus that is capable of inserting its genetic material into the DNA of a host cell.

rostral   An anatomical term that means "toward the head." The opposite is "caudal" (toward the tail). For the brain, "anterior" and "rostral" are synonymous. However, for other regions, "rostral" must be used to refer to the same place in different species. For example, "anterior parts of the spinal cord" obviously means something quite different in rats compared with humans, because of the postural difference.

Schwann cell   The cell type that forms myelin in the peripheral nervous system. Each individual axon of a peripheral nerve is mylelinated by a series of Schwann cells, each of which is devoted to myelinating that individual axon. Schwann cells, in addition to their structural role, produce a number of substances that are important for adherence (e.g., L1) or for growth and survival (e.g., nerve growth factor), of axons.

sciatic nerve   The main peripheral nerve that supplies innervation to the muscles of the lower leg.

semispecific   A term that, as used in this book, connotes an effect of transplantation which can be reproduced by several types of cells but requires the transplantation of some type of cells.

sham   An "imitation" surgical procedure, designed to mimic all effects of the surgery other than the manipulation per se. For example, a transplantation procedure might cause improvement, or behavioral changes of some sort, because of the anesthesia or drilling of the skull. "Sham" surgery usually consists of anesthetizing the animals, placing them in a stereotaxic apparatus, drilling an opening in the skull, and perhaps even inserting a needle into the brain. This is not the same as a control procedure. In the above example, control transplantation might involve inserting inactive tissue into the brain. Such a control procedure is not considered "sham" surgery.

soma   The cell body, as distinguished from processes that may extend some distance from the center of the cell. For neurons, this term is similar to "perikaryon," which means the part of the cell close to the nucleus.

somatic cells   All cells of the body other than those involved in reproduction.

somatic gene therapy   Gene therapy applied to somatic cells, as opposed to germ line therapy. Cells targeted by somatic gene therapy are not involved in the process of reproduction.

specific   This term has many meanings. In the context of this book, and particularly chapter 5, "specific" is used to mean a change produced by a graft that requires a particular type of cell. Thus, changes following transplantation that are caused by host brain reactions to the presence of foreign cells, or changes that are produced by chemical substances released by many different cell types, are not considered to be specific. Thus, in the context of tissue transplantation, an effect that is produced only by transplantation of a particular type of cell is said to be specific for that type of cell.

spiny neurons   The primary large output neurons of the striatum, which are noted for the characteristically numerous dendritic spines. These spiny neurons send axons to the substantia nigra pars reticulata or to the globus pallidus.

sprouting   A process of axonal growth that frequently occurs subsequent to CNS injury. When CNS axons are cut, they usually do not regrow. Axons near the injury, or near the area to which the cut axons had projected, often produce branches (collateral sprouts) that grow into the area vacated by the cut axons. This process is called "collateral sprouting," or simply "sprouting." Technically, sprouting may also take place via the growth of entirely new axons rather than collaterals.

stable integration   Incorporation of a transgene into the genomic DNA of the target cell.

statistical significance   A convention used in statistical evaluation of data, which indicates that the probability a difference is due to chance is less than 1 in 20 ($p < 0.05$).

stem cell   An undifferentiated cell that has the capacity for self-renewal and that can give rise to differentiated progeny. (See embryonic stem cell and neural stem cell.)

stereotaxic instrument   A device used for neurosurgery in both animals and humans. Essentially, these devices immobilize the head in a fixed position, allowing for remote placement of devices (such as the tip of a long injection needle) into specific locations in the brain. Animals are usually fixed in position by bars placed into the ears and under the front teeth. Specific sites in the brain are mapped in reference to the ears or other fixed locations. Such a map of brain locations is called a stereotaxic atlas. In humans, similar devices are used, but the position is fixed by using pins that are placed to touch particular spots on the skull (rather than ear bars and tooth bars). For subhuman primates (monkeys) and humans, dimensions of the brain are variable. Thus, accurate stereotaxic surgery generally requires the use of magnetic resonance imaging to determine brain coordinates prior to surgery.

striated muscle   Skeletal muscle.

striatum   A term for the caudate nucleus, putamen, and globus pallidus. Same as corpus striatum.

stroke   Neurological impairment resulting from an interruption in local blood supply. Also called "cerebrovascular accident."

subcortical   Refers to any part of the brain below the cerebral cortex and associated white matter. The cerebral cortex surrounds the upper part of the brain;

that is, the dorsal surface of the brain (in animals) or the superior surface of the brain (in humans), in a helmetlike fashion. Within the envelope formed by the cerebral cortex, the remainder of the brain is referred to as subcortical.

substantia nigra (SN)   The region of the brain that contains the dopaminergic neurons which degenerate in Parkinson's disease. In humans, these neurons are dark in color because they contain the pigment neuromelanin; hence the name substantia nigra. Parkinson's disease was first identified as a disorder involving the substantia nigra because of a loss of the pigmented cells. Other cell losses also occur in Parkinson's disease.

substantia nigra pars compacta   The upper, or more dorsal, part of the substantia nigra, where the dopaminergic cell bodies are located, roughly in a band running from the medial area to the lateral area.

substantia nigra pars reticulata   The part of the substantia nigra located ventrally (below) the pars compacta. This region contains dendrites of the dopaminergic neurons.

sulcus   One of the folds or fissures in the cerebral cortex. The plural form is sulci.

superior   An anatomical term meaning "above."

supersensitive   (or supersensitivity): A condition of a postsynaptic neuron in which the neuron develops an increased sensitivity to neurotransmitter. This condition generally develops when the normal synaptic input to the neuron is lost or removed. Also called denervation supersensitivity.

suprachiasmatic nucleus   A region of the hypothalamus that controls circadian rhythms.

SV40 large T antigen   A protein produced by the SV40 virus (simian virus 40) that stimulates cell division.

sympathetic neurons   Neurons of the sympathetic nervous system, a part of the autonomic nervous system involved in the control of involuntary muscles and release of catecholamines from the adrenal medulla. Sympathetic neurons employ norepinephrine as a neurotransmitter.

synapse   A connection between neurons. In most cases, a synapse is a connection between an axonal terminal and the dendrite or the body of a target cell, where communication takes place by the release of chemicals called neurotransmitters.

synaptic cleft   The space between two cells that occurs at a synapse.

syngraft   A graft between two genetically identical individuals (inbred animals of the same strain or monozygotic twins). Same as isograft.

syringomyelia   A degenerative disorder of the spinal cord that involves progressive development and extension of cavities and gliosis.

system   This term is used to describe a collection of neurons, their dendrites, their axons, and their synapses, and their interrelationships with other cells. The central nervous system includes the brain, spinal cord, and optic nerve. The peripheral nervous system includes peripheral nerves, peripheral ganglia, and innervation of peripheral organs. The dopaminergic system of the brain includes the dopaminergic cell bodies, their axons and dendrites, and the afferents to other cells that are derived from these neurons.

T cells   Immune system cells, also called thymocytes, are the primary mediators of cell-mediated immunity. T cells are the component of the immune system primarily responsible for graft rejection. Each T cell is specific to a particular antigen, but T cells require other cells (mainly microglia in the CNS) in order to recognize an antigen.

telomere   A repeated sequence of bases at the ends of each chromosome that becomes progressively shorter each time a cell divides.

telomerase   An enzyme that increases the length of telomeres.

teratoma   A growth formed by transplantation of embryonic stem cells into an animal.

teratocarcinoma   A tumor formed from embryonic stem cells. Such tumors can be formed by transplantation of embryonic stem cells into an animal (see teratoma). Teratocarcinomas occasionally form spontaneously, in animals and in humans, and are the only type of tumor that is not thought to be caused by mutation.

terminal differentiation   Acquisition of a final, mature cellular form and function.

TH   Abbreviation for tyrosine hydroxylase.

TH+   Used to indicate structures, for example, cells or fibers, that contain TH. In other words, they are positive for TH by immunostaining with antibodies that bind to TH (see immunoreactive).

thoracic   Pertaining to the area below the neck and above the diaphragm.

transcription   The cellular process of copying information from a DNA molecule; it results in the formation of a corresponding messenger RNA molecule.

transcription factor   A protein that promotes the initiation of transcription.

transgene   A gene that has been transferred into a cell from outside.

translation   The process through which the information contained in a messenger RNA molecule is used to produce the corresponding protein molecule.

transplant   The process of removing an organ, cell preparation, or tissue fragment from an organism and reinstalling (grafting) it into another organism or another location in the same organism.

trinucleotide repeat   A repeated sequence of three nucleotides, coding for a single amino acid (usually glutamine), that may occur in excess at the end of certain genes in several diseases, notably Huntington's disease.

trituration   Repeated aspiration and ejection of tissue from a small glass tube, in order to break tissue into individual cells.

trophic factor   A protein that promotes the growth or differentiation of cells. Indicates a "nourishing" effect that occurs through stimulation of internal cellular mechanisms, not by providing nutrients required for energy metabolism.

trophectoderm   The outer layer of cells in the earliest division of the developing embryo, which goes on to form supporting structures, such as the placenta and amnion (also trophoblast).

tyrosine hydroxylase   An enzyme involved in the biosynthesis of catecholamines. It catalyzes the synthesis of L-DOPA, the precursor for catecholamines, and thus is essential for their synthesis. Tyrosine hydroxylase, often abbreviated TH, is rate-limiting, which means that among the enzymes in the catecholamine biosynthetic pathway, its activity regulates the overall activity of catecholamine synthesis. The presence of this molecule indicates that a cell is a catecholamine-producing cell, often a dopamine neuron.

UPDRS   Unified Parkinson's Disease Rating Scale, used for measuring the severity of Parkinson's disease.

vascularization   The process of growth of blood vessels into a tissue.

vasopressin   See antidiuretic hormone (ADH).

vector   A molecule or construct, usually a structure made from DNA or a disabled virus, that is used to transfer DNA from one cell to another.

ventral   Opposite of dorsal.

ventral root   The spinal nerve root through which motor fibers pass from spinal cord to peripheral nerves, and then to skeletal muscles.

ventral tegmentum   A region of the ventral mesencephalon that contains a group of dopamine-containing neurons which project mainly to the limbic system, including the nucleus accumbens and the olfactory tubercle.

xenogeneic   Across species, or from two different species of animal.

xenograft   A graft from one species to another. In its older usage, "xenograft" connoted a graft between widely separated species (e.g., between different orders), as opposed to "heterograft," which might be used to describe a graft between closely related species.

zona reticularis   The innermost division of the adrenal cortex, where adrenal cortical cells may be intermixed with chromaffin cells characteristic of the adrenal medulla.

References

Abrous, D. N., and Dunnett, S. B. (1994). Paw reaching in rats: The staircase test. *Neurosci. Protocols* 10: 1–9.

Adams, R. D., and Victor, M. (1993). *Principles of Neurology.* Fifth ed. Mc Graw-Hill, New York.

Aebischer, P., Tresco, P. A., Winn, S. R., Greene, L. A., and Jaeger, C. B. (1991). Long-term cross-species brain transplantation of a polymer-encapsulated dopamine-secreting cell line. *Exp. Neurol.* 111: 269–275.

Aguayo, A. J., Benfey, M., and David, S. (1983). A potential for axonal regeneration in neurons of the adult mammalian nervous system. In *Nervous System Regeneration,* B. Haber and J. R. Perez-Polo (eds.), pp. 327–349. Alan R. Liss, New York. March of Dimes Birth Defects Foundation, Birth Defects: Original Article Series, 19.

Aguayo, A. J., Rasminsky, M., Bray, G. M., Carbonetto, S., McKerracher, L., Villegas-Perez, M. P., Vidal-Sanz, M., and Carter, D. A. (1991). Degenerative and regenerative responses of injured neurons in the central nervous system of adult mammals. *Philos. Trans. R. Soc. Lond. Ser. B,* 331: 337–343.

Aihara, H. (1970). Autotransplantation of the cultured cerebellar cortex for spinal cord reconstruction. *Brain and Nerve* 22: 769–784. (In Japanese with English abstract.) Cited in C. C. Kao, J. R. Wrathall, and K. Kyoshima, "Rationales and goals of spinal cord reconstruction." In *Spinal Cord Reconstruction,* C. C. Kao, R. P. Bunge, and P. J. Reier (eds.), pp. 1–6. Raven Press, New York, 1983.

Alberts, B., Bray, D., Lewis, J., Raff, M., Roberts, K., and Watson, J. D. (1994). *Molecular Biology of the Cell.* Third ed. Garland Publishing, New York and London.

Allen, G. S., Burns, R. S., Tulipan, N. B., and Parker, R. A. (1989). Adrenal medullary transplantation to the caudate nucleus in Parkinson's disease: Initial results in 18 patients. *Arch. Neurol.* 46: 487–491.

Aloe, L. (1987). Intracerebral pretreatment with nerve growth factor prevents irreversible brain lesions in neonatal rats injected with ibotenic acid. *Biotechnology* 5: 1085–1086.

Anderson, Poul. (1993). *Harvest of Stars.* Tom Doherty Associates, New York.

Anderson, Poul. (1994). *The Stars Are Also Fire.* Tom Doherty Associates, New York.

Annett, L. E., Dunnett, S. B., Martel, F. L., Rogers, D. C., Ridley, R. M., Baker, H. F., and Marsden, C. D. (1990). A functional assessment of embryonic dopaminergic grafts in the marmoset. In *Neural Transplantation: From Molecular Basis to Clinical Applications,* S. B. Dunnett and S.-J. Richards (eds.), pp. 535–542. Elsevier, Amsterdam. Prog. Brain Res. 82.

Annett, L. E., Martel, F. L., Rogers, D. C., Ridley, R. M., Baker, H. F., and Dunnett, S. B. (1993). Behavioral assessment of the effects of embryonic nigral grafts in marmosets with unilateral 6-OHDA lesions of the nigrostriatal pathway. *Exp. Neurol.* 125: 228–246.

Anton, R., Kordower, J. H., Maidment, N. T., Manaster, J. S., Kane, D. J., Rabizadeh, S., Schueller S. B., Yang, J., Rabizadeh, S., Edwards, R. H., et al. (1994). Neural-targeted gene therapy for rodent and primate hemiparkinsonism. *Exp. Neurol.* 127: 207–218.

Apostolides, C., Sanford, E., Hong, M., and Mendez, I. (1998). Glial cell line-derived neurotrophic factor improves intrastriatal graft survival of stored dopaminergic cells. *Neuroscience* 83: 363–372.

Aramant, R. B., and Seiler, M. J. (1994). Human embryonic retinal cell transplants in immunodeficient rat hosts. *Cell Transplant.* 3: 461–474.

Archer, D. R., Leven, S., and Duncan, I. D. (1994). Myelination by cryopreserved xenografts and allografts in the myelin-deficient rat. *Exp. Neurol.* 125: 268–277.

Arendt, T., Allen, Y., Sinden, J., Schugens, M. M., Marchbanks, R. M., Lantos, P. L., and Gray, J. A. (1988). Cholinergic-rich brain transplants reverse alcohol-induced memory deficits. *Nature* 332: 448–450.

Attwell, D., Barbour, B., and Szatkowski, M. (1993). Nonvesicular release of neurotransmitter. *Neuron* 11: 401–407.

Backlund, E.-O., Granberg, P.-O., Hamberger, B., Knutson, E., Martensson, A., Sedvall, G., Seiger, A., and Olson, L. (1985). Transplantation of adrenal medullary tissue to striatum in parkinsonism: First clinical trials. *J. Neurosurg.* 62: 169–173.

Bakay, R., and Kennedy, P. (1999). Update of cognitive engineering. *Program and Abstracts of the American Society for Neural Transplantation and Repair* 5/6: 25.

Bakay, R. A. E., Fiandaca, M. S., Barrow, D. L., Schiff, A., and Collins, D. C. (1985). Preliminary report on the use of fetal neural tissue transplantation to correct MPTP induced primate model of parkinsonism. *Appl. Neurophysiol.* 48: 358–361.

Bankiewicz, K. S., Oldfield, E. H., Chiueh, C. C., Doppman, J. L., Jacobowitz, D. M., and Kopin, I. J. (1986). Hemiparkinsonism in monkeys after unilateral internal carotid artery infusion of 1-methyl–4-phenyl–1,2,3,6-tetrahydropyridine (MPTP). *Life Sci.* 39: 7–16.

Bankiewicz, K. S., Plunkett, R. J., Jacobowitz, D. M., Kopin, I. J., and Oldfield, E. H. (1991). Fetal nondopaminergic neural implants in parkinsonian primates. *J. Neurosurg.* 74: 97–104.

Bankiewicz, K. S., Plunkett, R. J., Jacobowitz, D., Porrino, L., diPorzio, U., London, W. T., Kopin, I. J., and Oldfield, E. H. (1990). The effect of fetal mesencephalon implants on primate MPTP-induced parkinsonism. *J. Neurosurg.* 72: 231–244.

Baron, M. S., Vitek, J. L., Bakay, R. A., Green, J., Kaneoke, Y., Hashimoto, T., Turner, R. S., Woodard, J. L., Cole, S. A., McDonald, W. M., and DeLong, M. R. (1996). Treatment of advanced Parkinson's disease by posterior GPi pallidotomy: 1-year results of a pilot study. *Ann. Neurol.* 40: 355–366.

Barry, D. I., Kikvadze, I., Brundin, P., Bolwig, T. G., Bjorklund, A., and Lindvall, O. (1987). Grafted noradrenergic neurons suppress seizure development in kindling-induced epilepsy. *Proc. Natl. Acad. Sci. U.S.A.* 84: 8712–8715.

Barry, D. I., Wanscher, B., Kragh, J., Bolwig, T. G., Kokaia, M., Brundin, P., Bjorklund, A., and Lindvall, O. (1989). Grafts of fetal locus coeruleus neurons in rat amygdala-piriform cortex suppress seizure development in hippocampal kindling. *Exp. Neurol.* 106: 125–132.

Bartlett, J. S., and Samulski, R. J. (1995). Genetics and biology of adreno-associated virus vectors. In *Viral Vectors: Gene Therapy and Neuroscience Applications*, M. G. Kaplitt and A. D. Loewy (eds.). Academic Press, San Diego.

Beal, M. F., Ferrante, R. J., Swartz, K. J., and Kowall, N. W. (1991). Chronic quinolinic acid lesions in rats closely resemble Huntington's disease. *J. Neurosci.* 11: 1649–1659.

Becker, J. B., Robinson, T. E., Barton, P., Sintov, A., Siden, R., and Levy, R. J. (1990). Sustained behavioral recovery from unilateral nigrostriatal damage produced by the controlled release of dopamine from a silicone polymer pellet placed into the denervated striatum. *Brain Res.* 508: 60–64.

Bengzon, J., Brundin, P., Kalen, P., Kokaia, M., and Lindvall, O. (1991). Host regulation of noradrenaline release from grafts of seizure-suppressant locus coeruleus neurons. *Exp. Neurol.* 111: 49–54.

Bengzon, J., Kokaia, M., Brundin, P., and Lindvall, O. (1990). Seizure suppression in kindling epilepsy by intrahippocampal locus coeruleus grafts: Evidence for an alpha–2-adrenoreceptor mediated mechanism. *Exp. Brain Res.* 81: 433–437.

Berglin, L., Gouras, P., Sheng, Y., Lavid, J., Lin, P. K., Cao, H., and Kjeldbye, H. (1997). Tolerance of human fetal retinal pigment epithelium xenografts in monkey retina. *Graefes Arch. Clin. Exp. Ophthalmol.* 235: 103–110.

Bermudez-Rattoni, F., Fernandez, J., Sanchez, M. A., Aguilar-Roblero, R., and Drucker-Colin, R. (1987). Fetal brain transplants induce recuperation of taste aversion. *Brain Res.* 416: 147–152.

Bes, J. C., Tkaczuk, J., Czech, K., Tafani, M., Bastide, R., Caratero, C., Pappas, G. D., and Lazorthes, Y. (1998). One-year chromaffin cell allograft survival in cancer patients with chronic pain: Morphological and functional evidence. *Cell Transplant.* 7: 227–238.

Bing, G., Notter, M. F. D., Hansen, J. T., and Gash, D. M. (1988). Comparison of adrenal medullary, carotid body, and PC12 cell grafts in 6–OHDA lesioned rats. *Brain Res. Bull.* 20: 399–406.

Bischoff, S., Scatton, B., and Korf, J. (1979). Dopamine metabolism, spiperone binding and adenylate cyclase activity in the adult rat hippocampus after in-growth of dopaminergic neurons from embryonic implants. *Brain Res.* 179: 77–84.

Bjorklund, A., Campbell, K., Sirinathsinghji, D. J., Fricker, R. A., and Dunnett, S. B. (1994). Functional capacity of striatal transplants in the rat Huntington model. In *Functional Neural Transplantation,* S. B. Dunnett and A. Bjorklund (eds.), pp. 157–195. Raven Press, New York.

Bjorklund, A., Dunnett, S. B., Stenevi, U., Lewis, M. E., and Iversen, S. D. (1980). Reinnervation of the denervated striatum by substantia nigra transplants: Functional consequences as revealed by pharmacological and sensorimotor testing. *Brain Res.* 199: 307–333.

Bjorklund, A., Schmidt, R. H., and Stenevi, U. (1980). Functional reinnervation of the neostriatum in the adult rat by the use of intraparenchymal grafting of dissociated cell suspensions from the substantia nigra. *Cell Tissue Res.* 212: 39–45.

Bjorklund, A., and Stenevi, U. (1979). Reconstruction of the nigrostriatal dopamine pathway by intracerebral nigral transplants. *Brain Res.* 177: 555–560.

Bjorklund, A., and Stenevi, U. (1985). Intracerebral neural grafting: A historical perspective. In *Neural Grafting in the Mammalian CNS,* A. Bjorklund and U. Stenevi (eds.), pp. 3–14. Elsevier Science Publishers, Amsterdam.

Bjornson, C. R., Rietze, R. L., Reynolds, B. A., Magli, M. C., and Vescovi, A. L. (1999). Turning brain into blood: A hematopoietic fate adopted by adult neural stem cells in vivo. *Science* 283: 534–537.

Bodnar, A. G., Ouellette, M., Frolkis, M., Holt, S. E., Chiu, C. P., Morin, G. B., Harley, C. B., Shay, J. W., Lichtsteiner, S., and Wright, W. E. (1998). Extension of life-span by introduction of telomerase into normal human cells. *Science* 279: 349–352.

Bohn, M. C., Marciano, F., Cupit, L., and Gash, D. M. (1987). Adrenal medullary grafts promote recovery of striatal dopaminergic fibers in MPTP treated mice. *Science* 237: 913–916.

Bolam, J. P., Freund, T. F., Bjorklund, A., Dunnett, S. B., and Smith, A. D. (1987). Synaptic input and local output of dopaminergic neurons in grafts that functionally reinnervate the host neostriatum. *Exp. Brain Res.* 68: 131–146.

Borlongan, C. V., Tajima, Y., Trojanowski, J. Q., Lee, V. M.-Y., and Sanberg, P. R. (1998). Transplantation of cryopreserved human embryonic carcinoma-derived neurons (NT2N cells) promotes functional revcovery in ischemic rats. *Exp. Neurol.* 149: 310–321.

Bouvier, M. M., and Mytilineou, C. (1995). Basic fibroblast growth factor increases division and delays differentiation of dopamine precursors in vitro. *J. Neurosci.* 15: 7141–7149.

Bowers, W. J., Howard, D. F., and Federoff, H. J. (1997). Gene therapeutic strategies for neuroprotection: Implications for Parkinson's disease. *Exp. Neurol.* 144: 58–68.

Bray, G. M., Rasminsky, M., and Aguayo, A. J. (1981). Interactions between axons and their sheath cells. *Ann. Rev. Neurosci.* 4: 127–162.

Bray, G. M., Villegas-Perez, M. P., Vidal-Sanz, M., and Aguayo, A. J. (1987). The use of peripheral nerve grafts to enhance neuronal survival, promote growth and permit terminal reconnections in the central nervous system of adult rats. *J. Exp. Biol.* 132: 5–19.

Brecknell, J. E., Du, J. S., Muir, E., Fidler, P. S., Hlavin, M. L., Dunnett, S. B., and Fawcett, J. W. (1996). Bridge grafts of fibroblast growth factor–4-secreting schwannoma cells promote functional axonal regeneration in the nigrostriatal pathway of the adult rat. *Neuroscience* 74: 775–884.

Bredesen, D. E., Hisanaga, K., and Sharp, F. R. (1990). Neural transplantation using temperature-sensitive immortalized neural cells: A preliminary report. *Ann. Neurol.* 27: 205–207.

Bregman, B. S. (1994). Recovery of function after spinal cord injury: Transplantation strategies. In *Functional Neural Transplantation,* S. B. Dunnett and A. Bjorklund (eds.), pp. 489–529. Raven Press, New York.

Bregman, B. S., Bernstein-Goral, H., and Kunkel-Bagden, E. (1991). CNS transplants promote anatomical plasticity and recovery of function after spinal cord injury. *Res. Neurol. Neurosci.* 2: 327–338.

Bregman, B. S., Diener, P. S., McAtee, M., Dai, H. N., and James, C. (1997). Intervention strategies to enhance anatomical plasticity and recovery of function after spinal cord injury. *Adv. Neurol.* 72: 257–275.

Bregman, B. S., Kunkel-Bagden, E., Schnell, L., Dai, H. N., Gao, D., and Schwab, M. E. (1995). Recovery from spinal cord injury mediated by antibodies to neurite growth inhibitors. *Nature* 378: 498–501.

Bresler, D. E., and Bitterman, M. E. (1969). Learning in fish with transplanted brain tissue. *Science* 163: 590–592.

Brown, J. A. (1988). Statement by Mrs. Judie A. Brown, president, American Life League. In *Report of the Human Fetal Tissue Transplantation Research Panel, December 1988.* Vol. II, *Consultants to the Advisory Committee to the Director, National Institutes of Health,* pp. D37–D49.

Bruckner, M. K., and Arendt, T. (1992). Intracortical transplants of purified astrocytes ameliorate memory deficits in rats induced by chronic treatment with ethanol. *Neurosci. Letters* 141: 251–254.

Brundin, P., Barbin, G., Strecker, R. E., Isacson, O., Prochiantz, A., and Bjork-lund, A. (1988). Survival and function of dissociated rat dopaminergic neurons grafted at different developmental stages or after being cultured in vitro. *Dev. Brain Res.* 39: 233–293.

Brundin, P., Nilsson, O. G., Strecker, R. E., Lindvall, O., Astedt, B., and Bjork-lund, A. (1986). Behavioural effects of human fetal dopamine neurons grafted in a rat model of Parkinson's disease. *Exp. Brain Res.* 65: 235–240.

Brundin, P., Strecker, R. E., Clarke, D. J., Widner, H., Nilsson, O. G., Astedt, B., Lindvall, O., and Bjorklund, A. (1988). Can human fetal dopamine neuron grafts provide a therapy for Parkinson's disease? In *Transplantation into the Mammalian CNS,* D. M. Gash and J. R. Sladek, Jr. (eds.), pp. 441–448. Elsevier, Amsterdam. Prog. Brain Res. 78.

Brundin, P., Strecker, R. E., Widner, H., Clarke, D. J., Nilsson, O. G., Astedt, B., Lindvall, O., and Bjorklund, A. (1988). Human fetal dopamine neurons grafted in a rat model of Parkinson's disease: Immunological aspects, spontaneous and drug-induced behavior, and dopamine release. *Exp. Brain Res.* 70: 192–208.

Buchanan, J. T., and Nornes, H. O. (1986). Transplants of embryonic brainstem containing the locus coeruleus into spinal cord enhance the hindlimb flexion reflex in adult rats. *Brain Res.* 381: 225–236.

Buchser, E., Goddard, M., Heyd, B., Joseph, J. M., Favre, J., DeTrebolet, N., Lysacht, M., and Aebsicher, P. (1996). Immunoisolated xenogeneic chromaffin cell therapy for chronic pain: Initial clinical experience. *Anesthesiology* 85: 1005–1012.

Bunge, R. P. (1968). Glial cells and the central myelin sheath. *Physiol. Rev.* 48: 197–251.

Burns, R. S., Chiueh, C. C., Markey, S. P., Ebert, M. H., Jacobowitz, D. M., and Kopin, I. J. (1983). A primate model of parkinsonism: Selective destruction of the pars compacta of the substantia nigra by N-methyl–4-phenyl–1,2,3,6 tetrahy-dropyridine. *Proc. Natl. Acad. Sci. U.S.A.* 80: 4546–4550.

Caroni, P., and Schwab, M. E. (1988). Antibody against myelin-associated inhibi-tor of neurite growth neutralizes nonpermissive substrate properties of CNS white matter. *Neuron* 1: 85–96.

Carvey, P. M., Vu, T. Q., Ling, Z. D., Sortwell, C. E., Daley, B. F., and Collier, T. J. (1999). Dopamine progenitor cells can be clinically expanded and success-fully grafted in lesioned rats. *Program and Abstracts of the American Society for Neural Transplantation and Repair* 5/6: 28.

Cheng, H. (1996). Spinal cord repair strategies. Doctoral dissertation, Dept. of Neuroscience, Karolinska Institute, Stockholm.

Cheng, H., Almstrom, S., and Olson, L. (1995). Fibrin glue used as an adhesive agent in CNS tissues. *J. Neural Transplant. Plast.* 5: 233–244.

Cheng, H., Cao, Y., and Olson, L. (1996). Spinal cord repair in adult paraplegic rats: Partial restoration of hind limb function. *Science* 273: 510–513.

Cheng, H., and Olson, L. (1995). A new surgical technique that allows proximo-distal regeneration of 5-HT fibers after complete transection of the rat spinal cord. *Exp. Neurol.* 136: 149–161.

Cheng-Yuan, W., Xiu-Feng, B., Cheng, Z., and Qing-Lin, Z. (1992). Fetal tissue grafts for cerebellar atrophy in humans: A preliminary report. In *Surgery of the Spinal Cord,* R. N. N. Holtzman and B. M. Stein (eds.), pp. 219–234. Springer-Verlag, New York.

Choi, H. K., Won, L. A., Kontur, P. J., Hammond, D. N., Fox, A. P., Wainer, B. H., Hoffman, P. C., and Heller, A. (1991). Immortalization of embryonic mes-encephalic dopamine neurons by somatic cell fusion. *Brain Res.* 552: 67–86.

Choi-Lundberg, D. L., Lin, Q., Chang, Y.-N., Chiang, Y. L., Hay, C. M., Moha-jeri, H., Davidson, B. L., and Bohn, M. C. (1997). Dopaminergic neurons pro-tected from degeneration by GDNF gene therapy. *Science* 275: 838–841.

Clarke, D. J., Brundin, P., Strecker, R. E., Nilsson, O. G., Bjorklund, A., and Lindvall, O. (1988). Human fetal dopamine neurons grafted in a rat model of Parkinson's disease: Ultrastructural evidence for synapse formation using tyrosine hydroxylase immunocytochemistry. *Exp. Brain Res.* 73: 115–126.

Clough, R., Statnick, M., Maring-Smith, M., Wang, C., Eells, J., Browning, R., Dailey, J., and Jobe, P. (1996). Fetal raphe transplants reduce seizure severity in serotonin-depleted GEPRs. *Neuroreport* 8: 341–346.

Coffey, P. J., Lund, R. D., and Rawlins, J. N. P. (1989). Retinal transplant-mediated learning in a conditioned suppression test in rats. *Proc. Natl. Acad. Sci. U.S.A.* 86: 7248–7249.

Cohen, J. (1994). New fight over fetal tissue grafts. *Science* 263: 600–601.

Cooper, J. R., Bloom, F. E., and Roth, R. H. (1996). *The Biochemical Basis of Neuropharmacology.* Seventh ed. Oxford University Press, New York.

Coyle, J. T., and Schwarcz, R. (1976). Lesion of striatal neurones with kainic acid provides a model for Huntington's chorea. *Nature* 263: 244–246.

Craig, C. G., Tropepe, V., Morshead, C. M., Reynolds, B. A., Weiss, S., and van der Kooy, D. (1996). In vivo growth factor expansion of endogenous subependy-mal neural precursor cell populations in the adult mouse brain. *J. Neurosci.* 16: 2649–2658.

Crawford, G. D., Jr., Le, W.-D., Smith, R. G., Xie, W.-J., Stefani, E., and Appel, S. H. (1992). A novel N18Tg2 X mesencephalon cell hybrid expresses properties that suggest a dopaminergic cell line of substantia nigra origin. *J. Neurosci.* 12: 3392–3398.

Dahlstrom, A., and Fuxe, K. (1964). Evidence for the existence of monoamine-containing neurons in the central nervous system: I. Demonstration of mono-amines in the cell bodies of brain stem neurons. *Acta Physiol. Scand.* 62 (suppl. 232): 1–55.

The Dana Alliance for Brain Initiatives. (1995). *Delivering Results: A Progress Report on Brain Research.* Available from: Dana Alliance. 1001 G. St. N. W., Suite 1025, Washington, D.C., 20001.

Das, G. D. (1983). Neural transplantation in the spinal cord of adult rats. Conditions, survival, cytology and connectivity of the transplants. *J. Neurol. Sci.* 62: 191–210.

Das, G. D., and Altman, J. (1971). Transplanted precursors of nerve cells: Their fate in the cerebellums of young rats. *Science* 173: 637–638.

Date, I., Asari, S., and Ohmoto, T. (1995). Two-year follow-up study of a patient with Parkinson's disease and severe motor fluctuations treated by co-grafts of adrenal medulla and peripheral nerve into bilateral caudate nuclei: Case report. *Neurosurgery* 37: 515–519.

Date, I., Felten, S. Y., and Felten, D. L. (1990). Cografts of adrenal medulla with peripheral nerve enhance the survivability of transplanted adrenal chromaffin cells and recovery of the host nigrostriatal system in MPTP-treated young adult mice. *Brain Res.* 537: 33–39.

Date, I., Yohimoto, Y., Miyoshi, Y., Imaoka, T., Furuta, T., Asari, S., and Ohmoto, T. (1993). The influence of donor age on cografting of adrenal medulla with pretransected peripheral nerve. *Brain Res.* 624: 233–238.

Davidoff, L. M., and Ransohoff, J. (1948). Absence of spinal cord regeneration in the cat. *J. Neurophysiol.* 11: 9–11.

Davidson, B. L., Allen, E. D., Kozarski, K. F., Wilson, J. M., and Roessler, B. J. (1993). A model system for in vivo gene transfer into the central nervous system using an adenoviral vector. *Nature Genet.* 3: 219–223.

Davis, G. C., Williams, A. C., and Markey, S. P. (1979). Chronic parkinsonism secondary to intravenous injection of meperidine analogues. *Psychiatry Res.* 1: 249–254.

Deacon, T., Schumacher, J., Dinsmore, J., Thomas, C., Palmer, P., Kott, S., Edge, A., Penny, D., Kassissieh, S., Dempsey, P., and Isacson, O. (1997). Histological evidence of fetal pig neural cell survival after transplantation into a patient with Parkinson's disease. *Nature Medicine* 3: 350–353.

Deckel, A. W., Moran, T. H., Coyle, J. T., Sanberg, P. R., and Robinson, R. G. (1986). Anatomical predictors of behavioral recovery following striatal transplants. *Brain Res.* 365: 249–258.

Deckel, A. W., and Robinson, R. G. (1987). Receptor characteristics and behavioral consequences of kainic acid lesions and fetal transplants of the striatum. *Ann. N.Y. Acad. Sci.* 495: 556–580. *Cell and Tissue Transplantation into the Adult Brain*, E. C. Azmitia and A. Bjorklund (eds.).

Deckel, A. W., Robinson, R. G., Coyle, J. T., and Sanberg, P. R. (1983). Reversal of long-term locomotor abnormalities in the kainic acid model of Huntington's disease by day 18 fetal striatal transplants. *European J. Pharmacol.* 93: 287–288.

del Cerro, M. (1990). Retinal transplants. *Prog. Retina Res.* 9: 229–272.

del Cerro, M., Gash, D. M., Rao, G. N., Notter, M. F., Wiegand, S. J., and Gupta, M. (1985). Intraocular retinal transplants. *Invest. Ophthalmol. Vis. Sci.* 26: 1182–1185.

del Cerro, M., Gash, D. M., Rao, G. N., Notter, M. F., Wiegand, S. J., Sathi, S., and del Cerro, C. (1987). Retinal transplants into the anterior chamber of the rat eye. *Neuroscience* 21: 707–723.

del Cerro, M., Ison, J. R., Bowen, G. P., Lazar, E., and del Cerro, C. (1991). Intraretinal grafting restores visual function in light-blinded rats. *Neuroreport* 2: 529–532.

del Cerro, M., Das, T. P., Lazar, E., Jalali, S., DiLoreto, D., Jr., Little, C., Sreedharan, A., del Cerro, C., and Rao, G. N. (1996). Fetal neural retinal grafts into human retinitis pigmentosa. *Soc. Neurosci. Abs.* 131: 12.

del Cerro, M., Lazar, E. S., and Diloreto, D., Jr. (1997). The first decade of continuous progress in retinal transplantation. *Microsc. Res. Tech.* 36: 130–141.

Del Conte, G. (1907). Einpflanzungen von embryonalrem gewebe ins gehirn. *Beitrage zur Patholog. Anatomie* 42: 193–202.

Delgado, J. M. R. (1969). *Physical Control of the Mind.* Harper & Row, New York.

Diaz-Cintra, S., Rivas, P., Cintra, L., Aguilar, A., Gutierrez, G., Perez, E., Escobar, M., and Bermudez-Rattoni, F. (1995). Morphometric study of fetal brain transplants in the insular cortex and NGF effects on neuronal and glial development. *Cell Transplant* 4: 505–513.

Diener, P. S., and Bregman, B. S. (1998). Fetal spinal cord transplants support the development of target reaching and coordinated postural adjustments after neonatal cervical spinal cord injury. *J. Neurosci.* 18: 763–778.

DiLoreto, D., Jr., del Cerro, C., and del Cerro, M. (1996). Cyclosporine treatment promotes survival of human fetal neural retina transplanted to the subretinal space of the light-damaged Fisher 344 rat. *Exp. Neurol.* 140: 37–42.

Dobson, A. T., Margolis, T. P., Sedarati, F., Stevens, J. G., and Feldman, L. T. (1990). A latent, nonpathogenic HSV–1-derived vector stably expresses β-galactosidase in mouse neurons. *Neuron* 5: 353–360.

Dohan, F. C., Robertson, J. T., Feler, C., Schweitzer, J., Hall, C., and Robertson, J. H. (1988). Autopsy findings in a Parkinson's disease patient treated with adrenal medullary to caudate nucleus transplant. *Soc. Neurosci. Abs.* 14: 8.

Drasner, K., and Fields, H. F. (1988). Synergy between the antinociceptive effects of intrathecal clonidine and systemic morphine in the rat. *Pain* 32: 309–312.

Drucker-Colin, R., Aguilar-Roberlo, R., Garcia-Hernandez, F., Fernandez-Cancino, F., and Bermudez-Rattoni, F. (1984). Fetal suprachiasmatic nucleus transplants: Diurnal rhythm recovery of lesioned rats. *Brain Res.* 311: 353–357.

Drucker-Colin, R., Madrazo, I., Ostrosky-Solis, F., Shkurovich, M., Franco, R., and Torres, C. (1988). Adrenal medullary tissue transplants in the caudate nucleus of Parkinson's patients. In *Transplantation in the Mammalian CNS*, D. M. Gash and J. R. Sladek, Jr. (eds.), pp. 567–574. Elsevier, Amsterdam. Prog. Brain Res. 78.

Dubach, M., and German, D. C. (1990). Extensive survival of chromaffin cells in adrenal medulla "ribbon" grafts in the monkey neostriatum. *Exp. Neurol.* 110: 167–180.

Duncan, I. D. (1996). Glial cell transplantation and remyelination of the central nervous system. *Neuropathol. Appl. Neurobiol.* 22: 87–100.

Dunn, E. H. (1917). Primary and secondary findings in a series of attempts to transplant cerebral cortex in the albino rat. *J. Comp. Neurol.* 27: 565–582.

Dunnett, S. B., and Bjorklund, A. (1984). Exploring dopamine function with nigral transplants. *IBRO News* 11: 17–22.

Dunnett, S. B., Bjorklund, A., Schmidt, R. H., Stenevi, U., and Iversen, S. D. (1983a). Intracerebral grafting of neuronal cell suspensions. IV. Behavioral recovery in rats with unilateral 6–OHDA lesions following implantation of nigral cell suspensions in different forebrain sites. *Acta Physiol. Scand. suppl.* 522: 29–37.

Dunnett, S. B., Bjorklund, A., Schmidt, R. H., Stenevi, U., and Iversen, S. D. (1983b). Intracerebral grafting of neuronal cell suspensions. V. Behavioural recovery in rats with bilateral 6–OHDA lesions following implantation of nigral cell suspensions. *Acta Physiol. Scand. Suppl.* 522: 39–47.

Dunnett, S. B., Bjorklund, A., Stenevi, U., and Iversen, S. D. (1981a). Behavioural recovery following transplantation of substantia nigra in rats subjected to 6–OHDA lesions of the nigrostriatal pathway. I. Unilateral lesions. *Brain Res.* 215: 147–161.

Dunnett, S. B., Bjorklund, A., Stenevi, U., and Iversen, S. D. (1981b). Grafts of embryonic substantia nigra reinnervating the ventrolateral striatum ameliorate sensorimotor deficits in rats with 6–OHDA lesions of the nigrostriatal pathway. *Brain Res.* 229: 209–217.

Dunnett, S. B., Hernandez, T. D., Summerfield, A., Jones, G. H., and Arbuthnott, G. (1988). Graft-derived recovery from 6–OHDA lesions: Specificity of ventral mesencephalic graft tissues. *Exp. Brain Res.* 71: 411–424.

Dunnett, S. B., Isacson, O., Sirinathsinghji, D. J. S., Clark, D. J., and Bjorklund, A. (1988). Striatal grafts in rats with unilateral neostriatal lesions: III. Recovery from dopamine-dependent motor asymmetry and deficits in skilled paw reaching. *Neuroscience* 24: 813–820.

Dunnett, S. B., Rogers, D.C., and Richards, S.-J. (1989). Nigrostriatal reconstruction after 6–OHDA lesions in rats: Combination of dopamine-rich nigral grafts and nigrostriatal "bridge" grafts. *Exp. Brain Res.* 75: 523–535.

Dunnett, S. B., Ryan, C. N., Levin, P. D., Reynolds, M., and Bunch, S. T. (1987). Functional consequences of embryonic neocortex transplanted to rats with prefrontal cortex lesions. *Behav. Neurosci.* 101: 489–503.

Dunnett, S. B., Whishaw, I. Q., Rogers, D.C., and Jones, G. H. (1987). Dopamine-rich grafts ameliorate whole body motor asymmetry and sensory neglect but not independent limb use in rats with 6-hydroxydopamine lesions. *Brain Res.* 415: 63–88.

Dymecki, J., Poltorak, M., and Freed, W. J. (1990). The degree of genetic disparity between donor and host correlates with survival of intraventricular substantia nigra grafts. *Regional Immunol.* 3: 17–22.

Eaton, M. J., Lopez, T. F., Frydel, B. R., Martinez, M. A., and Sagen, J. (1999). Transplants of immortalized chromaffin cells for neuropathic pain. *Program and Abstracts of the American Society for Neural Transplantation and Repair* 5/6: 55.

Eaton, M. J., Plunkett, J. A., Martinez, M. A., Lopez, T., Karmally, S., Cejas, P., and Whittemore, C. R. (1999). Transplants of neuronal cells bioengineered to synthesize GABA alleviate chronic neuropathic pain. *Cell Transplant.* 8: 87–101.

Eaton M. J., Santiago, D. I., Dancausse, H. A., and Whittemore, S. R. (1997). Lumbar transplants of immortalized serotonergic neurons alleviate chronic neuropathic pain. *Pain* 72: 59–69.

Editorial. (1972). Psychosurgery. *Lancet,* July 8, pp. 69–80.

Eilam, R., Malach, R., Bergman, F., and Segal, M. (1991). Hypertension induced by fetal hypothalamic transplantation from genetically hypertensive to normotensive rats. *J. Neurosci.* 11: 401–411.

Emerich, D. F., Cain, C. K., Greco, C., Saydoff, J. A., Hu, Z. Y., Liu, H., and Lidner, M. D. (1997). Cellular delivery of human CNTF prevents motor and cognitive dysfunction in a rodent model of Huntington's disase. *Cell Transplant.* 6: 249–266.

Emerich, D. F., Hammang, J. P., Baetge, E. E., and Winn, S. R. (1994). Implantation of polymer-encapsulated human nerve growth factor-secreting fibroblasts attenuates the behavioral and neuropathological consequences of quinolinic acid injections into rodent striatum. *Exp. Neurol.* 130: 141–150.

Emerich, D. F., Lidner, M. D., Winn, S. R., Chen, E. Y., Frydel, B. R., and Kordower, J. H. (1996). Implants of encapsulated human CNTF-producing fibroblasts prevent behavioral deficits and striatal degeneration in a rodent model of Huntington's disease. *J. Neurosci.* 16: 5168–5181.

Emerich, D. F., Winn, S. R., Hantraye, P. M., Peschanski, M., Chen, E. Y., Chu, Y., McDermott, P., Baetge, E. E., and Kordower, J. H. (1997). Protective effect of encapsulated cells producing neurotrophic factor CNTF in a monkey model of Huntington's disease. *Nature* 386: 395–399.

Ernfors, P., Ebendal, T., Olson, L., Mouton, P., Stromberg, I., and Persson, H. (1989). A cell line producing recombinant nerve growth factor evokes growth responses in intrinsic and grafted central cholinergic neurons. *Proc. Natl. Acad. Sci. U.S.A.* 86: 4756–4760.

Ervin, F. R., and Mark, V. H. (1969). Behavioral and affective responses to brain stimulation in man. In *Neurobiological Aspects of Psychopathology,* J. Zubin and C. Shagass (eds.), pp. 54–65. Grune and Stratton, New York.

Escobar, M., Fernandez, J., Guevara-Aguilar, R., and Bermudez-Rattoni, F. (1989). Fetal brain grafts induce recovery of learning deficits and connectivity in rats with gustatory neocortical lesion. *Brain Res.* 478: 368–374.

Everett, N. B., Sundsten, J. W., and Lund, R. D. (1971). *Functional Neuroanatomy*, 6th ed. Lea & Febiger, Philadelphia.

Fackelmann, K. (1998). Stroke rescue: Can cells injected into the brain reverse paralysis? *Sci. News* 154: 120–122.

Fazzini, E., Dwork, A. J., Blum, C., Burke, R., Cote, L., Goodman, R. R., Jacobs, T. P., Naini, A. B., Pezzoli, G., Pullman, S., et al. (1991). Stereotaxic implantation of autologous adrenal medulla into caudate nucleus in four patients with parkinsonism. One-year follow-up. *Arch. Neurol.* 48: 813–820.

Federoff, H. J., Brooks, A., Muhkerjee, B., and Corden, T. (1997). Somatic gene transfer approaches to manipulate neural networks. *J. Neurosci. Meth.* 71: 133–142.

Federoff, H. J., Geschwind, M. D., Geller, A. I., and Kessler, J. A. (1992). Expression of nerve growth factor in vivo from a defective herpes simplex virus I vector prevents effects of axotomy on sympathetic ganglia. *Proc. Natl. Acad. Sci. U.S.A.* 89: 1636–1640.

Fernandez-Ruiz, J., Escobar, M. L., Pina, A. L., Diaz-Cintra, S., Cintra-McClone, F. L., and Bermudez-Rattoni, F. (1991). Time-dependent recovery of taste aversion learning by fetal brain transplants in gustatory neocortex-lesioned rats. *Behav. Neural Biol.* 55: 179–193.

Ferrari, F. K., Xiao, X., McCarty, D., and Samulski, R. J. (1997). New developments in the generation of Ad-free, high-titer rAAV gene therapy vectors. *Nat. Med.* 3: 1295–1297.

Fiandaca, M. S., Kordower, J. H., Hansen, J. T., Jiao, S.-S., and Gash, D. M. (1988). Adrenal medullary autografts into the basal ganglia of cebus monkeys: Injury-induced regeneration. *Exp. Neurol.* 102: 76–91.

Finch, C. (1985). Comments on review by Gash et al.: Applications of recombinant DNA techniques. *Neurobiol. Aging* 6: 156–158.

Fine, A., Hunt, S. P., Oertel, W. H., Nomoto, M., Chuong, P. N., Bond, A., Waters, C., Temlett, J. A., Annett, L., Dunnett, S., Jenner, P., and Marsden, C. D. (1988). Transplantation of embryonic marmoset dopaminergic neurons to the corpus striatum of marmosets rendered parkinsonian by l-methyl–4-phenyl–1,2,3,6-tetrahydropyridine. In *Transplantation in the Mammalian CNS*, D. M. Gash and J. R. Sladek, Jr. (eds.), pp. 479–489. Elsevier, Amsterdam. Prog. Brain Res. 78.

Fisher, L. J., Jinnah, H. A., Kale, L. C., Higgins, G. A., and Gage, F. H. (1991). Survival and function of intrastriatal grafts of primary fibroblasts genetically modified to produce L-DOPA. *Neuron* 6: 371–380.

Flax, J. D., Aurora, S., Yang, C., Simonin, C., Willis, A. M., Billinghurst, L. L., Jendoubi, M., Sidman, R. L., Wolfe, J. H., Kim, S. U., and Snyder, E. Y. (1998). Engraftable human neural stem cells respond to developmental cues, replace neurons, and express foreign genes. *Nature Biotechnol.* 16: 1–7.

Foley, K. M., and Yaksh, T. L. (1993). Another call for patience instead of patients: Developing novel therapies for chronic pain. *Anesthesiology* 79: 637–640.

Folkerth, R. D., and Durso, R. (1996). Survival and proliferation of nonneural tissues, with obstruction of cerebral ventricles, in a parkinsonian patient treated with fetal allografts. *Neurology* 46: 1219–1225.

Folstein, S. E. (1989). *Huntington's Disease.* Johns Hopkins University Press, Baltimore.

Forno, L. S., and Langston, J. W. (1989). Adrenal medullary transplant to the brain for Parkinson's disease. Neuropathological report of an unsuccessful case. *J. Neuropathol. Exp. Neurol.* 48: 339.

Forssberg, H., and Grillner, S. (1973). The locomotion of the acute spinal cat injected with clonidine i.v. *Brain Res.* 50: 184–186.

Forssman, J. (1900). Zur kenntniss des neurotropismus. *Beitrage zur Patholog. Anat.* 27: 407–430.

Frankensteins "R" Us. (1998). *Time,* May 11, p. 19.

Freed, C. R., Breeze, R. E., Greene, P. E., Tsai, W.-Y., Eidelberg, D., Trojanowski, J. O., Rosenstein, J. M., and Fahn, S. (1999). Double-blind controlled trial of human embryonic dopamine cell transplants in advanced Parkinson's disease. *Program and Abstracts of the American Society for Neural Transplantation and Repair* 5/6: 20.

Freed, C. R., Breeze, R. E., Leehey, M. A., Schneck, S. A., O'Brien, C. F., Thompson, L. L., Ramig, L. O., McRae, C. A., Mazziotta, J. C., Miletich, R. S., and Eidelberg, D. (1998). Ten years experience with fetal neurotransplantation in patients with advanced Parkinson's disease. *Soc. Neurosci. Abs.* 24: 559.

Freed, C. R., Breeze, R. E., Rosenberg, N. L., Schneck, S. A., Kriek, E., Qi, J.-X., Lone, T., Zhang, Y.-B., Snyder, J. A., Wells, T. H., Ramig, L. O., Thompson, L., Mazziotta, J. C., Huang, S. C., Grafton, S. T., Brooks, D., Sawle, G., Schroter, G., and Ansari, A. A. (1992). Survival of implanted fetal dopamine cells and neurologic improvement 12 to 46 months after transplantation for Parkinson's disease. *New Eng. J. Med.* 327: 1549–1555.

Freed, C. R., Breeze, R. E., Rosenberg, N. L., Schneck, S. A., Schroter, G., Lafferty, K., Talmage, D. W., Barrett, J. N., Wells, T., Mazziotta, J. C., Huang, S. C., Eidelberg, D., and Rottenberg, D. A. (1991). Fetal neural implants for Parkinson's disease: Results at 15 months. In *Intracerebral Transplantation in Movement Disorders,* O. Lindvall, A. Bjorklund, and H. J. Widner (eds.), pp. 69–77. Elsevier, Amsterdam.

Freed, C. R., Breeze, R. E., Rosenberg, N. L., Schneck, S. A., Wells, T. H., Barrett, J. N., Grafton, S. T., Huang, S. C., Eidelberg, D., and Rottenberg, D. A. (1990). Transplantation of human fetal dopamine cells for Parkinson's disease: Results at 1 year. *Arch. Neurol.* 47: 505–512.

Freed, C. R., Richards, J. B., Hutt, C. J., Kriek, E. H., and Reite, M. L. (1988). Rejection of fetal substantia nigra allografts in monkeys with MPTP-induced Parkinson's syndrome. *Soc. Neurosci. Abs.* 14: 9.

Freed, C. R., Richards, J. B., Sabol, K. E., and Reite, M. L. (1988). Fetal substantia nigra transplants lead to dopamine cell replacement and behavioral improvement in Bonnet monkeys with MPTP-induced Parkinsonism. In *Pharmacology and Functional Regulation of Dopaminergic Neurons*, P. M. Beart, G. Woodruff, and D. M. Jackson (eds.), pp. 353–360. Macmillan, New York.

Freed, W. J. (1983). Functional brain tissue transplantation: Reversal of lesion-induced rotation by intraventricular substantia nigra and adrenal medulla grafts, with a note on intracranial retinal grafts. *Biol. Psychiat.* 18: 1205–1267.

Freed, W. J. (1985). Repairing neuronal circuits with brain grafts: Where can brain grafts be used as a therapy? *Neurobiol. Aging* 6: 153–156.

Freed, W. J. (1990). Fetal brain grafts and Parkinson's disease. *Science* 250: 1434.

Freed, W. J. (1991a). Comments on brain tissue transplantation without immunosuppression. *Arch. Neurol.* 48: 259–260.

Freed, W. J. (1991b). Editorial: Brain tissue grafting and human applications. *J. Neurosurg. Anesthesiol.* 3: 167–169.

Freed, W. J. (1993). Neural transplantation: Prospects for clinical use. *Cell Transplant.* 2: 13–31.

Freed, W. J. (1994). Tissue transplants for Parkinson's disease. "Special correspondence." *Neurology* 44: 573–577.

Freed, W. J., and Cannon-Spoor, H. E. (1988). Cortical lesions increase reinnervation of the dorsal striatum by substantia nigra grafts. *Brain Res.* 446: 133–143.

Freed, W. J., and Cannon-Spoor, H. E. (1989). Cortical lesions interfere with behavioral recovery from unilateral substantia nigra lesions induced by brain grafts. *Behav. Brain Res.* 32: 279–288.

Freed, W. J., Cannon-Spoor, H. E., and Krauthamer, E. (1985). Intrastriatal adrenal medulla grafts in rats: Long-term survival and behavioral effects. *J. Neurosurg.* 65: 664–670.

Freed, W. J., de Medinaceli, L., and Wyatt, R. J. (1985). Promoting functional plasticity in the damaged nervous system. *Science* 227: 1544–1552.

Freed, W. J., Geller, H. M., Poltorak, M., Cannon-Spoor, H. E., Cottingham, S. L., Lamarca, M. E., Schultzberg, M., Rehavi, M., Paul, S., and Ginns, E. I. (1990). Genetically altered and defined cell lines for transplantation in animal models of Parkinson's disease. In *Proceeedings of the IIIrd International Symposium on Neural Transplantation*, S. B. Dunnett and S. J. Richards (eds.), pp. 11–21. Elsevier, Amsterdam. Prog. Brain Res. 82.

Freed, W. J., Karoum, F., Spoor, H. E., Morihisa, J. M., Olson, L., and Wyatt, R. J. (1983). Catecholamine content of intracerebral adrenal medulla grafts. *Brain Res.* 269: 184–189.

Freed, W. J., Ko, G. N., Niehoff, D. L., Kuhar, M. J., Hoffer, B. J., Olson, L., Cannon-Spoor, H. E., Morihisa, J. M., and Wyatt, R. J. (1983). Normalization of spiroperidol binding in the denervated rat striatum by homologous grafts of substantia nigra. *Science* 222: 937–939.

Freed, W. J., Morihisa, J., Spoor, E., Hoffer, B., Olson, L., Seiger, A., and Wyatt, R. J. (1981). Transplanted adrenal chromaffin cells in rat brain reduce lesion-induced rotational behavior. *Nature* 292: 351–352.

Freed, W. J., Olson, L., Ko, G. N., Morihisa, J. M., Niehoff, D., Stromberg, I., Kuhar, M., Hoffer, B. J., and Wyatt, R. J. (1985). Intraventricular substantia nigra and adrenal medulla grafts: Mechanisms of action and [3H]spiroperidol autoradiography. In *Neural Grafting in the Mammalian CNS*, A. Bjorklund and U. Stenevi (eds.), pp. 471–489. Elsevier, Amsterdam.

Freed, W. J., Perlow, M. J., Karoum, F., Seiger, A., Olson, L., Hoffer, B. J., and Wyatt, R. (1980). Restoration of dopaminergic function by grafting of fetal rat substantia nigra to the caudate nucleus: Long term behavioral, biochemical, and histochemical studies. *Ann. Neurol.* 8: 510–519.

Freed, W. J., Poltorak, M., and Becker, J. B. (1990). Intracerebral adrenal medulla grafts: A review. *Exp. Neurol.* 110: 139–166.

Freeman, T. B., Deacon, T., Cicchetti, F., Hauser, R., and Sanberg, P. (1999). Histological evaluation of human fetal striatal transplants in a patient with Huntington's disease. *Program and Abstracts of the American Society for Neural Transplantation and Repair 5/6*: 21.

Freeman, T. B., Olanow, C. W., Hauser, R. A., Nauert, G. M., Smith, D. A., Borlongan, C. V., Sanberg, P. R., Holt, D. A., Kordower, J. H., Vingerhoets, F. J. G., Snow, B. J., Calne, D., and Gauger, L. L. (1995). Bilateral fetal nigral transplantation into the postcommissural putamen in Parkinson's disease. *Ann. Neurol.* 38: 379–388.

Freeman, T. B., Sanberg, P. R., Nauert, G. M., Boss, B. D., Spector, D., Olanow, C. W., and Kordower, J. H. (1995). Influence of donor age on the survival of solid and suspension intraparenchymal human embryonic nigral grafts. *Cell Transplant.* 4: 141–154.

Freeman, T. B., Spence, M. S., Boss, B. D., Spector, D. H., Strecker, R. E., Olanow, C. W., and Kordower, J. H. (1991). Development of dopaminergic neurons in the human substantia nigra. *Exp. Neurol.* 113: 344–353.

Freeman, T. B., Wojak, J. C., Brandeis, L., Michel, J. P., Pearson, J., and Flamm, E. S. (1988). Cross-species intracerebral grafting of embryonic swine dopaminergic neurons. In *Transplantation in the Mammalian CNS*, D. M. Gash and J. R. Sladek, Jr. (eds.), pp. 473–477. Elsevier, Amsterdam. Prog. Brain Res. 78.

Freund, T. F., Bolam, J. P., Bjorklund, A., Stenevi, U., Dunnett, S. B., Powell, J. F., and Smith, A. D. (1985). Efferent synaptic connections of grafted dopaminergic neurons reinnervating the host neostriatum: A tyrosine hydroxylase immunocytochemical study. *J. Neurosci.* 5: 603–616.

Frim, D. M., Short, M. P., Rosenberg, W. S., Simpson, J., Breakefield, X. O., and Isacson, O. (1993). Local protective effects of nerve growth factor-secreting fibroblasts against excitotoxic lesions in the rat striatum. *J. Neurosurg.* 78: 267–273.

Frim, D. M., Simpson, J., Uhler, T. A., Short, M. P., Bossi, S. R., Breakefield, X. O., and Isacson, O. (1993). Striatal degeneration induced by mitochondrial blockade is prevented by biologically delivered NGF. *J. Neurosci. Res.* 35: 452–458.

Gage, F. H., Coates, P. W., Palmer, T. D., Kuhn, H. G., Fisher, L. J., Suhonen, J. O., Peterson, D. A., Suhr, S. T., and Ray, J. (1995). Survival and differentiation of adult neuronal progenitor cells transplanted to the adult brain. *Proc. Natl. Acad. Sci. U.S.A.* 92: 11879–11883.

Gage, F. H., Wolff, J. A., Rosenberg, M. B., Xu, L., Yee, J.-K., Shults, C., and Friedmann, T. (1987). Grafting genetically modified cells to the brain: Possibilities for the future. *Neuroscience* 23: 795–807.

Gash, D. M. (1984). Neural transplants in mammals: A historical overview. In *Neural Transplants: Development and Function,* J. R. Sladek and D. M. Gash (eds.), pp. 1–12. Plenum Press, New York.

Gash, D. M., Notter, M. F. D., Okawara, S. H., Kraus, A. L., and Joynt, R. J. (1986). Amitotic neuroblastoma cells used for neural implants in monkeys. *Science* 233: 1420–1422.

Gash, D. M., Sladek, J. R., Jr., and Sladek, C. D. (1980). Functional development of grafted vasopressin neurons. *Science* 210: 1367–1369.

Gash, D. M., Zhang, Z., Cass, W. A., Oviada, A., Simmerman, L., Martin, D., Russell, D., Collins, F., Hoffer, B. J., and Gerhardt, G. A. (1995). Morphological and functional effects of intranigrally administered GDNF in normal rhesus monkeys. *J. Comp. Neurol.* 363: 345–358.

Gash, D. M., Zhang, Z., Oviada, A., Cass, W. A., Yi, A., Simmerman, L., Russell, D., Martin, D., Lapchak, P. A., Collins, F., Hoffer, B. J., and Gerhardt, G. A. (1996). Functional recovery in parkinsonian monkeys treated with GDNF. *Nature* 380: 252–255.

Geller, A. I., Keyomarski, K., Bryan, J., and Pardee, A. B. (1990). An efficient deletion mutant packaging system for defective HSV–1 vectors: Potential applications to neuronal physiology and human gene therapy. *Proc. Natl. Acad. Sci. U.S.A.* 87: 8950–8954.

Geller, H. M., and Dubois-Dalcq, M. (1988). Antigenic and functional characterization of a rat central nervous system-derived cell line immortalized by a retroviral vector. *J. Cell. Biol.* 107: 1977–1986.

Geller, H. M., Quinones-Jenab, V., Poltorak, M., and Freed, W. J. (1991). Applications of immortalized cells in basic and clinical neurology. *J. Cell. Biochem.* 45: 279–283.

Gervais, K. G., Vawter, D. E., and Caplan, A. L. (1992). Fetal tissue guidelines depart from the cadaver donor framework. *J. Neural Transplant. Plast.* 3: 259–260.

Gibson, M. J., Krieger, D. T., Charlton, H. M., Zimmerman, E. A., Silverman, A. J., and Perlow, M. J. (1984). Mating and pregnancy can occur in genetically hypogonadal mice with preoptic area brain grafts. *Science* 225: 949–951.

Giordano, M., Ford, L. M., Shipley, M. T., and Sanberg, P. R. (1990). Neural grafts and pharmacological intervention in a model of Huntington's disease. *Brain Res. Bull.* 25: 453–465.

Giordano, M., Hagenmeyer-Houser, S. H., and Sanberg, P. R. (1988). Intraparenchymal fetal striatal transplants and recovery in kainic acid lesioned rats. *Brain Res.* 446: 183–188.

Giordano, M., Takashima, H., Herranz, A., Poltorak, M., Geller, H. M., Marone, M., and Freed, W. J. (1993). Immortalized GABAergic cell lines derived from rat striatum using a temperature-sensitive allele of the SV40 large T antigen. *Exp. Neurol.* 124: 395–400.

Giordano, M., Takashima, H., Poltorak, M., Geller, H. M., and Freed, W. J. (1994). Development of immortalized cell lines for transplantation in central nervous system injury and degeneration models. In *Providing Pharmacological Access to the Brain: Alternate Approaches,* T. R. Flanagan, D. F. Emerich, and S. R. Winn (eds.), pp. 308–325. Academic Press, New York.

Giordano, M., Takashima, H., Poltorak, M., Geller, H. M., and Freed, W. J. (1996). Constitutive expression of glutamic acid decarboxylase (GAD) by striatal cell lines immortalized using the tsA58 allele of the SV40 large T antigen. *Cell Transplant.* 5: 563–575.

Goddard, G. V., McIntyre, D.C., and Leech, C. K. (1969). A permanent change in brain function resulting from daily electrical stimulation. *Exp. Neurol.* 25: 295–330.

Goetz, C. G., Olanow, C. W., Koller, W. C., Penn, R. D., Cahill, D., Morantz, R., Stebbins, G., Tanner, C. M., Klawans, H. L., Shannon, K. M., Comella, C. L., Witt, T., Cox, C., Waxman, M., and Gauger, L. (1989). Multicenter study of autologous adrenal medullary transplantation of the corpus striatum in patients with advanced Parkinson's disease. *N. Eng. J. Med.* 320: 337–341.

Goetz, C. G., Stebbins G. T. III, Klawans, H. L., Koller, W. C., Grossman, R. G., Bakay, R. A. E., and Penn, R. D., and the United Parkinson Foundation Neural Transplantation Registry. (1991). United Parkinson Foundation neurotransplantation registry on adrenal medullary transplants: Presurgical, and 1- and 2-year follow-up. *Neurology* 41: 1719–1722.

Goetz, C. G., Tanner, C. M., Penn, R. D., Stebbins, G. T., Gilley, D. W., Shannon, K. M., Klawans, H. L., Comella, C. L., Wilson, R. S., and Witt, T. (1990). Adrenal medullary transplant to the striatum of patients with advanced Parkinson's disease: 1-year motor and psychomotor data. *Neurology* 40: 273–276.

Goldsmith, H. S., Steward, E., Chen, W. F., and Duckett, S. (1983). Application of intact omentum to the normal and traumatized spinal cord. In *Spinal Cord Reconstruction,* C. C. Kao, R. P. Bunge, and P. J. Reier (eds.), pp. 235–244. Raven Press, New York.

Goodfellow, P. N. (1993). Planting alfalfa and cloning the Huntington's disease gene. *Cell* 72: 817–818.

Gouras, P., and Algvere, P. (1996). Retinal cell transplantation in the macula: New techniques. *Vision Res.* 36: 4121–4125.

Greene, H. S. N., and Arnold, H. (1945). The homologous and heterologous transplantation of brain and brain tumors. *J. Neurosurg.* 2: 315–321.

Greene, L. A., and Tischler, A. S. (1976). Establishment of a noradrenergic clonal line of rat adrenal pheochromocytoma cells which respond to nerve growth factor. *Proc. Natl. Acad. Sci. U.S.A.* 73: 2424–2428.

Grossman, S. P. (1979). The biology of motivation. *Ann. Rev. Psychol.* 30: 209–242.

Grothe, C., Hofmann, H.-D., Verhofstad, A. A. J., and Unsicker, K. (1985). Nerve growth factor and dexamethasone specify the catecholaminergic phenotype of cultured rat chromaffin cells: Dependence on developmental stage. *Dev. Brain Res.* 21: 125–132.

Groves, A. K., Barnett, S. C., Franklin, R. J. M., Crang, A. J., Mayer, M., Blakemore, W. F., and Noble, M. (1993). Repair of demyelinated lesions by transplantation of purified O–2A progenitor cells. *Nature* 362: 453–455.

Halasz, B., Pupp, L., Uhlarik, S., and Tima, L. (1965). Further studies on the hormone secretion of the anterior pituitary transplanted into the hypophysiotrophic area of the rat hypothalamus. *Endocrinology* 77: 343–355.

Hama, A. T., and Sagen, J. (1993). Reduced pain-related behavior by adrenal medullary transplants in rats with peripheral neuropathy. *Pain* 52: 223–231.

Hantraye, P., Riche, D., Maziere, M., and Isacson, O. (1992). Intrastriatal transplantation of cross-species fetal striatal cells reduced abnormal movements in a primate model of Huntington disease. *Proc. Natl. Acad. Sci. U.S.A.* 89: 4187–4191.

Harrison, R. G. (1929). Correlation in the development and growth of the eye studied by means of heterotopic transplantation. *Arch. Entw. Mech. Org.* 120: 1–55.

Harrison, R. G. (1933–1934). Heteroplastic grafting in embryology. *The Harvey Lectures 1933–1934,* ser. no. 29: 116–157.

Harwood, D. D., Hanumanthu, S., and Stoudemire, A. (1992). Pathophysiology and management of phantom limb pain. *Gen. Hospital Psychiatry* 14: 107–118.

Hayflick, J. (1965). The limited in vitro lifetime of diploid cell strains. *Exp. Cell Res.* 37: 614–636.

Heath, R. G. (1963). Electrical self-stimulation of the brain in man. *Am. J. Psychiat.* 120: 571–577.

Heath, R. G. (ed.). (1964). *The Role of Pleasure in Behavior.* Hoeber Press, New York.

Hefti, F. (1986). Nerve growth factor promotes survival of septal cholinergic neurons after fimbrial transections. *J. Neurosci.* 6: 2155–2162.

Hefti, F., Dravid, A., and Hartikka, J. (1984). Chronic intraventricular injections of nerve growth factor elevate hippocampal choline acetyltransferase activity in adult rats with partial septo-hippocampal lesions. *Brain Res.* 293: 305–311.

Henderson, B. T. H., Clough, C. G., Hughes, R. C., Hitchcock, E. R., and Kenny, B. G. (1991). Implantation of human fetal ventral mesencephalon to the right caudate nucleus in advanced Parkinson's disease. *Arch. Neurol.* 48: 822–827.

Hirsch, E. C., Duyckaerts, C., Javoy-Agid, F., Hauw, J.-J., and Agid, Y. (1990). Does adrenal graft enhance recovery of dopaminergic neurons in Parkinson's disease? *Ann. Neurol.* 27: 676–682.

Hitchcock, E. R., Clough, C. G., Hughes, R. C., and Kenny, B. G. (1988). Embryos and Parkinson's disease. *Lancet* 1: 1274.

Hitchcock, E. R., Henderson, B. T. H., Kenny, B. G., Clough, C. G., Hughes, R. C., and Detta, A. (1991). Stereotaxic implantation of foetal mesencephalon. In *Intracerebral Transplantation in Movement Disorders,* O. Lindvall, A. Bjorklund, and H. Widner (eds.), pp. 79–86. Elsevier, Amsterdam.

Hitchcock, E. R., Kenny, B. G., Clough, C. G., Hughes, R. C., Henderson, B. T. H., and Detta, A. (1990). Stereotaxic implantation of foetal mesencephalon (STIM): The UK experience. In *Neural Transplantation: From Molecular Basis to Clinical Applications,* S. B. Dunnett and S.-J. Richards (eds.), pp. 723–728. Elsevier, Amsterdam. Prog. Brain Res. 82.

Hitchcock, E. R., Whitwell, H. L., Sofroniew, M. Y., and Bankiewicz, K. S. (1994). Survival of TH-positive and neuromelanin-containing cells in patients with Parkinson's disease after intrastriatal grafting of fetal ventral mesencephalon. In American Society for Neural Transplantation, *Program and Abstracts of the First Annual Conference,* vol. 1, p. 28, abstract S33. (*Exp. Neurol.* 129: 3.)

Hoehn, M. D., and Yahr, M. M. (1967). Parkinsonism: Onset, progression, and mortality. *Neurology* 17: 427–442.

Horellou, P., Brundin, P., Kalen, P., Mallet, J., and Bjorklund, A. (1990). In vivo release of DOPA and dopamine from genetically engineered cells grafted to the denervated rat striatum. *Neuron* 5: 393–402.

Horellou, P., Guibert, B., Leviel, V., and Mallet, J. (1989). Retroviral transfer of a human tyrosine hydroxylase cDNA in various cell lines: Regulated release of dopamine in mouse anterior pituitary AtT–20 cells. *Proc. Natl. Acad. Sci. U.S.A.* 86: 7233–7237.

Horellou, P., Marlier, L., Privat, A., and Mallet, J. (1990). Behavioral effect of engineered cells that synthesize L-DOPA or dopamine after grafting into the rat neostriatum. *Eur. J. Neurosci.* 2: 116–119.

Horellou, P., Sabate, O., Buc-Caron, M. H., and Mallet, J. (1997). Adenovirus-mediated gene transfer to the central nervous system for Parkinson's disease. *Exp. Neurol.* 144: 131–138.

Hornykiewicz, O. (1966). Metabolism of brain dopamine in human parkinsonism: Neurochemical and clinical aspects. In *Biochemistry and Pharmacology of the Basal Ganglia,* E. Costa, L. J. Cote, and M. D. Yahr (eds.), pp. 171–181. Hewlett Press, New York.

Hoshimaru, M., Ray, J., Sah, D. W., and Gage, F. H. (1996). Differentiation of the immortalized adult neuronal progenitor cell line HC2S2 into neurons by regulatable suppression of the v-myc oncogene. *Proc. Natl. Acad. Sci. U.S.A.* 20: 1518–1523.

Houle, J. D. (1991). Demonstration of the potential for chronically injured neurons to regenerate axons into intraspinal peripheral nerve grafts. *Exp. Neurol.* 113: 1–9.

Howland, D. R., Bregman, B. S., Tessler, A., and Goldberger, M. E. (1995). Transplants enhance locomotion in neonatal kittens whose spinal cords are transected: A behavioral and anatomical study. *Exp. Neurol.* 135: 123–145.

The Huntington's Disease Collaborative Research Group. (1993). A novel gene containing a trinucleotide repeat that is expanded and unstable on Huntington's disease chromosomes. *Cell* 72: 971–983.

Hurtig, H., Joyce, J., Sladek, J. R., and Trojanowski, J. Q. (1989). Postmortem analysis of adrenal-medulla-to-caudate autograft in a patient with Parkinson's disease. *Ann. Neurol.* 25: 607–614.

Hynes, M., Porter, J. A., Chiang, C., Chang, D., Tessier-Lavigne, M., Beachy, P. A., and Rosenthal, A. (1995). Induction of midbrain dopaminergic neurons by Sonic hedgehog. *Neuron* 15: 35–44.

Hynes, M., Poulsen, K., Tessier-Lavigne, M., and Rosenthal, A. (1995). Control of neuronal diversity by the floor plate: Contact-mediated induction of midbrain dopaminergic neurons. *Cell* 80: 95–101.

Iadarola, M. J., and Gale, K. (1982). Substantia nigra: Site of anticonvulsant activity mediated by γ-aminobutyric acid. *Science* 218: 1237–1240.

Isacson, O., Dunnett, S. B., and Bjorklund, A. (1986). Graft-induced behavioral recovery in an animal model of Huntington disease. *Proc. Natl. Acad. Sci. U.S.A.* 83: 2728–2732.

Isacson, O., Hantraye, P., Maziere, M., Sofroniew, M. V., and Riche, D. (1990). Apomorphine-induced dyskinesias after excitotoxic caudate-putamen lesions and the effects of neural transplantation in non-human primates. In *Neural Transplantation: From Molecular Basis to Clinical Applications,* S. B. Dunnett and S.-J. Richards (eds.), pp. 523–533. Elsevier, Amsterdam. Prog. Brain Res. 82.

Isacson, O., Hantraye, P., Riche, D., Schmuacher, J. M., and Maziere, M. (1991). The relationship between symptoms and functional anatomy in the chronic neurodegenerative diseases: From pharmacological to biological replacement therapy in Huntington's disease. In *Intracerebral Transplantation in Movement Disorders,* O. Lindvall, A. Bjorklund, and H. Widner (eds.), pp. 245–258. Elsevier, Amsterdam.

Itoh, Y., Waldeck, R. F., Tessler, A., and Pinter, M. J. (1996). Regenerated dorsal root fibers form functional synapses in embryonic spinal cord transplants. *J. Neurophysiol.* 76: 1236–1245.

Iversen, S. D., and Iversen, L. L. (1981). *Behavioral Pharmacology.* Second ed. Oxford University Press, New York.

Iwashita, Y., Kawaguchi, S., and Murata, M. (1994). Restoration of function by replacement of spinal cord segments in the rat. *Nature* 367: 167–170.

Jacobson, L. (1997). A mind is a terrible thing to waste. *Lingua Franca,* August, pp. 6–8.

Jankovic, J., Grossman, R., Goodman, C., Pirozzolo, F., Schneider, L., Zhu, Z., Scardino, P., Garber, A. J., Jhingran, S. G., and Martin, S. (1989). Clinical, biochemical, and neuropathological findings following transplantation of adrenal medulla to the caudate nucleus for treatment of Parkinson's disease. *Neurology* 39: 1227–1234.

Jat, P. S., and Sharp, P. A. (1989). Cell lines established by a temperature-sensitive simian virus 40 large-T-antigen gene are growth restricted at the nonpermissive temperature. *Mol. Cell Biol.* 9: 1672–1681.

Jat, P. S., Cepko, C. L., Mulligan, R. C, and Sharp, P. A. (1986). Recombinant retroviruses encoding simian virus 40 large T antigen and polyomavirus large and middle T antigens. *Mol. Cell Biol.* 6: 1204–1217.

Jat, P. S., Noble, M. D., Ataliotis, P., Tanaka Y., Yannoutsos, N., Larsen, L., and Kioussis, D. (1991). Direct derivation of conditionally immortal cell lines from an H-2k^b-tsA58 transgenic mouse. *Proc. Natl. Acad. Sci. U.S.A.* 88: 5096–5100.

Jellinger, K., and Seitelberger, F. (1958). Akute todlische enmarkungs-encephalitis nach wiederholten hirntrockenzellen-injektionen. *Klin. Wochenschr.* 36: 437–441.

Jiang, X. R., Jimenez, G., Chang, E., Frolkis, M., Kusler, B., Sage, M., Beeche, M., Bodnar, A. G., Wahl, G. M., Tisty, T. D., and Chiu, C. P. (1999). Telomerase expression in human somatic cells does not induce changes associated with a transformed phenotype. *Nat. Genet.* 21: 111–114.

Johnson, P. A., Yoshida, K., Gage, F. H., and Friedman, T. (1992). Effects of gene transfer into cultured CNS neurons with a replication-defective herpes simplex type I vector. *Mol. Brain Res.* 12: 95–102.

Johnston, R. E., and Becker, J. B. (1997). Intranigral grafts of fetal ventral mesencephalic tissue in adult 6-hydroxydopamine lesioned rats can induce behavioral recovery. *Cell Transplant.* 6: 267–276.

Kang, U. J. (1998). Potential of gene therapy for Parkinson's disease: Neurobiologic issues and new developments in gene transfer methodologies. *Movement Disorders* 13, Suppl. 1: 59–82.

Kang, U. J., Fisher, L. J., Joh, T. H., O'Malley, K. L., and Gage, F. H. (1993). Regulation of dopamine production by genetically modified primary fibroblasts. *J. Neurosci.* 13: 5203–5211.

Kao, C. C. (1974). Comparison of healing process in transected spinal cords grafted with autogenous brain tissue, sciatic nerve, and nodose ganglion. *Exp. Neurol.* 44: 424–439.

Kao, C. C., Bunge, R. P., and Reier, P. J. (eds.). (1983). *Spinal Cord Reconstruction.* Raven Press, New York.

Kao, C. C., Chang, L. W., and Bloodworth, J. M. B., Jr. (1977). Axonal regeneration across transected mammalian spinal cords: An electron microscopic study of delayed microsurgical nerve grafting. *Exp. Neurol.* 54: 591–615.

Kao, C. C., Fariello, R. G., Qualieri, C. E., Messert, B., and Bloodworth, J. M. B., Jr. (1977). Functional recovery of contused spinal cords repaired by delayed nerve grafting. *Proc. Am. Assn. Neurol. Surgeons,* article 7.

Kao, C. C., Shimizu, Y., Perkins, L. C., and Freeman, L. W. (1970). Experimental use of cultured cerebellar cortical tissue to inhibit the collagenous scar following spinal cord transection. *J. Neurosurg.* 33: 127–139.

Kaplan, H. J., Tezel, T. H., Berger, A. S., Wolf, M. L., and Del Priore, L. V. (1997). Human photoreceptor transplantation in retinitis pigmentosa. A safety study. *Arch. Ophthalmol.* 115: 1168–1172.

Kawaja, M. D., Rosenberg, M. B., Yoshida, K., and Gage, F. H. (1992). Somatic gene transfer of nerve growth factor promotes the survival of axotomized septal neurons and the regeneration of their axons in adult rats. *J. Neurosci.* 12: 2849–2864.

Kelly, P. J., Ahlskog, J. E., van Heerden, J. A., Carmichael, S. W., Stoddard, S. L., and Bell, G. N. (1989). Adrenal medullary autograft transplantation into the striatum of patients with Parkinson's disease. *Mayo Clin. Proc.* 64: 282–290.

Kennedy, P. R., and Bakay, R. A. (1998). Restoration of neural output from a paralyzed patient by a direct brain connection. *Neuroreport* 9: 1707–1711.

Kesslak, J. P., Brown, L., Steichen, C., and Cotman, C. W. (1986). Adult and embryonic frontal cortex transplants after frontal cortex ablation enhance recovery on a reinforced alternation task. *Exp. Neurol.* 94: 615–626.

Kesslak, J. P., Nieto-Sampedro, M., Globus, J., and Cotman, C. W. (1986). Transplants of purified astrocytes promote behavioral recovery after frontal cortex ablation. *Exp. Neurol.* 92: 377–390.

Kessler, R. C., McGonagle, K. A., Zhao, S., Nelson, C. B., Hughes, M., Eshleman, S., Wittchen, H.-U., and Kendler, K. S. (1994). Lifetime and 12-month prevalence of DSM-III-R psychiatric disorders in the United States. *Arch. Gen. Psychiat.* 51: 8–19.

Kish, S. J., Shannak, K., and Hornykiewicz, O. (1988). Uneven pattern of dopamine loss in the striatum of patients with Parkinson's disease. *N. Eng. J. Med.* 318: 876–880.

Klassen, H., and Lund, R. D. (1987). Retinal transplants can drive a pupillary reflex in host rat brains. *Proc. Natl. Acad. Sci. U.S.A.* 84: 6958–6960.

Knorr-Held, S., Brendel, W., Kiefer, H., Paal, G., and von Sprecht, B. U. (1986). Sensitization against brain gangliosides after therapeutic swine brain implantation in a multiple sclerosis patient. *J. Neurol.* 233: 54–56.

Kokaia, M., Aebischer, P., Elmer, E., Bengzon, J., Kalen, P., Kokaia, Z., and Lindvall, O. (1994). Seizure suppression in kindling epilepsy by intracerebral implants of GABA- but not noradrenaline-releasing polymer matrices. *Exp. Brain Res.* 100: 385–395.

Kolarik, J., Nadvornik, P., Tabarka, K., Dvorak, M., and Rozhold, O. (1988). Transplantation of human embryonic nerve tissue into a schizophrenic's brain. *Zentralbl. Neurochir.* 49: 147–150.

Kolb, B., and Fantie, B. (1994). Cortical graft function in adult and neonatal rats. In *Functional Neural Transplantation,* S. B. Dunnett and A. Bjorklund (eds.), pp. 415–436. Raven Press, New York.

Kolb, B., Reynolds, B., and Fantie, B. (1988). Frontal cortex grafts have different effects at different post-operative recovery times. *Behav. Neural Biol.* 50: 193–206.

Koller, W. C., Morantz, R., Vetere-Overfield, B., and Waxman, M. (1989). Autologous adrenal medullary transplant in progressive supranuclear palsy. *Neurology* 39: 1066–1068.

Kondziolka, D., Wechsler, L., Goldstein, S., Jannetta, P., DeCesare, S., Meltzer, C., Thulborn, K., Rakela, J., Elder, E., and Thompson, T. P. (1999). Cerebral transplantation of cultured neuronal cells in patients with fixed motor deficits after basal ganglia stroke: A phase I clinical trial. *Program and Abstracts of the American Society for Neural Transplantation and Repair* 5/6: 21.

Kopov, O. V., Jacques, S., Lieberman, A., Duma C. M., and Eagle, K. S. (1998). Safety of intrastriatal neurotransplantation for Huntington's disease patients. *Exp. Neurol.* 149: 97–108.

Kordower, J. H., Cochran, E., Penn, R. D., and Goetz, C. G. (1991). Putative chromaffin cell survival and enhanced host-derived TH-fiber innervation following a functional adrenal medulla autograft for Parkinson's disease. *Ann. Neurol.* 29: 405–412.

Kordower, J. H., Freeman, T. B., Chen, E. Y., Mufson, E. J., Sanberg, P. R., Hauser, R. A., Snow, B., and Olanow, C. W. (1998). Fetal nigral grafts survive and mediate clinical benefit in a patient with Parkinson's disease. *Movement Disorders* 13: 383–393.

Kordower, J. H., Freeman, T. B., Snow, B. J., Vingerhoets, F. J. G., Mufson, E. J., Sanberg, P. R., Hauser, R. A., Smith, D. A., Nauert, G. M., Perl, D. P., and Olanow, C. W. (1995). Neuropathological evidence of graft survival and striatal reinnervation after the transplantation of fetal mesencephalic tissue in a patient with Parkinson's disease. *N. Eng. J. Med.* 332: 1118–1124.

Kordower, J. H., Rosenstein, J. M., Collier, T. J., Burke, M. A., Chen, E.-Y., Li, J. M., Martel, L., Levey, A. E., Mufson, E. J., Freeman, T. B., and Olanow, C. W. (1996). Functional fetal nigral grafts in a patient with Parkinson's disease: Chemoanatomic, ultrastructural, and metabolic studies. *J. Comp. Neurol.* 370: 203–230.

Kordower, J. H., Styren, S., Clarke, M., DeKosky, S. T., Olanow, C. W., and Freeman, T. B. (1997). Fetal grafting for Parkinson's disease: Expression of immune markers in two patients with functional fetal nigral implants. *Cell Transplant.* 6: 213–219.

Korsching, S., Auburger, G., Heumann, R., Scott, J., and Thoenen, H. (1985). Levels of nerve growth factor and its mRNA in the central nervous system of the rat correlate with cholinergic innervation. *EMBO J.* 4: 1389–1393.

Koutouzis, T. K., Emerich, D. F., Borlongan, C. V., Freeman, T. B., Cahill, D. W., and Sanberg, P. R. (1994). Cell transplantation for central nervous system disorders. *Crit. Rev. Neurobiol.* 8: 125–162.

Kramer, P. D. (1993). *Listening to Prozac.* Penguin Books, New York.

Krieglstein, K., Deimling, F., Suter-Crazzolara, C., and Unsicker, K. (1996). Expression and localization of GDNF in developing and adult adrenal chromaffin cells. *Cell Tissue Res.* 286: 263–268.

Krieger, D. T., Perlow, M. J., Gibson, M. J., Davies, T. F., Zimmerman, E. A., Ferin, M., and Charlton, H. M. (1982). Brain transplants reverse hypogonadism of gonadotropin releasing hormone deficiency. *Nature* 298: 468–471.

Kromer, L. F. (1987). Nerve growth factor treatment after brain injury prevents neuronal death. *Science* 235: 214–216.

Kunkel-Bagden, E., and Bregman, B. S. (1990). Spinal cord transplants enhance the recovery of locomotor function after spinal cord injury at birth. *Exp. Brain Res.* 81: 25–34.

Kurlan, R., Kim, M. H., and Gash, D. M. (1991). The time course and magnitude of spontaneous recovery of parkinsonism produced by intracarotid administration of 1-methyl–4-phenyl–1,2,3,6-tetrahydropyridine to monkeys. *Ann. Neurol.* 29: 677–679.

Labbe, R., Firl, A., Jr., Mufson, E. J., and Stein, D. G. (1983). Fetal brain transplants: Reduction of cognitive deficits in rats with frontal cortex lesions. *Science* 221: 470–472.

Landau, W. (1993). Clinical Neuromythology. X. Faithful fashion: Survival status of the brain transplant cure for parkinsonism. *Neurology* 43: 644–649.

Landau, W. M. (1990). Clinical neuromythology. VII. Artificial intelligence: The brain transplant cure for parkinsonism. *Neurology* 40: 733–840.

Langston, J. W., Ballard, P., Tetrud, J. W., and Irwin, I. (1983). Chronic parkinsonism in humans due to a product of meperidine-analog synthesis. *Science* 219: 979–980.

Le Gal La Salle, G., Robert, J. J., Berrard, S., Ridoux, V., Stratford-Perricaudet, L. D., Perricaudet, M., and Mallet, J. (1993). An adenoviral vector for gene transfer into neurons and glia in the brain. *Science* 259: 988–990.

Le Gros Clark, W. E. (1940). Neuronal differentiation in implanted foetal cortical tissue. *J. Neurol. Psychiat.* 3: 263–284.

Lehman, M. N., and Ralph, M. R. (1994). Modulation and restitution of circadian rhythms. In *Functional Neural Transplantation*, S. B. Dunnett and A. Bjorklund (eds.), pp. 467–487. Raven Press, New York.

Lehman, M. N., Silver, R., Gladstone, W. R., Kahn, R. M., Gibson, M., and Bittman, E. L. (1987). Circadian rhythmicity restored by neural transplant. Immunocytochemical characterization of the graft and its integration with the host brain. *J. Neurosci.* 7: 1626–1638.

Levi-Montalcini, R. (1987). The nerve growth factor 35 years later. *Science* 237: 1154–1162.

Levi-Montalcini, R., Dal Toso, R., della Valle, F., Skaper, S. D., and Leon, A. (1995). Update of the NGF saga. *J. Neurol. Sci.* 130: 119–127.

Levi-Montalcini, R., Skaper, S. D., Dal Toso, R., Petrelli, L., and Leon, A. (1996). Nerve growth factor: From neurotrophin to neurokine. *Trends Neurosci.* 19: 514–520.

Levivier, M., Gash, D. M., and Przedborski, S. (1995). Time course of the neuroprotective effect of transplatation on quinolinic acid-induced lesions of the striatum. *Neuroscience* 69: 43–50.

Lewin, R. (1988). Research news: Brain graft puzzles. *Science* 240: 879.

Li, W. J., Li, S. H., Sharp, S. H., Nucifora, F. C., Jr., Schilling, G., Lanahan, A., Worley, P., Snyder, S. H., and Ross, C. A. (1995). A Huntington-associated protein enriched in brain with implications for pathology. *Nature* 378: 398–402.

Li, Y., Field, P. M., and Raisman, G. (1997). Repair of adult rat corticospinal tract by transplants of olfactory ensheathing cells. *Science* 277: 2000–2002.

Lindvall, O., Backlund, E. O., Farde, L., Sedvall, G., Freedman, R., Hoffer, B., Nobin, A., Seiger, A., and Olson, L. (1987). Transplantation in Parkinson's disease: Two cases of adrenal medullary grafts to the putamen. *Ann. Neurol.* 22: 457–468.

Lindvall, O., Brundin, P., Widner, H., Rehncrona, S., Gustavii, B., Frackowiak, R., Leenders, K. L., Sawle, G., Rothwell, J. C., Marsden, C. D., and Bjorklund, A. (1990). Grafts of fetal dopamine neurons survive and improve motor function in Parkinson's disease. *Science* 247: 574–577.

Lindvall, O., Rehncrona, S., Brundin, P., Gustavii, B., Astedt, B., Widner, H., Lindholm, T., Bjorklund, A., Leenders, K. L., Rothwell, J. C., Frackowiak, R., Marsden, C. D., Johnels, B., Steg, G., Freedman, R., Hoffer, B. J., Seiger, A., Bygdeman, M., Stromberg, I., and Olson, L. (1989). Human fetal dopamine neurons grafted into the striatum in two patients with severe Parkinson's disease: A detailed account of methodology and a 6-month follow-up. *Arch. Neurol.* 46: 615–631.

Lindvall, O., Sawle, G., Widner, H., Rothwell, J. C., Bjorklund, A., Brooks, D., Brundin, P., Frackowiak, R., Marsden, C. D., Odin, P., and Rehncrona, S. (1994). Evidence for long-term survival and function of dopaminergic grafts in progressive Parkinson's disease. *Ann. Neurol.* 35: 172–180.

Lindvall, O., Widner, H., Rehncrona, S., Brundin, P., Odin, P., Gustavii, B., Frackowiak, R., Leenders, K. L., Sawle, G., Rothwell, J. C., Bjorklund, A., and Marsden, C. D. (1992). Transplantation of fetal dopaminergic neurons in Parkinson's disease: One-year clinical and neurophysiological observations in two patients with putaminal implants. *Ann. Neurol.* 31: 155–165.

Ling, Z. D., Potter, E. D., Lipton, J. W., and Carvey, P. M. (1998). Differentiation of mesencephalic progenitor cells into dopaminergic neurons by cytokines. *Exp. Neurol.* 149: 411–413.

Little, C. W., Castillo, B., DiLoreto, D. A., Cox, C., Wyatt, J., del Cerro, C., and del Cerro, M. (1996). Transplantation of human fetal retinal pigment epithelium rescues photoreceptor cells from degeneration in the Royal College of Surgeons rat retina. *Invest. Ophthalmol. Vis. Sci.* 37: 204–211.

Lois, C., and Alvarez-Buylla, A. (1993). Long-distance neuronal migration in the adult mammalian brain. *Science* 264: 1145–1148.

Lopez-Garcia, J. C., Fernandez-Ruiz, J., Bermudez-Rattoni, F., and Tapia, R. (1990). Correlation between acetylcholine release and recovery of conditioned taste aversion induced by fetal neocortex grafts. *Brain Res.* 523: 105–110.

Lopez-Lozano, J. J., Bravo, G., Abascal, J., and the Clinica Puerta de Hierro Neural Transplantation Group. (1991). Grafting of perfused adrenal medullary tissue into the caudate nucleus of patients with Parkinson's disease. *J. Neurosurg.* 75: 234–243.

Lopez-Lozano, J. J., Bravo, G., Brera, B., Uria, J., Dargallo, J., Salmean, J., Insausti, J., Cerrolaza, J., and CPH Neural Transplantation Group. (1991). Can an analogy be drawn between the clinical evolution of Parkinson's patients who undergo autoimplantation of adrenal medulla and those of fetal ventral mesencephalon transplant recipients? In *Intracerebral Transplantation in Movement Disorders*, O. Lindvall, A. Bjorklund, and H. Widner (eds.), pp. 87–98. Elsevier, Amsterdam.

Loscher, W., Ebert, U., Lehmann, H., Rosenthal, C., and Nikkah, G. (1998). Seizure suppression in kindling epilepsy by grafts of fetal GABAergic neurons in rat substantia nigra. *J. Neurosci. Res.* 51: 196–209.

Luine, V., Renner, K., Frankfurt, M., and Azmitia, E. (1985). Raphe transplants into hypothalamus reverse facilitation of sexual behavior in 5,7-dihydroxytryptamine-treated female rats: Immunocytochemical, neurochemical, and behavioral studies. In *Neural Grafting in the Mammalian CNS*, A. Bjorklund and U. Stenevi (eds.), pp. 655–662. Elsevier, Amsterdam.

Lund, R. D., Coffey, P. J., Sauve, Y., and Lawrence, J. M. (1997). Intraretinal transplantation to prevent photoreceptor degeneration. *Ophthalmic Res.* 29: 305–319.

Lund, R. D., and Hankin, M. H. (1995). Pathfinding by retinal ganglion cell axons: Transplantation studies in genetically and surgically blind mice. *J. Comp. Neurol.* 356: 481–489.

Lund, R. D., and Hauschka, S. D. (1976). Transplanted neural tissue develops connections with host rat brain. *Science* 193: 582–584.

Macias, A. E., Valencia, A., and Vilana, M. (1989). Long-lasting dementia following brain grafting for the treatment of Parkinson's disease. *Transplantation* 48: 348.

Macklis, J. D. (1993). Transplanted neocortical neurons migrate selectively into regions of neuronal degeneration produced by chromophore-targeted laser photolysis. *J. Neurosci.* 13: 3848–3863.

Madrazo, I., Drucker-Colin, R., Diaz, V., Martinez-Marta, J., Torres, C., and Becerril, J. J. (1987). Open microsurgical autograft of adrenal medulla to the right caudate nucleus in Parkinson's disease: A report of two cases. *N. Eng. J. Med.* 316: 831–834.

Madrazo, I., Franco-Bourland, R., Aguilera, M., Ostrosky-Solis, F., Cuevas, C., Castrejon, H., Velazquez, D., Grijalva, E., Guizar-Zahagun, G., Magallon, E., and Madrazo, M. (1991). Fetal ventral mesencephalon brain homotransplantation in Parkinson's disease: The Mexican experience. In *Intracerebral Transplantation in Movement Disorders,* O. Lindvall, A. Bjorklund, and H. Widner (eds.), pp. 123–130. Elsevier, Amsterdam.

Madrazo, I., Franco-Bourland, R., Aguilera, M., Ostrosky-Solis, F., Madrazo, M., Cuevas, C., Castrejon, H., Guizar-Zahagun, G., and Magallon, E. (1991). Autologous adrenal medullary, fetal mesencephalic, and fetal adrenal brain transplantation in Parkinson's disease: A long-term postoperative follow-up. *J. Neural Transplant. Plast.* 2:157–164.

Madrazo, I., Franco-Bourland, R. E., Castrejon, H., Cuevas, C., Ostrosky-Solis, F., Aguilera, M., Magallon, E., Grijalva, E., and Guizar-Sahagun, G. (1993). Fetal striatal brain homografting in two patients with Huntington's disease. *Soc. Neurosci. Abs.* 19: 864 (no. 357.7).

Madrazo, I., Franco-Bourland, R. E., Cuevas, C., Aguilera, M. C., Ostrosky-Solis, F., Santiago, N., Castrejon, H., Magallon, E., and Guizar-Sahagun, G. (1991). Fetal neural grafting for the treatment of Huntington's disease: Report of the first case. *Soc. Neurosci. Abs.* 17: 902 (no. 359.1).

Madrazo, I., Franco-Bourland, R., Ostrosky-Solis, F., Aguilera, M., Cuevas, C., Castrejon, H., Guizar, G., and Magallon, E. (1990). Dementia following brain grafting. *Transplantation* 49: 1026–1027.

Madrazo, I., Franco-Bourland, R., Ostrosky-Solis, F., Aguilera, M., Cuevas, C., Zamorano, C., Morelos, A., Magallan, E., and Guizar-Sahagun, G. (1990). Fetal homotransplants (ventral mesencephalon and adrenal tissue) to the striatum of parkinsonian subjects. *Arch. Neurol.* 47: 1285–1291.

Mahalik, T. J., Finger, T. E., Stromberg, I., and Olson, L. (1985). Substantia nigra transplants into denervated striatum of the rat: Ultrastructure of graft and host connections. *J. Comp. Neurol.* 240: 60–80.

Mahalik, T. J., Stromberg, I., Gerhardt, G. A., Granholm, A.-C., Seiger, A., Bygdeman, M., Olson, L., Hoffer, B. J., and Finger, T. E. (1989). Human ventral mesencephalic xenografts to the catecholamine-depleted striata of athymic rats: Ultrastructure and immunocytochemistry. *Synapse* 4: 19–29.

Major, E. O., Miller, A. E., Mourrain, P., Traub, R. G., and De Widt, E. (1985). Establishment of a line of human fetal glial cells that supports JC virus multiplication. *Proc. Natl. Acad. Sci. U.S.A.* 82: 1257–1261.

Mamelak, A. N., Eggerding, F. A., Oh, D. S., Wilson, E., Davis, R. L., Spitzer, R., Hay, J. A., and Caton, W. L. III. (1998). Fatal cyst formation after fetal mesencephalic allograft transplant for Parkinson's disease. *J. Neurosurg.* 89: 592–598.

Mandel, R. J., Brundin, P., and Bjorklund, A. (1990). The importance of graft placement and task complexity for transplant-induced recovery of simple and complex sensorimotor deficits in dopamine denervated rats. *Eur. J. Neurosci.* 2: 888–894.

Mandel, R. J., Rendahl, K. G., Spratt, S. K., Snyder, R. O., Cohen, L. K., and Leff, S. E. (1998). Characterization of intrastriatal recombinant adeno-associated virus-mediated gene transfer of human tyrosine hydroxylase and human GTP-cyclohydrolase I in a rat model of Parkinson's disease. *J. Neurosci.* 18: 4271–4284.

Mandel, R. J., Spratt, S. K., Snyder, R. O., and Leff, S. E. (1997). Midbrain injection of recombinant adeno-associated virus encoding rat glial cell line-derived neurotrophic factor protects nigral neurons in a progressive 6-hydroxydopamine-induced degeneration model of Parkinson's disease in rats. *Proc. Natl. Acad. Sci. U.S.A.* 94: 14083–14088.

Marciano, F. F., Wiegand, S. J., Sladek, J. R., and Gash, D. M. (1989). Fetal hypothalamic transplants promote survival and functional regeneration of axotomised adult supraoptic magnocellular neurons. *Brain Res.* 483: 135–142.

Mark, V. H., and Ervin, F. R. (1970). *Violence and the Brain.* Harper & Row, New York.

Mark, V. H., and Neville, R. (1973). Brain surgery in aggressive epileptics: Social and ethical implications. *J. Am. Med. Assn.* 226: 765–872.

Marshall, J. F., and Ungerstedt, U. (1977). Striatal efferent fibers play a role in maintaining rotational behavior in the rat. *Science* 198: 62–64.

Martindale, D., Hackam, A., Wieczorek, A., Ellerby, L., Wellington, C., McCutcheon, K., Singaraja, R., Kazemi-Esfarjani, P., Devon, R., Kim, S. U., Bredesen, D. E., Tufaro, F., and Hayden, M. R. (1998). Length of huntingtin and its polyglutamine tract influences localization and frequency of intracellular aggregates. *Nature Genet.* 18: 150–154.

Mattson, M. P., and Ryuchlik, B. (1990). Glia protect hippocampal neurons against excitatory amino acid-induced degeneration: Involvement of fibroblast growth factor. *Int. J. Dev. Neurosci.* 8: 399–415.

May, R. M. (1955). Cerebral transplantation in mammals. *Transplant. Bull.* 2: 62–66.

Mayer, E., Dunnett, S. B., and Fawcett, J. W. (1993). Mitogenic effect of basic fibroblast growth factor on embryonic ventral mesencephalic dopaminergic neuron precursors. *Dev. Brain Res.* 72: 253–258.

McCown, T. J., Xiao, X., Li, J., Breese, G. R., and Samulski, R. J. (1996). Differential and persistent expression patterns of CNS gene transfer by an adeno-associated virus (AAV) vector. *Brain Res.* 713: 99–107.

McGeer, E. G., and McGeer, P. L. (1976). Duplication of biochemical changes of Huntington's chorea by intrastriatal injection of glutamic and kainic acids. *Nature* 263: 517–519.

McIntyre, D. C., Saari, M., and Pappas, B. A. (1979). Potentiation of amygdala kindling in adult or infant rats by injections of 6-hydroxydopamine. *Exp. Neurol.* 63: 527–544.

McNamara, J. O. (1984). Kindling: An animal model of complex partial epilepsy. *Ann. Neurol.* 16 (suppl.): 72–86.

McNeill, W. H. (1976). *Plagues and Peoples.* Doubleday, New York.

Mendez, I., and Hong, M. (1997). Reconstruction of the striato-nigro-striatal circuitry by simultaneous double dopaminergic grafts: A tracer study using fluorogold and horseradish peroxidase. *Brain Res.* 778: 194–205.

Mendez, I., Sadi, D., and Hong, M. (1996). Reconstruction of the nigrostriatal pathway by simultaneous intrastriatal and intranigral dopaminergic transplants. *J. Neurosci.* 16: 7216–7227.

Miranda, M. I., Lopez-Colome, A. M., and Bermudez-Rattoni, F. (1997). Recovery of taste aversion learning induced by fetal neocortex grafts: Correlation with in vivo extracellular acetylcholine. *Brain Res.* 759: 141–148.

Misiewicz, B., Poltorak, M., Raybourne, R. B., Gomez, M., Listwak, S., and Sternberg, E. M. (1997). Intracerebroventricular transplantation of embryonic neuronal tissue from inflammatory resistant into inflammatory susceptible rats suppresses specific components of inflammation. *Exp. Neurol.* 146: 305–314.

Molina, H. (1990). Neurotransplantation in Parkinson's disease—the Cuban experience. *Restorative Neurol. Neurosci.* 1: 164.

Molina, H., Quinones, R., Alvarez, L., Galarraga, J., Piedra, J., Suarez, C., Rachid, M., Garcia, J. C., Perry, T. L., Santana, A., Carmenate, H., Macias, R., Torres, O., Rojas, M. J., Cordova, F., and Munoz, J. L. (1991). Transplantation of human fetal ventral mesencephalic tissue in caudate nucleus as treatment for Parkinson's disease: The Cuban Experience. In *Intracerebral Transplantation in Movement Disorders,* O. Lindvall, A. Bjorklund, and H. Widner (eds.), pp. 99–110. Elsevier, Amsterdam.

Money offered in spinal surgical trial. (1994). *Science* 264: 667.

Monroe, R., and Heath, R. G. (1954). Psychiatric observations. In *Studies in Schizophrenia,* R. G. Heath (ed.), pp. 345–386. Harvard University Press, Cambridge, Mass.

Montoya, C. P., Astell, S., and Dunnett, S. B. (1990). Effects of nigral and striatal grafts on skilled forelimb use in the rat. In *Neural Transplantation: From Molecular Basis to Clinical Applications,* S. B. Dunnett and S.-J. Richards (eds.), Prog. Brain Res., 82, pp. 459–466. Elsevier, Amsterdam.

Morshead, C. M., and van der Kooy, D. (1992). Postmitotic death is the fate of constitutively proliferating cells in the subependymal layer of the adult mouse brain. *J. Neurosci.* 12: 249–256.

Mouradian, M. M., Heuser, I. J. E., Baronti, F., and Chase, T. N. (1990). Modification of central dopaminergic mechanisms by continuous levodopa therapy for advanced Parkinson's disease. *Ann. Neurol.* 27: 18–23.

Murphy, C. A., Canbeyli, R., and Yongue, B. G. (1992). The development of hypertension in rats with intraventricular grafts of fetal SHR or WKY hypothalamus. *J. Neural Transplant. Plast.* 3: 301–302.

Murphy, J. E., and Sturm, E. (1923). Conditions determining the transplantability of tissue in the brain. *J. Exp. Med.* 38: 183–197.

Nakao, N., Kokaia, Z., Odin, P., and Lindvall, O. (1995). Protective effects of BDNF and NT-3 but not PDGF against hypoglycemic injury to cultured striatal neurons. *Exp. Neurol.* 131: 1–10.

National Foundation for Brain Research. (1992). *The Cost of Disorders of the Brain.* Available from: National Foundation for Brain Research, 1250 24th St. N. W., Suite 300, Washington, D.C., 20037.

Nesmeyanova, T. (1977). *Experimental Studies of Regeneration of Spinal Neurons.* V. H. Winston and Sons, Washington, D.C.

Nicholas, M. K., and Arnason, B. G. W. (1989). Immunologic considerations in transplantation to the central nervous system. In *Neural Regeneration and Transplantation,* F. J. Seil (ed.), pp. 239–284. Alan R. Liss, New York.

Nieto-Sampedro, M., Lewis, E. R., Cotman, C. W., Manthorpe, M., Skaper, S. D., Barbin, G., Longo, F. M., and Varon, S. (1982). Brain injury causes a time-dependent increase in neuronotrophic activity at the lesion site. *Science* 217: 860–861.

Nikkhah, G., Bentlage, C., Cunningham, M. G., and Bjorklund, A. (1994). Intranigral fetal dopamine grafts induce behavioral compensation in the rat Parkinson model. *J. Neurosci.* 14: 3449–3461.

Nikkhah, G., Cunningham, M. G., Cenci, M. A., McKay, R. D., and Bjorklund, A. (1995). Dopaminergic microtransplants into the substantia nigra of neonatal rats with bilateral 6-OHDA lesions. I. Evidence for anatomical reconstruction of the nigrostriatal pathway. *J. Neurosci.* 15: 3548–3561.

Nikkhah, G., Cunningham, M. G., Jodicke, A., Knappe, U., and Bjorklund, A. (1994). Improved graft survival and striatal reinnervation by microtransplantation of fetal nigral cell suspensions in the rat Parkinson model. *Brain Res.* 633: 133–143.

Nikkhah, G., Duan, W.-M., Knappe, U., and Bjorklund, A. (1993). Restoration of complex sensorimotor behavior and skilled forelimb use by a modified nigral cell transplantation approach in the rat Parkinson model. *Neuroscience* 56: 33–43.

Niven, L. (1966). Jigsaw man. In his *Three Books of Known Space*, pp. 62–83. Ballantine Books, New York.

Niven, L. (1995). *Flatlander*. Ballantine Books, New York.

No, D., Yao, T.-P., and Evans, R. M. (1996). Ecdysone-inducible gene expression in mammalian cells and transgenic mice. *Proc. Natl. Acad. Sci. U.S.A.* 93: 3346–3351.

Norman, A. B., Calderon, S. F., Giordano, M., and Sanberg, P. R. (1988). Striatal tissue transplants attenuate apomorphine-induced rotational behavior in rats with unilateral kainic acid lesions. *Neuropharmacology* 27: 333–336.

Olanow, C. W., Koller, W., Goetz, C. G., Stebbins, G. T., Cahill, D. W., Gauger, L. L., Morantz, R., Penn, R. D., Tanner, C. M., Klawans, H. L., Shannon, K. M., Comella, C. L., and Witt, T. (1990). Autologous transplantation of adrenal medulla in Parkinson's disease: 18 month results. *Arch. Neurol.* 47: 1286–1289.

Olds, J., and Milner, P. (1954). Positive reinforcement produced by electrical stimulation of septal area and other regions of the rat brain. *J. Comp. Physiol. Psychol.* 47: 419–427.

Olson, L. (1970). Fluorescence histochemical evidence for axonal growth and secretion from transplanted adrenal medullary tissue. *Histochemie* 22: 1–8.

Olson, L., Backlund, E. O., Ebendal, T., Freedman, R., Hamberger, B., Hansson, P., Hoffer, B., Lindblom, U., Meyerson, B., Stromberg, I., Sydow, O., and Seiger, A. (1991). Intraputaminal infusion of nerve growth factor to support adrenal medullary autografts in Parkinson's disease. One-year follow-up of first clinical trial. *Arch. Neurol.* 48: 373–381.

Olson, L., and Malmfors, T. (1970). Growth characteristics of adrenergic nerves in the adult rat. Fluorescence histochemical and ^{3}H-noradrenaline uptake studies using tissue transplantation to the anterior chamber of the eye. *Acta Physiol. Scand.* (suppl.) 348: 1–112.

Olson, L., and Seiger, A. (1972). Brain tissue transplanted to the anterior chamber of the eye. I. Fluorescence histochemistry of immature catecholamine and 5-hydroxytryptamine neurons innervating the rat iris. *Z. Zellforsch.* 195: 175–194.

Olsson, M., Bentlage, C., Wictorin, K., Campbell, K., and Bjorklund, A. (1997). Extensive migration and target innervation by striatal precursors after grafting into the neonatal striatum. *Neuroscience* 79: 57–88.

Onifer, S. M., Whittemore, S. R., and Holets, V. R. (1993). Variable morphological differentiation of a raphe-derived neuronal cell line following transplantation into the adult rat CNS. *Exp. Neurol.* 122: 130–142.

Otto, D., and Unsicker, K. (1990). Basic FGF reverses chemical and morphological deficits in the nigrostriatal system of MPTP treated mice. *J. Neurosci.* 10: 1912–1921.

Pacheco-Cano, M. T., Garcia-Hernandez, F., Hiriart, M., Komisaruk, B. R., and Drucker-Colin, R. (1990). Dibutyryl cAMP stimulates analgesia in rat bearing a ventricular adrenal medulla transplant. *Brain Res.* 531: 290–293.

Paino, C. L., and Bunge, M. B. (1991). Induction of axon growth into Schwann cell implants grafted into lesioned adult rat spinal cord. *Exp. Neurol.* 114: 254–257.

Palmer, T. D., Rosman, G. J., Osborne, W. R. A., and Miller, A. D. (1991). Genetically modified skin fibroblasts persist long after transplantation but gradually inactivate introduced genes. *Proc. Natl. Acad. Sci. U.S.A.* 88: 1330–1334.

Pappas, G. D., Lazorthes, Y., Bes, J. C., Tafani, M., and Winnie, A. P. (1997). Relief of intractable cancer pain by human chromaffin cell transplants: Experience at two medical centers. *Neurolog. Res.* 19: 71–87.

Pearlman, S., Levivier, M., Collier, T. J., Sladek, J. R., Jr., and Gash, D. M. (1993). Striatal implants protect the host striatum against quinolinic acid toxicity. *Exp. Brain Res.* 84: 303–310.

Pearlman, S., Levivier, M., and Gash, D. M. (1993). Striatal implants of fetal striatum protect against quinolinic acid lesions of the striatum. *Brain Res.* 613: 203–211.

Perlow, M. J., Freed, W. J., Hoffer, B. J., Seiger, A., Olson, L. and Wyatt, R. J. (1979). Brain grafts reduce motor abnormalities produced by destruction of nigrostriatal dopamine system. *Science* 204: 643–647.

Perlow, M. J., Kokoris, G., Gibson, M. J., Silverman, A. J., Krieger, D. T., and Zimmerman, E. A. (1987). Accessory olfactory bulb transplants correct hypogonadism in mutant mice. *Brain Res.* 415: 158–162.

Peterson, D. I., Price, M. L., and Small, C. S. (1989). Autopsy findings in a patient who had an adrenal-to-brain transplant for Parkinson's disease. *Neurology* 39: 235–238.

Pezzoli, G., Fahn, S., Dwork, A., Truong, D. D., de Yebenes, J. G., Jackson-Lewis, V., Herbert, J., and Cadet, J. L. (1988). Non-chromaffin tissue plus nerve growth factor reduces experimental parkinsonism in aged rats. *Brain Res.* 459: 398–403.

Plunkett, R. J., Bankiewicz, K. S., Cummins, A. C., Miletich, R. S., Schwartz, J. P., and Oldfield, E. H. (1990). Long-term evaluation of hemiparkinsonian monkeys after adrenal medulla grafting or cavitation alone. *J. Neurosurg.* 73: 918–926.

Poltorak, M., and Freed, W. J. (1990). Cell adhesion molecules in adrenal medulla grafts: Enhancement of chromaffin cell L1/Ng-CAM expression and reorganization of extracellular matrix following transplantation. *Exp. Neurol.* 110: 73–85.

Poltorak, M., Shimoda, K., and Freed, W. J. (1990). Cell adhesion molecules (CAMs) in adrenal medulla in situ and in vitro: Enhancement of chromaffin cell L1/Ng-CAM expression by NGF. *Exp. Neurol.* 110: 52–82.

Poltorak, M., Shimoda, K., and Freed, W. J. (1992). L1 substrate enhances outgrowth of tyrosine hydroxylase-immunoreactive neurites in mesencephalic cell culture. *Exp. Neurol.* 117: 176–184.

Poltorak, M., Williams, J. R., and Freed, W. J. (1993). Degradation fragments of L1 antigen enhance tyrosine hydroxylase-immunoreactive neurite outgrowth in mesencephalic cell culture. *Brain Res.* 619: 255–262.

Pons, T. P., Garraghty, P. E., Ommaya, A. K., Kaas, J. H., Taub, E., and Mishkin, M. (1991). Massive cortical reorganization after sensory deafferentation in adult macaques. *Science* 252: 1857–1860.

Postone, N. (1987). Phantom limb pain: A review. *Int. J. Psychiatry Med.* 17: 57–70.

Price, L. H., Spencer, D. D., Marek, K. L., Robbins, R. J., Leranth, C., Farhi, A., Naftolin, F., Roth, R. H., Bunney, B. S., Hoffer, P. B., Makuch, R., and Redmond, D. E. (1995). Psychiatric status after human fetal mesencephalic tissue transplantation in Parkinson's disease. *Biolog. Psychiatry* 38: 498–505.

Privat, A., Mansour, H., Rajaofetra, N., and Geffard, M. (1989). Intraspinal transplants of serotonergic neurons in the adult rat. *Brain Res. Bull.* 22: 123–129.

Przedborski, S., Levivier, M., Kostic, V., Jackson-Lewis, V., Kollison, A., Gash, D. M., Fahn, S., and Cadet, J. L. (1991). Sham transplantation protects against 6-hydroxydopamine-induced dopaminergic toxicity in rats: Behavioral and morphological evidence. *Brain Res.* 550: 231–238.

Ptak, L. R., Hart, K. R., Lin, D., and Carvey, P. M. (1995). Isolation and manipulation of rostral mesencephalic tegmental progenitor cells fom rat. *Cell Transplant.* 4: 335–342.

Ralph, M. R., Foster, R. G., Davis, F. C., and Menaker, M. (1990). Transplanted suprachaismatic nucleus determines circadian photoperiod. *Science* 247: 975–978.

Ralph, M. R., and Lehman, M. N. (1991). Transplantation: A new tool in the analysis of the mammalian hypothalamic circadian pacemaker. *Trends Neurosci.* 14: 362–366.

Ramon y Cajal, S. (1906). Mechanismo de la regeneracion de los nervios. *Trab. Lab. Invest. Biol. Univ. Madrid* 4: 119–155.

Ramon y Cajal, S. (1928). Cajal's *Degeneration and Regeneration of the Nervous System*. Translated by R. M. May and edited by J. DeFelipe and E. G. Jones. Facsimile of the 1928 edition, Oxford University Press, New York, 1991.

Redmond, D. E., Jr., Leranth, C., Spencer, D. D., Robbins, R., Vollmer, T., Kim, J. H., Roth, R., Dwork, A. J., and Naftolin, F. (1990). Fetal neural graft survival. *Lancet* 336: 820–822.

Redmond, D. E., Jr., Marek, K. L., Naftolin, F., Leranth, C., Robbins, R. J., Bunney, B. S., Elsworth, J. D., Vollmer, T., Hoffer, P. B., Roth, R. H., Makuch, R., Chen, Y.-T., and Spencer, D. D. (1998). Outcome of fetal mesencephalic grafts placed into the striatum of 15 patients with parkinsonism: Site of placement and extended functional effects. *Program and Abstracts of the American Society for Neural Transplantation.* 4: 19.

Redmond, D. E., Sladek, J. R., Jr., Roth, R. H., Collier, T. J., and Elsworth, J. D. (1986). Fetal neuronal grafts in monkeys given methylphenyltetrahydropyridine. *Lancet* 1: 1125–1127.

Reier, P. J., Anderson, D. K., Young, W., Michel, M. E., and Fessler, R. (1994). Workshop on intraspinal transplantation and clinical application. *J. Neurotrauma* 11: 369–377.

Renfranz, P. J., Cunningham, M. G., and McKay, R. D. G. (1991). Region-specific differentiation of the hippocampal stem cell line HiB5 upon implantation into the developing mammalian brain. *Cell* 66: 713–729.

Reynolds, B. A., and Weiss, S. (1992). Generation of neurons and astrocytes from isolated cells of the adult mammalian central nervous system. *Science* 255: 1707–1710.

Richardson, P. M., McGuinness, U. M., and Aguayo, A. J. (1980). Axons from CNS neurones regenerate into PNS grafts. *Nature* 284: 264–265.

Robertson, G. S., Fine, A., and Robertson, H. A. (1991). Dopaminergic grafts in the striatum reduce D1 but not D2 receptor-mediated rotation in 6-OHDA-lesioned rats. *Brain Res.* 539: 304–311.

Rose, G., Gerhardt, G., Stromberg, I., Olson, L., and Hoffer, B. J. (1985). Monoamine release from dopamine-denervated rat caudate nucleus reinnervated by substantia nigra transplants: An "in vivo" electrochemical study. *Brain Res.* 341: 92–100.

Rosenberg, M. B., Friedmann, T., Robertson, R. C., Tuszynski, M., Wolff, J. A., Breakefield, X. O., and Gage, F. (1988). Grafting genetically modified cells to the damaged brain: Restorative effects of NGF expression. *Science* 242: 1575–1578.

Rosenblad, C., Martinez-Serrano, A., and Bjorklund, A. (1996). Glial cell line-derived neurotrophic factor increases survival, growth, and function of intrastriatal dopaminergic grafts. *Neuroscience* 75: 979–985.

Rosenstein, J. M., and Brightman, M. W. (1978). Intact cerebral ventricle as a site for tissue transplantation. *Nature* 276: 83–85.

Ruppert, C., Sandrasagra, A., Anton, B., Evans, C., Schweitzer, E. S., and Tobin, A. J. (1993). Rat-1 fibroblasts engineered with GAD65 and GAD67 cDNAs in retroviral vectors produce and release GABA. *J. Neurochem.* 61: 768–771.

Ryder, E. F., Snyder, E. Y., and Cepko, C. L. (1990). Establishment and characterization of multipotent neural cell lines using retrovirus vector-mediated oncogene transfer. *J. Neurobiol.* 21: 356–375.

Sagen, J., Kemmler, J. E., and Wang, H. (1991). Adrenal medullary transplants increase spinal cord cerebrospinal fluid catecholamine levels and reduce pain sensitivity. *J. Neurochem.* 56: 623–627.

Sagen, J., Pappas, G. D., and Ortega, J. D. (1990). Host-graft relationships of isolated bovine chromaffin cells in rat periaqueductal grey. *J. Neurocytol.* 19: 697–707.

Sagen, J., Pappas, G. D., and Perlow, M. J. (1986). Adrenal medullary tissue transplants in the rat spinal cord reduce pain sensitivity. *Brain Res.* 384: 189–194.

Sagen, J., Pappas, G. D., and Pollard, H. B. (1986). Analgesia induced by isolated bovine chromaffin cells implanted in rat spinal cord. *Proc. Natl. Acad. Sci. U.S.A.* 83: 7522–7526.

Sagen, J., Pappas, G. D., and Winnie, A. P. (1993). Alleviation of pain in cancer patients by adrenal medullary transplants in the spinal subarachnoid space. *Cell Transplant.* 2: 259–266.

Sagen, J., and Wang, H. (1990). Prolonged analgesia by enkephalinase inhibition in rats with spinal cord adrenal medullary transplants. *Eur. J. Pharmacol.* 179: 427–433.

Sagen, J., Wang, H., and Pappas, G. D. (1990). Adrenal medullary implants in the rat spinal cord reduce nociception in a chronic pain model. *Pain* 42: 69–89.

Saltykow, S. (1905). Versüche über gehirnplantation, zugleich ein beitrag zur kenntniss der vorgange an den zellingen gehirnelementen. *Arch. Psychiatr. Nervenkr.* 40: 329–388.

Sanberg, P. R., Borlongan, C. V., Othberg, A. I., Saporta, S., Freeman, T. B., and Cameron, D. I. (1997). Testis-derived Sertoli cells have a trophic effect on dopamine neurons, and alleviate hemiparkinsonism in rats. *Nature Med.* 3: 1129–1132.

Sanberg, P. R., Borlongan, C. V., Saporta, S., and Cameron, D. I. (1996). Testis-derived Sertoli cells survive and provide localized immunoprotection for xenografts in rat brain. *Nature Biotechnol.* 14: 1692–1695.

Sanberg, P. R., Calderon, S. F., Giordano, M., Tew, J. M., and Norman, A. B. (1989). The quinolinic model of Huntington's disease: Locomotor abnormalities. *Exp. Neurol.* 105: 45–53.

Sanberg, P. R., Giordano, M., Henault, M. A., Nash, D. R., Ragozzino, M., and Hagenmeyer-Houser, S. H. (1989). Intraparenchymal striatal transplants required for maintenance of behavioral recovery in an animal model of Huntington's disease. *J. Neural Transplant.* 1: 23–31.

Sanberg, P. R., Koutouzis, T. K., Freeman, T. B., Cahill, D. W., and Norman, A. B. (1993). Behavioral effects of fetal neural transplants: Relevance to Huntington's disease. *Brain Res. Bull.* 32: 493–496.

Sanberg, P. R., and Norman, A. B. (1988). Adrenal transplants for Huntington's disease? *Nature* 335: 122.

Santa-Olalla, J., and Covarrubias, L. (1995). Epidermal growth factor (EGF), transforming growth factor-alpha (TGF-alpha), and basic fibroblast growth factor (bFGF) differentially influence neural precursor cells of mouse embryonic mesencephalon. *J. Neurosci. Res.* 42: 172–183.

Sauer, H., and Brundin, P. (1991). Effects of cool storage on survival and function of intrastriatal mesencephalic tissue grafts. *Res. Neurol. Neurosci.* 2: 123–135.

Savio, T., and Schwab, M. E. (1990). Lesioned corticospinal tract axons regenerate in myelin-free rat spinal cord. *Proc. Natl. Acad. Sci. U.S.A.* 87: 4130–4133.

Sawle, G. V., Bloomfield, P. M., Bjorklund, A., Brooks, D. J., Brundin, P., Leenders, K. L., Lindvall, O., Marsden, C. D., Rehncrona, S., Widner, H., and Frackowiak, S. J. (1992). Transplantation of fetal dopamine neurons in Parkinson's disease: PET [^{18}F]-6-fluorodopa studies in two patients with putaminal implants. *Ann. Neurol.* 31: 166–173.

Schnell, L., Schnelder, R., Kolbeck, R., Barde, Y.-A., and Schwab, M. E. (1994). Neurotrophin–3 enhances sprouting of corticospinal tract during development and after spinal cord lesion. *Nature* 367: 170–172.

Schnell, L., and Schwab, M. E. (1990). Axonal regeneration in the rat spinal cord produced by an antibody against myelin-associated neurite growth inhibitors. *Nature* 343: 269–272.

Schnistine, M., and Gage, F. H. (1993). Factors affecting proviral expression in primary cells grafted into the CNS. *Res. Pub. Assoc. Nerv. Ment. Dis.* 71: 311–323.

Schumacher, J. M., Isacson, O., Weiss, R. A., Patience, C., and Takeuchi, Y. (1997). Neuronal xenotransplantation in Parkinson's disease. *Nature Medicine* 3: 474–475.

Schumacher, J. M., Short, M. P., Hyman, B. T., Breakefield, X. O., and Isacson, O. (1991). Intracerebral implantation of nerve growth factor secreting fibroblasts protects striatum against neurotoxic levels of excitatory amino acids. *Neuroscience* 45: 561–570.

Schwab, M. E. (1996). Bridging the gap in spinal cord regeneration. *Nat. Med.* 2: 976–977.

Schwab, R. S., and England, A. C. (1969). Projection technique for evaluating surgery in Parkinson's disease. In *Third Symposium on Parkinson's Disease*, F. J. Gillingham and I. M. L. Donaldson (eds.), pp. 152–157. E. & S. Livingstone, Edinburgh.

Schwarz, E. J., Alexander, G. M., Prockop, D. J., and Azizi, S. A. (1999). Rat marrow stromal cells can be transduced to synthesize L-DOPA. *Program and Abstracts of the American Society for Neural Transplantation and Repair 5/6*: 48.

Schwarz, S., and Freed, W. J. (1987). Brain tissue transplantation in neonatal rats prevents a lesion-induced syndrome of adipsia, aphagia, and akinesia. *Exp. Brain Res.* 65: 449–454.

Seiger, A., Bygdeman, M., Goldstein, M., Almqvist, P., Hoffer, B., Stromberg, I., and Olson, L. (1988). Human fetal catecholamine-containing tissues grafted intraocularly and intracranially to immuno-compromised rodent hosts. In *Transplantation into the Mammalian CNS*, D. M. Gash and J. R. Sladek, Jr. (eds.), pp. 449–455. Elsevier, Amsterdam. Prog. Brain Res. 78.

Seiger, A., and Olson, L. (1977). Quantitation of fiber growth in transplanted monoaminergic neurons. *Cell Tissue Res.* 179: 285–316.

Seiler, M. J., and Aramant, R. B. (1995). Transplantation of embryonic retinal donor cells labelled with BrdU or carrying a genetic marker to adult retina. *Exp. Brain Res.* 105: 59–66.

Sherman, R. A., Arena, J. G., Sherman, C. J., and Ernst, J. L. (1989). The mystery of phantom pain: Growing evidence for psychophysiological mechanisms. *Biofeedback Self Regulation* 14: 267–280.

Shibayama, M., Matsui, N., Himes, B. T., Murray, M., and Tessler, A. (1998). Critical interval for rescue of axotomized neurons by transplants. *Neuroreport* 9: 11–14.

Shihabuddin, L. S., Brunschwig, J. P., Holets, V. R., Bunge, M. B., and Whittemore, S. R. (1996). Induction of mature neuronal properties in immortalized neuronal precursor cells following grafting into the neonatal CNS. *J. Neurocytol.* 25: 101–111.

Shihabuddin, L. S., Hertz, J. A., Holets, V. R., and Whittemore, S. R. (1995). The adult CNS retains the potential to direct region-specific differentiation of a transplanted neuronal precursor cell line. *J. Neurosci.* 15: 6666–6678.

Shimohama, S., Rosenberg, M. B., Fagan, A. M., Wolff, J. A., Short, M. P., Breakefield, X. O., Friedmann, T., and Gage, F. H. (1989). Grafting genetically modified cells into the rat brain: Characteristics of *E. coli* beta-galactosidase as a reporter gene. *Mol. Brain Res.* 5: 271–278.

Silver, R., LeSauter, J., Tresco, P. A., and Lehman, M. N. (1996). A diffusable coupling signal from the transplanted superchiasmatic nucleus controlling circadian locomotor rhythms. *Nature* 382: 810–813.

Simonds, G. R., and Freed, W. J. (1990). Effects of intraventricular substantia nigra allografts as a function of donor age. *Brain Res.* 530: 12–19.

Sladek, J. R., Collier, T. J., Haber, S. N., Roth, R. H., and Redmond, D. E. (1986). Survival and growth of fetal catecholamine neurons transplanted into primate brain. *Brain Res. Bull.* 17: 809–818.

Snyder, E. Y., Deitcher, D. L., Walsh, C., Arnold-Aldea, S., Hartweig, E. A., and Cepko, C. L. (1992). Multipotent neural cell lines can engraft and participate in development of mouse cerebellum. *Cell* 68: 33–51.

Snyder, E. Y., Taylor, R. M., and Wolfe, J. H. (1995). Neural progenitor cell engraftment corrects lysosomal storage throughout the MPS VII mouse brain. *Nature* 374: 367–370.

Snyder, E. Y., and Wolfe, J. H. (1996). Central nervous system cell transplantation: A novel therapy for storage diseases? *Curr. Opin. Neurol.* 9: 126–136.

Snyder, S. H., and Childers, S. (1979). Opiate receptors and opioid peptides. *Ann. Rev. Neurosci.* 2: 35–64.

Snyder, S. H., Sabatini, D. M., Lai, M. M., Steiner, J. P., Hamilton, G. S., and Suzdak, P. D. (1998). Neural actions of immunophilin ligands. *Trends Pharmacol. Sci.* 19: 21–26.

Spencer, D. D., Robbins, R. J., Naftolin, F., Marek, K. L., Vollmer, T., Leranth, C., Roth, R. H., Price, L. H., Gjedde, A., Bunney, B. S., Sass, K. J., Elsworth, J. D.,

Kier, E. L., Makuch, R., Hoffer, P., and Redmond, D. E., Jr. (1992). Unilateral transplantation of human fetal mesencephalic tissue into the caudate nucleus of patients with Parkinson's disease. *New Eng. J. Med.* 327: 1541–1548.

Stein, D. G. (1991). Fetal brain tissue grafting as therapy for brain dysfunctions: Unanswered questions, unknown factors and practical concerns. *J. Neurosurg. Anesthesiol.* 3: 170–189.

Stein, D. G., Labbe, R., Firl, A., Jr., and Mufson, E. (1985). Behavioral recovery following implantation of fetal brain tissue into mature rats with bilateral, cortical lesions. In *Neural Grafting in the Mammalian CNS*, A. Bjorklund and U. Stenevi (eds.), pp. 605–614. Elsevier, Amsterdam.

Stemple, D. L., and Mahanthappa, N. K. (1997). Neural stem cells are blasting off. *Neuron* 18: 1–4.

Stenevi, U., Bjorklund, A., and Svendgaard, N.-A. (1976). Transplantation of central and peripheral monoamine neurons to the adult rat brain: Techniques and conditions for survival. *Brain Res.* 114: 1–20.

Stevens, J. R. (1990). Psychiatric consequences of temporal lobectomy for intractable seizures: A 20–30-year follow up of 14 cases. *Psychol. Med.* 20: 529–545.

Stevens, J. R. (1992). Abnormal reinnervation as a basis for schizophrenia: A hypothesis. *Arch. Gen. Psychiatry* 49: 238–243.

Stokes, B., and Reier, P. (1992). Fetal grafts alter chronic behavioral outcome after contusion damage to the adult rat spinal cord. *Exp. Neurol.* 116: 1–12.

Street, D. M. (1967). Traumatic paraplegia treated by vertebral resection, excision of spinal cord lesion, and interbody fusion. In *Proceedings of Veterans Administration Spinal Cord Injury Conference*. Cited in C. C. Kao, J. R. Wrathall, and K. Kyoshima, "Rationales and goals of spinal cord reconstruction." In *Spinal Cord Reconstruction*, C. C. Kao, R. P. Bunge, and P. J. Reier (eds.), pp. 1–6. Raven Press, New York, 1983.

Stromberg, I., Almqvist, P., Bygdeman, M., Finger, T. E., Gerhardt, G., Granholm, A.-Ch., Mahalik, T. J., Seiger, A., Hoffer, B., and Olson, L. (1988). Intracerebral xenografts of human mesencephalic tissue into athymic rats: Immunochemical and in vivo electrochemical studies. *Proc. Natl. Acad. Sci. U.S.A* 85: 8331–8334.

Stromberg, I., Almqvist, P., Bygdeman, M., Finger, T. E., Gerhardt, G., Granholm, A.-Ch., Mahalik, T. J., Seiger, A., Olson, L., and Hoffer, B. (1989). Human fetal mesencephalic tissue grafted to dopamine-denervated striatum of athymic rats: Light- and electron-microscopical histochemistry and in vivo chronoamperometric studies. *J. Neurosci.* 9: 614–624.

Stromberg, I., Bygdeman, M., Goldstein, M., Seiger, A., and Olson, L. (1986). Human fetal substantia nigra grafted to the dopamine-denervated striatum of immunosuppressed rats: Evidence for functional reinnervation. *Neurosci. Letters* 71: 271–276.

Stromberg, I., Ebendal, T., Olson, L., and Hoffer, B. (1990). Chromaffin grafts: Survival and nerve fiber formation as a function of donor age, nerve growth factor and host sympathetic denervation. *Prog. Brain Res.* 82: 87–94.

Stromberg, I., Herrera-Marschitz, M., Hultgren, L., Ungerstedt, U., and Olson, L. (1984). Adrenal medullary implants in the dopamine-denervated rat striatum. I. Acute catecholamine levels in grafts and host caudate as determined by HPLC-electrochemistry and fluorescence histochemical image analysis. *Brain Res.* 297: 41–51.

Stromberg, I., Herrera-Marschitz, M., Ungerstedt, U., Ebendal, T., and Olson, L. (1985). Chronic implants of chromaffin tissue into the dopamine-denervated rat striatum. Effects of NGF on graft survival, fiber growth, and rotational behavior. *Exp. Brain Res.* 60: 335–349.

Stromberg, I., van Horne, C., Bygdeman, M., Weiner, N., and Gerhardt, G. A. (1991). Function of intraventricular human mesencephalic xenografts in immunosuppressed rats: An electrophysiological and neurochemical analysis. *Exp. Neurol.* 112: 140–152.

Studer, L., Tabar, V., and McKay, R. D. G. (1998). Transplantation of expanded mesencephalic precursors leads to recovery in parkinsonian rats. *Nature Neurosci.* 1: 290–295.

Sugar, O., and Gerard, R. W. (1940). Spinal cord regeneration in the rat. *J. Neurophysiol.* 3: 1–19.

Sullivan, W. (1981). New tissue will be implanted in brain to treat Parkinson's. *New York Times,* Nov. 24, pp. C1, C3.

Suri, C., Fung, B. P., Tischler, A. S., and Chikaraishi, D. M. (1993). Catecholaminergic cell lines from the brain and adrenal glands of tyrosine hydroxylase-SV40 T antigen transgenic mice. *J. Neurosci.* 13: 1280–1291.

Svendsen, C. N., Fawcett, J. W., Bentlage, C., and Dunnett, S. B. (1995). Increased survival of rat EGF-generated CNS precursor cells using B27 supplemented medium. *Exp. Brain Res.* 102: 407–414.

Svendsen, C. N., and Rosser, A. E. (1995). Neurones from stem cells? *Trends Neurosci.* 18: 465–467.

Takashima, H., Poltorak, M., Becker, J. B., and Freed, W. J. (1992). Effects of adrenal medulla grafts on plasma catecholamines and rotational behavior. *Exp. Neurol.* 118: 24–34.

Takashima, H., Walker, B. R., Cannon-Spoor, H. E., and Freed, W. J. (1993). Kainic acid lesions increase reafferentation of the striatum by substantia nigra grafts. *Brain Res.* 621: 71–88.

Taylor, J. R. , Elsworth, J. D., Roth, R. H., Collier, T. J., Sladek, J. R., Jr., and Redmond, D. E., Jr. (1990). Improvements in MPTP-induced object retrieval deficits and behavioral deficits after fetal nigral grafting in monkeys. In *Neural Transplantation: From Molecular Basis to Clinical Applications,* S. B. Dunnett and S.-J. Richards (eds.), pp. 543–559. Elsevier, Amsterdam. Prog. Brain Res. 82.

Taylor, J. R., Elsworth, J. D., Roth, R. H., Sladek, J. R., Jr., Collier, T. J., and Redmond, D. E., Jr. (1991). Grafting of fetal substantia nigra to striatum reverses behavioral deficits induced by MPTP in primates: A comparison with other types of grafts as controls. *Exp. Brain Res.* 85: 335–348.

Taylor, J. R., Elsworth, J. D., Sladek, J. R., Jr., Collier, T. J., Roth, R. H., and Redmond, D. E., Jr. (1995). Sham surgery does not ameliorate MPTP-induced behavioral deficits in monkeys. *Cell Transplant.* 4: 13–26.

Teitelbaum, P. (1971). The encephalization of hunger. In *Progress in Physiological Psychology,* vol. 4, E. Stellar and J. M. Sprague (eds.), pp. 319–350. Academic Press, New York.

Tello, F. (1911). La influencia del neurotropismo en la regeneracion de los centros nervisosos. *Trab. Lab. Invest. Biol. Univ. Madrid* 9: 123–159.

Tessler, A. (1991). Intraspinal transplants. *Ann. Neurol.* 29: 115–123.

Thompson, F. J., Uthman, B., Mott, S., Remson, E. J., Wirth, E. D. III, Fessler, R. G., Reier, P. J., Behrman, A., Trimble, M., and Anderson, D. K. (1998). Neural tissue transplantation in syringomyelia patients: Neurophysiological assessments. Paper presented at the fifth Annual Conference of the American Society for Neural Transplantation. vol. 4, pp. 33.

Thompson, W. G. (1890). Successful brain grafting. *N.Y. Med. J.,* June 28, pp. 701–702.

Tomac, A., Lindqvist, E., Lin, L. F., Ogren, S. O., Young, D., Hoffer, B. J., and Olson, L. (1995). Protection and repair of the nigrostriatal system by GDNF in vivo. *Nature* 373: 335–339.

Tontsch, U., Archer, D. R., Dubois-Dalcq, M., and Duncan, I. D. (1994). Transplantation of an oligodendrocyte cell line leading to extensive myelination. *Proc. Natl. Acad. Sci. U.S.A.* 91: 11616–11620.

Tornatore, C., Baker-Cairns, B., Yadid, G., Hamilton, R., Meyers, K., Atwood, W., Cummins, A., Tanner, V., and Major, E. (1996). Expression of tyrosine hydroxylase in an immortalized human astrocyte cell line: In vitro characterization and engraftment into the rodent striatum. *Cell Transplant.* 5: 145–163.

Tresco, P. A., Winn, S. R., Tan, S., Jaeger, C. B., Greene, L. A., and Aebischer, P. (1992). Polymer-encapsulated PC12 cells: Long-term survival and associated reduction in lesion-induced rotational behavior. *Cell Transplant.* 1: 255–264.

Triarhou, L. C. (1996). The cerebellar model of neural grafting: Structural integration and functional recovery. *Brain Res. Bull.* 39: 127–138.

Triarhou, L. C., Zhang, W., and Lee, W. H. (1995). Graft-induced restoration of function in hereditary cerebellar ataxia. *Neuroreport* 6: 1827–1832.

Truckenmiller, M. E., Tornatore, C., Wright, R. D., Dillon-Carter, O., Meiners, S., Geller, H. M., and Freed, W. J. (1998). A truncated SV40 large T antigen lacking the p53 binding domain overcomes p53-induced growth arrest and immortalizes primary mesencephalic cells. *Cell Tissue Res.* 291: 175–189.

Tweedle, C. D., Smithson, K. G., and Hatton, G. I. (1993). Rapid synaptic changes and bundling in the supraoptic dendritic zone of the perfused rat brain. *Exp. Neurol.* 124: 200–207.

Twitty, V. C. (1966). *Of Scientists and Salamanders*. W. H. Freeman, San Francisco.

Ungerstedt, U. (1971a). Adipsia and aphagia after 6-hydroxydopamine induced degeneration of the nigro-striatal dopamine system. *Acta Physiol. Scand.* 367 (suppl.): 95–122.

Ungerstedt, U. (1971b). Postsynaptic supersensitivity after 6-hydroxydopamine induced degeneration of the nigro-striatal dopamine system. *Acta Physiol. Scand.* 367 (suppl.): 69–93.

Ungerstedt, U. (1971c). Stereotaxic mapping of the monoamine pathways in the rat brain. *Acta Physiol. Scand.* 367 (suppl.): 1–48.

Ungerstedt, U. (1971d). Striatal dopamine release after amphetamine or nerve degeneration revealed by rotational behaviour. *Acta Physiol. Scand.* 367 (suppl.): 49–68.

Ungerstedt, U., and Arbuthnott, G. W. (1970). Quantitative recording of rotational behavior in rats after 6-hydroxy-dopamine lesions of the nigrostriatal dopamine system. *Brain Res.* 24: 485–493.

Unsicker, K. (1993). The trophic cocktail made by adrenal chromaffin cells. *Exp. Neurol.* 123: 167–173.

Unsicker, K., and Krieglstein, K. (1996). Growth factors in chromaffin cells. *Prog. Neurobiol.* 48: 307–324.

Unsicker, K., Krisch, B., Otten, U., and Thoenen, H. (1978). Nerve growth factor-induced fiber outgrowth from isolated rat adrenal chromaffin cells: Impairment by glucocorticoids. *Proc. Natl. Acad. Sci. U.S.A.* 75: 3498–3502.

Utzschneider, D. A., Archer, D. R., Kocsis, J. D., Waxman, S. G., and Duncan, I. D. (1994). Transplantation of glial cells enhances action potential conduction of amyelinated spinal cord axons in the myelin-deficient rat. *Neurobiology* 91: 53–57.

Valenstein, E. S. (1973). *Brain Control*. John Wiley & Sons, New York.

Van der Zee, C. E., Rashid, K., Le, K., Moore, K. R., Stanisz, J., Diamond, J., Racine, R. J., and Fahnestock, M. (1995). Intraventricular administration of antibodies to nerve growth factor retards kindling and blocks mossy fiber sprouting in adult rats. *J. Neurosci.* 15: 5316–5323.

van Horne, C., Mahalik, T., Hoffer, B., Bygdeman, M., Almqvist, P., Stieg, P., Seiger, A., Olson, L. and Stromberg, I. (1990). Behavioral and electrophysiological correlates of human mesencephalic dopaminergic xenograft function in the rat striatum. *Brain Res. Bull.* 25: 325–334.

van Menen, J., and Speelman, J. D. (1988). Caudate lesions as surgical treatment in Parkinson's disease. *Lancet* 1: 175.

Vaquero, J., Martinez, R., Oya, S., Coca, S., Salazar, F. G., and Colado, M. I. (1988). Transplantation of adrenal medulla into spinal cord for pain relief: Disappointing outcome. *Lancet* 2: 1315.

Vawter, M. P., Basaric-Keys, J., Li, Y., Lester, D. S., Lebovics, R. S., Lesch, K. P., Kulaga, H., Freed, W. J., Sunderland, T., and Wolozin, B. (1996). Human olfactory neuroepithelial cells: Tyrosine phosphorylation and process extension are increased by the combination of IL–1beta, IL–6, NGF, and bFGF. *Exp. Neurol.* 142: 179–194.

Vitek, J. L., Bakay, R. A., and DeLong, M. R. (1997). Microelectrode-guided pallidotomy for medically intractable Parkinson's disease. *Adv. Neurol.* 74: 183–198.

Vogelbaum, M. A., and Menaker, M. (1992). Temporal chimeras produced by hypothalamic transplants. *J. Neurosci.* 12: 3619–3627.

Wachtel, S. R., Bencsics, C., and Kang, U. J. (1997). Role of aromatic L-amino acid decarboxylase for dopamine replacement by genetically modified fibroblasts in a rat model of Parkinson's disease. *J. Neurochem.* 69: 2055–2063.

Wang, Y., Tien, L. T., Lapchak, P. A., and Hoffer, B. J. (1996). GDNF triggers fiber outgrowth of fetal ventral mesencephalic grafts from nigra to striatum in 6-OHDA lesioned rats. *Cell Tissue Res.* 286: 225–233.

Waters, C., Itabashi, H. H., Apuzzo, M. L. J., and Weiner, L. P. (1990). Adrenal to caudate transplantation—postmortem study. *Movement Disorders* 5: 248–250.

Weiss, S., Dunne, C., Hewson, J., Wohl, C., Wheatley, M., Peterson, A. C., and Reynolds, B. A. (1996). Multipotent stem cells are present in the adult mammalian spinal cord and ventricular neuraxis. *J. Neurosci.* 16: 7599–7609.

Welner, S. A., Koty, Z. C., and Boska, P. (1990). Chromaffin cell grafts to rat cerebral cortex reverse lesion-induced memory deficits. *Brain Res.* 527: 163–166.

Wenning, G. K., Odin, P., Morrish, P., Rehncrona, S., Widner, H., Brundin, P., Rothwell, J. C., Brown, R., Gustavii, B., Hagell, P., Jahanshahi, M., Sawle, G., Bjorklund, A., Brooks, D. J., Marsden, C. D., Quinn, N. P., and Lindvall, O. (1997). Short- and long-term survival and function of unilateral intrastriatal dopaminergic grafts in Parkinson's disease. *Ann. Neurol.* 42: 95–107.

Westerman, K. A., and Leboulch, P. (1996). Reversible immortalization of mammalian cells mediated by retroviral transfer and site-specific recombination. *Proc. Natl. Acad. Sci. U.S.A.* 93: 8971–8976.

Whitaker-Azmitia, P., Clarke, C., and Azmitia, E. (1993). Localization of 5-HT$_{1A}$ receptors to astroglial cells in adult rats: Implications for neuronal-glial interactions and psychoactive drug mechanisms of action. *Synapse* 14: 201–205.

White, R. J. (1968). Experimental transplantation of the brain. In *Human Transplantation,* F. T. Rapaport and J. Dausset (eds.), pp. 692–809. Grune and Stratton, New York.

Whittemore, S. R., Neary, J. T., Kleitman, N., Sanon, H. R., Benigno, A., Donahue, R. P., and Norenberg, M. D. (1994). Isolation and characterization of conditionally immortalized astrocyte cell lines from adult human spinal cord. *Glia* 10: 211–226.

Whittemore, S. R., and Snyder, E. Y. (1996). Physiological relevance and functional potential of central nervous system-derived cell lines. *Mol. Neurobiol.* 12: 13–38.

Whittemore, S. R., and White, L. A. (1993). Target regulation of neuronal differentiation in a temperature-sensitive cell line derived from medullary raphe. *Brain Res.* 615: 27–40.

Wictorin, K., Simerly, R. B., Isacson, O., Swanson, L. W., and Bjorklund, A. (1989). Connectivity of striatal grafts implanted into the ibotenic acid-lesioned striatum. III. Efferent projecting neurons and their relation to host afferents within the grafts. *Neuroscience* 30: 313–330.

Widner, H. (1994). NIH neural transplantation funding. *Science* 263: 737.

Widner, H., Tetrud, J., Rehncrona, S., Snow, B., Brundin, P., Gustavii, B., Bjorklund, A., Lindvall, O., and Langston, J. W. (1992). Bilateral fetal mesencephalic grafting in two patients with parkinsonism induced by 1-methyl-4-phenyl–1,2,3,6-tetrahydropyridine (MPTP). *N. Eng. J. Med.* 327: 1556–1563.

Willing, A. E., Othberg, A. I., Saporta, S., Anton, A., Sinibaldi, S., Poulos, S. G., Cameron, D. F., Freeman, T. B., and Sanberg, P. R. (1999). Sertoli cells enhance the survival of co-transplanted dopamine neurons. *Brain Res.* 822: 246–250.

Winnie, A. P., Pappas, G. D., Das Gupta, T. K., Wang, H., Ortega, J. D., and Sagen, J. (1993). Subarachnoid adrenal medullary transplants for terminal cancer pain: A report of preliminary studies. *Anesthesiology* 79: 644–653.

Wirth, E. D. III, Fessler, R. G., Reier, P. J., Thompson, F. J., Uthman, B., Behrman, A., Beard, J., and Anderson, D. K. (1999). Neural tissue transplantation in patients with syringomyelia: Update on feasibility and safety. *Program and Abstracts of the American Society for Neural Transplantation and Repair* 5/6: 22.

Wolff, J. A., Fisher, L. J., Jinnah, H. A., Langlais, P. J., Iuvone, P. M., O'Malley, K. L., Rosenberg, M. B., Shimohama, S., Friedman, T., and Gage, F. H. (1989). Grafting fibroblasts genetically modified to produce L-dopa in a rat model of Parkinson's disease. *Proc. Natl. Acad. Sci. U.S.A.* 86: 9011–9014.

Woolf, N. J. (1991). Cholinergic systems in mammalian brain and spinal cord. *Prog. Neurobiol.* 37: 475–524.

Woolsey, D., Mineckler, J., Rezende, N., and Klemme, R. (1944). Human spinal cord transplant. *Exp. Med. Surg.* 2: 93–111.

Wrathall, J. R., Kapoor, V., and Kao, C. C. (1984). Observation of cultured peripheral nonneuronal cells implanted into the transected spinal cord. *Acta Neuropathol.* 64: 203–212.

Wrathall, J. R., Rigamonte, D. D., Bradford, M. R., and Kao, C. C. (1982). Reconstruction of the contused cat spinal cord by the delayed nerve graft technique and cultured peripheral nonneuronal cells. *Acta Neuropathol.* 57: 59–69.

Wu, D. K., and Cepko, C. L. (1994). The stability of endogenous tyrosine hydroxylase protein in PC–12 cells differs from that expressed in mouse fibroblasts by gene transfer. *J. Neurochem.* 62: 863–872.

Wyatt, R. J., Henter, I., Leary, M. C., and Taylor, E. (1995). An economic evaluation of schizophrenia—1991. *Soc. Psychiatry Psychiatric Epidemiol.* 30: 196–205.

Xiao, X., Li, J., McCown, T. J., and Samulski, R. J. (1997). Gene transfer by adeno-associated virus vectors into the central nervous system. *Exp. Neurol.* 144: 113–124.

Xiao, X., Li, J., and Samulski, R. J. (1998). Production of high-titer recombinant adeno-associated virus vector in the absence of helper adenovirus. *J. Virol.* 72: 2224–2232.

Yakovleff, A., Roby-Brami, A., Guezard, B., Mansour, H., Bussel, B., and Privat, A. (1989). Locomotion in rats transplanted with noradrenergic neurons. *Brain Res. Bull.* 22: 115–121.

Yaksh, T. L., and Reddy, S. V. (1981). Studies in the primate on the analgesic effects associated with intrathecal actions of opiates, alpha-adrenergic agonists, and baclofen. *Anesthesiology* 54: 451–467.

Yongue, B. G., and Canbeyli, R. (1994). Fetal brain grafts from normotensive (WKY) rats reduce blood pressure in borderline hypertensive rats. *Abs. Intl. Behav. Neurosci. Soc.* 3: 77.

Young, W. (1993). Secondary injury mechanisms in acute spinal cord injury. *J. Emerg. Med.* 11(suppl 1): 13–22.

Yuen, E. C., and Mobley, W. C. (1996). Therapeutic potential of neurotrophic factors for neurological disorders. *Ann. Neurol.* 40: 346–354.

Zabek, M., Mazurowski, W., Dymecki, J., Stelmachow, J., and Zawada, E. (1994). A long term follow-up of fetal dopaminergic neuron transplantation into the brain of three parkinsonian patients. *Res. Neurol. Neurosci.* 6: 97–106.

Zetterstrom, R. H., Solomin, L., Jansson, L., Hoffer, B. J., Olson, L., and Perlmann, T. (1997). Dopamine neuron agenesis in Nurr1-deficient mice. *Science* 276: 248–250.

Zhou, F. C., Chiang, Y. H., and Wang, Y. (1996). Constructing a new nigrostriatal pathway in the parkinsonian model with bridged neural transplantation in substantia nigra. *J. Neurosci.* 16: 6965–6974.

Index